AUTONOMY AND PATIENTS' DECISIONS

AUTONOMY AND PATIENTS' DECISIONS

Merle Spriggs

LEXINGTON BOOKS
Lanham • Boulder • New York • Toronto • Oxford

LEXINGTON BOOKS
An imprint of The Rowman & Littlefield Publishing Group, Inc.
4501 Forbes Boulevard, Suite 200
Lanham, MD 20706

PO Box 317
Oxford
OX2 9RU, UK

British Library Cataloguing in Publication Information Available

Library of Congress Cataloging-in-Publication Data

Spriggs, Merle.
Autonomy and patients' decisions / Merle Spriggs.
p. cm.
Includes bibliographical references and index.
ISBN 0-7391-0918-9 (cloth : alk. paper)
1. Autonomy (Philosophy). 2. Human Behavior I. Title.
R724.S675 2005
174.2—dc22 2004025431

Printed in the United States of America

The paper used in this publication meets the minimum requirements of American National Standard for Information Sciences—Permanence of Paper for Printed Library Materials, ANSI/NISO Z39.48–1992.

To Owen

CONTENTS

ACKNOWLEDGMENTS

This book is a revised version of my Ph.D. thesis *Autonomy and Patients' Decisions*, which I worked on at the Centre for Human Bioethics, Monash University, from 1996 to 2001. I gratefully acknowledge the assistance of Peter Singer who supervised my Ph.D. thesis. It was a privilege to have him as a supervisor and to benefit from his comments and his clear thinking. I thank him also for his continued supervision, support, and encouragement after he left Monash for Princeton in 1999.

I am also grateful to and would like to thank Justin Oakley for his comments on early drafts of the work. Part of this work has also benefited from the helpful comments of Robert Young. Early drafts benefited from the comments of Lynn Gillam, Julian Savulescu, Ani Satz, Udo Schuklenk, and those attending the Murdoch Childrens Research Institute and the Monash, Bioethics Journal Club. An early draft of chapter 3 (previously titled "Contemporary Muddle in Concepts of Autonomy") was presented at the Sixth National Conference of the Australasian Bioethics Association in Hobart, Australia, and profited from the comments of those attending. I would also like to thank Megan Clayton.

I am grateful to Bob Williamson, Director of the Murdoch Childrens Research Institute, and Julian Savulescu, Director of the Ethics Unit of the Murdoch Childrens Research Institute, for allowing me to revise my manuscript while working in the MCRI Ethics Unit.

For their encouragement and support while writing this book, I would like to thank Owen and Ron Harris and Ann Coote. I would also like to thank Robert Carley at Lexington Books for his help in preparing this manuscript.

Quotations from Albert R. Jonsen are used with his permission. Quotations from Robert Young, *Personal Autonomy: Beyond Negative and Positive Liberty*, are used with the author's permission. The quotations from Howard Klepper are used with his permission. The quotation from Tony Hope, "Personal Identity and Psychiatric Illness" in A. Phillips Griffiths (ed.) *Philosophy, Psychology and Psychiatry*, is used with the author's permission. Quotations from *The Theory and Practice of Autonomy* by Gerald Dworkin are used with the permission of the author and the publishers, Cambridge University Press, New York. Quotations from Ravi Savarirayan are used with his permission. Quotations from Immanuel Kant, *Groundwork of the Metaphysic of Morals*, in H. J. Paton trans. *The Moral Law*, 3rd ed. (London: Hutchinson of London, 1956), are used with the permission of the publisher, Thomson Publishing Services on behalf of Taylor and Francis Books Ltd. Permission to use the quotation from *The Death of Ivan Ilyich and Other Stories* by Leo Tolstoy, translated with an introduction by Rosmary Edmonds (Penguin Classics, 1960) was granted by the publishers, Penguin Group (United Kingdom).

The extract from *Cancer Ward* by Aleksandr Solzhenitsyn, published by Bodley Head, is used by permission of the Random House Group Limited. Quotations from J. S. Mill, *On Liberty* in *On Liberty and Considerations on Representative Government*, edited by R. B. McCallum, (Oxford: Basil Blackwell, 1948), are used with the permission of the publisher. Quotations from *The Silent World of Doctor and Patient*, by Jay Katz, are used with the permission of the author.

INTRODUCTION

In an earlier work I looked at the way in which standard theories of autonomy in contemporary bioethics discussions rely on the idea that people have some kind of life plan, or at least a stable set of values. I discussed the fact that when someone receives a devastating diagnosis they may act in ways that could be interpreted as a departure from a previously held life plan or stable values. I also looked at examples of people who were to some extent self-determining despite having suffered a traumatic life event.[1] In these kinds of situations it is difficult for doctors to know whether a patient's decision is autonomous or not. Now I am exploring some of the issues more systematically.

One of the issues I give considerable attention to is whether the idea of autonomy that has been around in philosophical discussions for some centuries is the same idea that people are referring to when they talk about autonomy in the medical setting. My approach is a chronological one. I describe the history and the development of the contemporary idea of autonomy. This involves looking closely at the ideas of Rousseau, Kant, and Mill. Many discussions of autonomy provide some historical background but I am doing more than that. I set out to actually trace the modern concept from its historical roots.

I also trace the way in which the principle of respect for autonomy got into contemporary American bioethics. Then, because of the wide influence of Beauchamp and Childress's *Principles of Biomedical Ethics*[2] in the field of bioethics I look at the changes that take place in their chapter on autonomy in successive editions of their work. This shows us how many in the field view the concept of autonomy. One conclusion I reach is that our support for the idea of persons as ends in themselves, which is commonly linked to the notion of autonomy, does not need any notion of autonomy. We think it is a good thing even without reference to notions of autonomy.

I identify different notions of autonomy and look at a variety of theories, but I am doing more than a survey. I am presenting an argument that current usage is muddled and I am proposing a clearer and better account of autonomy. First, I am trying to work out what we are really referring to when we talk of autonomy—hence the need to look at the historical development of the contemporary idea. Secondly, I am trying to find a theory of autonomy that is applicable and useful for the clinical setting. The theory needs to be useful in the sense that we need criteria for doctors and relevant others to decide when patients' decisions should be respected or when intervention is justified.

In contemporary discussions of autonomy, it seems that different ideas are often run together. There are quite different things that we may be referring to when we speak of autonomy. I identify four distinct notions of autonomy.[3] To begin with, there is the notion of autonomy derived from Kant, which depends on a specific metaphysics about the world and the kind of beings humans are. There is another view in which autonomy is a psychological ideal. Preferences, desires, capacities, competencies and notions of the self, life plans and rationality are central to this theory. In another view, autonomy is seen as a constraint on action. Here, the focus is on the regulation of the consent-seeker's behavior and the underlying value at work is something other than autonomy. There is also an evaluative notion of autonomy. In this view, when we say someone is autonomous we are making a judgment. We are not saying what it means to be autonomous but saying that this person or this person's decision qualifies as deserving respect.

Disentangling these different ideas is an essential preliminary to a clear and coherent discussion about the role of autonomy. It is important that we are clear about the kind of concept we are using and that we use it in a consistent way. Only when that is done can we have a meaningful discussion about autonomy in the clinical context—and decide what kind of notion is a useful one.

The question of the value of autonomy is *not* something I will be discussing at the outset. I cannot discuss its value until I clarify what autonomy is. Further, it is important to understand that the notion of what it is to be autonomous and the question of whether or why we ought to respect autonomy are separate issues.

Finally, I will test likely theories of autonomy in light of some different clinical situations. These include situations faced by someone who receives a devastating diagnosis, a question about consent given by a Jehovah's Witness, the case of Mr. M who suffers from manic depression and the possible enhancement of autonomy brought about by taking a drug such as Prozac. This analysis may help us to see the value of autonomy. But also, I am trying to find whether there is an account of autonomy that can assist physicians in deciding whether a patient's decision should be respected or intervention justified. In addition, I am trying to find an account of autonomy that is both philosophically defensible and relevant to the clinical context.

Some readers may prefer to skip the chapters on Rousseau, Kant, and Mill and begin with the development of the contemporary idea of autonomy—with the chapter that introduces the *Belmont Report*[4] and *Principles of Biomedical Ethics*. Readers can refer back to the earlier historical chapters as desired.

NOTES

1. Merle Spriggs, *Autonomy and Shattered Assumptions,* (unpublished manuscript, submitted for Master of Bioethics, Centre for Human Bioethics Monash University, 1995); Merle Spriggs, "Autonomy in the Face of a Devastating Diagnosis," *Journal of Medical Ethics* 24, (April 1998): 123–26.
2. Tom L. Beauchamp and James F. Childress, *Principles of Biomedical Ethics,* (New York: Oxford University Press, 1st ed., 1979).
3. Two of the 'notions' of autonomy I identify are approaches to autonomy rather than 'notions' because they are not substantive notions of autonomy. Nevertheless, I will sometimes refer to them as 'notions' of autonomy because this is how they are sometimes perceived in contemporary discussions.
4. The National Commission for the Protection of Human Subjects of Biomedical and Behavioral Research, *The Belmont Report: Ethical Principles and Guidelines for the Protection of Human Subjects Research.* (DHEW Publication No (OS) 78-0012, 1978).

I

HISTORICAL BACKGROUND

1

KANT'S IDEA OF AUTONOMY

ROUSSEAU'S INFLUENCE ON KANT: THE GENERAL WILL

Rousseau's writings inspired Kant and had an influence on the development of the idea of autonomy. Although Rousseau's main concern was political theory, there are parallels between his notion of the general will and Kant's notion of reason.

Rousseau's interest was in finding a form of association that defends and protects each person while allowing each to retain their freedom. This requires securing the collective strength of the group, but there is a difficulty in securing that without putting restrictions on individual freedom. Rousseau saw value in maintaining that individual freedom:

> Such a sum of forces can be produced only by the collaboration of a group of men. But since each man's strength and freedom are his primary means of self-preservation, how can he pledge them without harming himself, without neglecting the care he owes to himself?[1]

This situation involves a conflict between individuals and society and between freedom and moral obligations. Rousseau's solution is in the idea of the general will; each individual makes a complete surrender of all his or her rights to the whole community. According to Rousseau, this is not the same thing as giving away one's freedom:

> in giving himself to all, each man gives himself to no one, and since he acquires the same right over all the other associates as they acquire over him, he gains the equivalent of everything he loses, plus greater power to preserve what he has.[2]

In this give-and-take situation, if we surrender to the general will, we exchange natural freedom for civil freedom. In other words, although we may not be able to have anything we want or can take, we are able to secure 'ownership' of what we possess.[3]

According to Rousseau, there is a further gain attached to this. In surrendering to the general will we also gain moral freedom. Choosing to surrender to the general will is choosing obedience to a self-imposed law that is an expression of our moral or higher self. When physical impulses yield to the voice of duty, we demonstrate that we are intelligent beings who use reason as opposed to beings driven by appetite or inclination. This gives our acts the morality they lack when we are motivated solely by instinct.[4]

Surrendering to the general will amounts to freedom—freedom of a special kind. When we consult our reason rather than listening to inclination we substitute equality and justice for physical impulses and instinct.[5] This is freedom and the nature of the freedom we gain is moral freedom. From this, we associate the idea of reason with goodness or value.

To be driven by appetite alone is slavery according to Rousseau. Surrendering to the general will on the other hand is freedom in the sense that a person is truly his own master. He is choosing for himself rather than being determined by outside forces. It is what distinguishes an intelligent being from a 'stupid, short-sighted animal.'[6] For this reason, Rousseau holds that a person who renounces freedom also renounces his or her humanity and thus removes 'all morality' from his or her acts.[7]

The condition we are in when we are controlled by our passions had been likened to slavery by others prior to this, but Rousseau's idea that we make our own law and impose it on ourselves was new and different. It was an alternative to the idea that we must follow the laws of an external authority such as God or nature and that morality must be imposed on us. Rousseau held that the way to create a free and just society was through obedience to a law we have imposed on our selves.[8]

Rousseau makes some distinctions about the social pact—the form of association that describes the general will. This collective is called the 'people' and they are individually both 'citizens' and 'subjects.' As a citizen the individual benefits from the protections and rights that the general will provides and as a subject has duties and owes obedience to certain laws.[9] The general will is concerned with the common good and tends toward equality. It is different from the sum of individual wills and it is not the 'will of all' nor what the majority wills.[10] Individuals can have a private will which may be different from or in conflict with the general will which the same individual has as a citizen. Private individual wills may be selfish and may come into conflict with the common interest. There is a 'reciprocal commitment,' however, between individuals and the collective to which they belong and this circumvents possible conflict. Individuals need to fulfill the duties they have as subjects so they can benefit as citizens:

> In order . . . that the social pact shall not be an empty formality, it tacitly includes one stipulation without which all the others would be ineffectual: that anyone who refuses to obey the general will shall be compelled to do so by the whole body. This means nothing else than that he shall be forced to be free.[11]

For Rousseau, surrendering to the general will is the sense in which yielding to force is a duty and an act of will. It is to be distinguished from acts of prudence or acts of necessity (in the sense of being caused).[12] Obedience to the general will is the only thing that legitimizes civil obligations. This also includes situations where an individual is coerced (forced to be free) as well as when it is voluntarily chosen. Surrendering to the general will is to accept a self-imposed law and 'obedience to self-imposed law is freedom.'[13]

According to Isaiah Berlin, Rousseau's view of freedom means that he must eventually consider the wills of others in society, not just the inner life of a particular individual. His belief in freedom as 'rational self-direction' raises the question: 'If I am rational, I cannot deny that what is right for me must, for the same reasons, be right for others who are rational like me.'[14] This shows that there is something universal in all of us and it is distinct from mere wants or desires. Rousseau's idea of freedom which comes with surrender to the general will is, as Onora O'Neill claims: 'no mere matter of wilfulness or independence from others or from social conventions.' It is to take into account and respect the 'like moral status' of others. It is to act morally.[15]

There is some suggestion in Rousseau that surrendering to or choosing the general will is grounds for valuing human nature. Rousseau claims that in yielding to the voice of duty and by consulting reason a person may miss some advantages but gains in other ways: 'his faculties are exercised and developed, his ideas are broadened, his feeling are ennobled, his whole soul is uplifted.'[16]

Rousseau separates reason from human nature by distinguishing the general or rational will from an individual's particular will. We get the idea that persons reason disinterestedly, in so far as they exercise their reason. Surrendering to the general will connects freedom with duty. It is what makes us free rather than a slave to our selfish and particular desires. This foreshadows the ideas of Kant.

KANT

I am tracing the roots of the idea of autonomy because we want to know if the idea of autonomy that has figured in philosophical discussions for some centuries is the same idea that people are referring to in contemporary discussions in the medical setting. I am presenting the aspects of Kant's thinking that seem crucial to understanding his idea of autonomy and I am dealing strictly with the views expressed by Kant in his central texts, not with so-called Kantian ethics.[17]

I emphasize Kant's *The Groundwork of the Metaphysic of Morals* and *Critique of Practical Reason*, which contain the essentials of Kant's distinctive view of morality in which he came to think that a 'formal principle of avoiding practical self-contradiction must be at the centre of morality.'[18] Some of Kant's earlier writings appeal to human feeling[19] but, by 1770 he did not accept this view of morality. He wrote in a letter that year:

> I have resolved . . . this winter . . . to put in order and complete my investigations of pure moral philosophy, in which no empirical principles are to be found, the "Metaphysics of Morals." It will in many respects pave the way for the most important views involved in the reconstruction of metaphysics.[20]

TWO PLANES OF EXISTENCE: THE PHYSICAL AND THE INTELLECTUAL WORLDS

Rousseau's influence on Kant is unmistakable. For both Rousseau and Kant, freedom is more than the common sense idea of freedom to do as we like or political freedom. It is a 'symptom of reason's dominance' and because of this it is inseparable from duty or moral obligation.[21] As we shall see, Kant's idea of the will which generates moral action is anticipated in Rousseau's general will. For Rousseau, surrendering to the general will 'makes a man truly his own master' whereas choosing on the basis of individual private interest is 'impulsion by appetite.' It is 'slavery.'[22] Kant separates reason from empirical human nature and his view of our desires enslaving us is similar to Rousseau's.

For Kant, it is because we are members of both the physical world and the intelligible world that we use the 'moral "I ought".' If reason was in control and we were not subject to the encumbrance of the sensuous desires of the physical world we could simply say 'I will.'[23] Instead, because we exist in the sensible world as well as the intelligible world, we 'do not always act as reason by itself would act.'[24] We are always divided between our physical, desiring selves, and our rational selves.

Kant claims that knowledge gained through our senses is deficient because it is only 'knowledge of *appearances*.' We receive this knowledge passively in the sense that the ideas are given to us 'from without.'[25] We only know things to the extent that we are affected by them rather than as they are 'in themselves.' The knowledge we gain through the senses is also not reliable because it can vary according to the differences in different observers. Furthermore, it follows that we only know ourselves in this same superficial way because we acquire our self concepts empirically. According to Kant reality does not comprise just the physical world. There is something more than, or beyond, the world of sense and appearance. There are also ideas that come into consciousness that are not caused by objects outside of us. They are 'something' that is left over when we exclude from the grounds determining our will, everything that belongs to the world of sense.[26]

Kant refers to a kind of immediacy or spontaneity in our thinking and connects that with what he calls the intellectual world.[27] Reason belongs to that world also. This may seem somewhat incomprehensible, but that is the nature of reason and the intellectual world according to Kant. We cannot have knowledge of it because it is not part of the physical world and not accessible to our senses. We can, however, know it in the sense that we can comprehend the incomprehensibility of it.[28]

Kant claims that reason is 'a power which distinguishes us from all other things,' even from ourselves so far as we are affected by objects.[29] What is more, rational beings have two viewpoints:

> He can consider himself *first*—so far as he belongs to the sensible world—to be under laws of nature (heteronomy); and *secondly*—so far as he belongs to the intelligible world—to be under laws which, being independent of nature, are not empirical but have their ground in reason alone.[30]

This leads to a kind of divided notion of what we are like. It seems that in each of us there is a higher or moral self that reasons and chooses disinterestedly. For Kant, insofar as we are rational we act in accordance with principles and that leads to the notion of the good will.[31]

When we act on the basis of reason this is autonomy. Kant also claims that autonomy is a property of the will of any rational being.[32] To have a will does not mean that there exists an internal part of the self called the will—it is to be capable of being moved by reason. It is 'the power' to act 'in accordance with principles' or 'practical reason'—to choose what is good independently of inclination and desire.[33] Rational beings are therefore autonomous whereas nonrational beings are not.

Kant claims that a good will is not the only good but it is the 'highest good.'[34] He claims that the only thing that is intrinsically good is a good will and a will that is not autonomous cannot be good. The manifestation of a good will is an act of respect for the moral law. As we shall see, this has a central place in Kant's approach to the role of reason. It is what gives actions their moral worth. The distinction between an act done 'from duty' (out of respect for the law) and one that only conforms with duty illustrates this. Kant uses the example of a grocer who does not overcharge his customers. Although the grocer's action may be honest, it is self-interest that motivates it, so the grocer is acting prudently rather than from the motive of duty. It is the existence of competitors, rather than principles of fair dealing that moves the grocer to act in this way.[35] His will is not autonomous, because it is affected by outside influences.

Duty, for Kant, is not duty in the sense that we have to adhere to certain laws because we believe that they are good or worthwhile. Rather, duty is something we cannot escape if reason is in control. To go against our duty would be to act in a way we know is unreasonable. Our actions gain moral worth because they are grounded in pure reason rather than our empirical natures or our circumstances.[36] There is no moral worth when we act on laws in which our interest is merely extrinsic. Actions of this kind may have legality but no morality.[37]

AUTONOMY AND HETERONOMY

From Kant, like Rousseau, we get the idea that we make laws or give the law to ourselves rather than having it imposed on us. This is what makes us autonomous and the opposite of autonomy is heteronomy. Kant distinguishes between being self-directed and being directed by outside forces and claims we are self-directed in the sense that we are moved by our intellect when we act on reason rather than instinct. When we act on instinct or desire, we are being directed by the physical world.

For Kant we are not autonomous when we are at the mercy of outside forces such as inclinations and desires. These outside forces are responses to, or originate in things, outside ourselves. When we act from desire or inclination our action is conditioned or determined by the object that our will focuses on. For instance, a desire for a cool drink on a hot day is conditioned by the heat and our feeling of thirst. These are both outside forces. This is the kind of thing Kant refers to as heteronomy. It is something that is somehow not our choice. He would say that the same is true when we are driven by feelings such as sympathy or compassion:

> there are many spirits of so sympathetic a temper that, without any further motive of vanity or self-interest, they find an inner pleasure in spreading happiness around them and can take delight in the contentment of others as their own work. Yet I maintain that in such a case an action of this kind, however right and however amiable it may be, has still no genuinely moral worth. It stands on the same footing as other inclinations.[38]

Kant claims that it is a duty to help others where we can, but when that is a response to an outside force rather than something I choose autonomously, the action may be morally good in letter but it is not morally good in spirit.[39] He contrasts this with the situation where a man helps a friend out of duty:

> Suppose then that the mind of this friend of man were overclouded by sorrows of his own which extinguished all sympathy with the fate of others, but that he still had power to help those in distress, though no longer stirred by the need of others because sufficiently occupied with his own; and suppose that, when no longer moved by any inclination, he tears himself out of this deadly insensibility and does the action without any inclination for the sake of duty alone; then for the first time his action has its genuine moral worth.[40]

Further to this, reason and desire create a divide between the intellectual and the physical world. Everything in the physical world is under the law of nature that involves causes and effects while things in the physical world are determined. Kant does not allow determinism by things outside ourselves to count as autonomy. As rational beings we are autonomous because we have freedom of the will and we are able to follow reason. We can act for reasons rather than being caused and because of this, we are able to escape the determinism that is the fate of every nonrational being.

Kant claims that autonomy is 'the ground of the dignity of human nature and of every rational being.'[41] The autonomy of our will elevates our worth and as we shall see, enables us to share in the making of universal law. We have dignity because we have an intellect and that means we can act from principles of reason rather than instinct or self-interest

THE FUNCTION OF REASON

According to Kant, a good will is the only thing which is 'good without qualification.'[42] It demonstrates the true function of reason. The value of a good will does not lie in attaining particular ends or in its usefulness. It is 'good in itself' in the sense that the 'willing alone'; the submitting to obligation is what makes it good. This means it has value even when it accomplishes nothing.[43] Kant holds a purposive view of nature and argues that if results were paramount, instinct could do the job more efficiently than the use of reason:

> Suppose now that for a being possessed of reason and a will the real purpose of nature were his *preservation*, his *welfare*, or in a word his *happiness*. In that case nature would have hit on a very bad arrangement. . . . For all the actions he has to perform with this end in view . . . the end in question could have been maintained far more surely by instinct than it ever can be by reason.[44]

The role Kant gives reason is fundamental in his account of autonomy. It emphasizes the idea that autonomy does not consist in acting for the sake of ends or any goal except respect for the moral law. For Kant, it is not the ends of our actions that have value but the principle of the will (the principle we act on). When we act out of duty or reverence for the law we are free from the influence of anything but our own reason: 'although reverence is a feeling, it is not a feeling received through outside influence, but one self-produced by a rational concept'[45] To the extent that we are autonomous or free in Kant's sense of the term, we are subject to the moral law, our actions have moral worth and we have dignity. Our heteronomous self is not in control and our actions are based in reason.

FREEDOM

Kant links the notion of freedom to autonomy but does not suggest that it is the same concept. Autonomy means acting on laws that we give ourselves.

In Kant's view, freedom can only consist in acting autonomously. As already noted, it differs from the common sense idea of freedom that suggests we are free when we can do what we like. For Kant, freedom 'insofar as it is not restrained' is the 'most terrible thing there ever could be.' The result is 'much savage disorder.'[46] A lawless freedom is at best a superficial kind of freedom in which we may only think that we are free. If we do not give laws to ourselves, they will be imposed from outside. For Kant, we always act under laws of some sort. Even if we drift along aimlessly, we are not free from the laws of nature. Even then—especially then—we are determined by any thing that we meet or anything that confronts us and this is not freedom, but determinism. Kant claims that reason governs the will of rational beings, and it is precisely for this reason that freedom is not lawlessness.

Kant is not suggesting that rational beings act only according to reason. He recognizes that we are also subject to desires and that we can consider ourselves also 'under the laws of nature (heteronomy).'[47] For Kant, we are free from the causal laws of the physical world when we are acting in accordance with the laws of the intelligible world which are grounded in reason. Reason distinguishes us from other things—and from our heteronomous selves. There is a parallel here with Rousseau who found moral worth only in those actions in which our duty overruled our physical impulses.

DUTY

For Kant, autonomy, reason, and morality are linked. It is through our morality, our ability to rise above our nature and our own self interest, that we reveal our dignity. As we have already seen, autonomy is the expression of a free will that uses reason rather than instinct or desire. A free will is also a will under moral laws. Kant suggests that when confronted with a choice of action there is an option that has a certain irresistibility or compulsion for a being with reason. That option is our duty and when we act on that, we give our actions moral worth. Kant seems to think that it is a compulsion or necessity of the same kind as that which takes our mind through the steps of a logical proof. There is something in the law and something in us that responds to it, and it is that which produces the obligation:

> Therefore nothing but the *idea of the law* in itself, *which admittedly is present only in a rational being* . . . can constitute that preeminent good which we call moral, a good which is already present in the person acting on this idea and has not to be awaited merely from the result.[48]

Kant gives duty an a priori character in the sense that it involves necessity and because we are not dependent on outside objects or experience to tell us what our duty is. According to Kant, duty is not derived from 'the special characteristics of human nature'; it is an 'unconditioned necessity of action.'[49] It is the 'necessity to act out of reverence for the law.'[50] Kant seems to be suggesting that there is something, (the law), which directs us to act even though at times 'our every propensity, inclination, and natural bent [are] opposed to it.'[51] The connection with morality is to do with the compulsion or necessity we feel when faced with some options. Our duty exerts this 'pull' on us because it is in accordance with our reason. Kant argues that reverence is not merely an effect but an activity of the will. Our duty is a choice we make but it is not simply a matter of choosing between alternatives. It involves making a choice, but there is also something more than that. Reverence does not serve inclination; it outweighs it or at least leaves inclination out of account in our choice. Reverence is consciousness of 'immediate determination of the will by the law.'[52] The necessity for us to act out of respect for the law (and reason compels our immediate reverence) is what 'constitutes duty.'[53] We are autonomous in the sense that we can act for reasons rather than inclination and there is moral worth in acting for the law or duty alone.[54]

AUTONOMY AND CHOICE

For Kant, acting autonomously involves more than making choices. It is worth looking at Kant's view of animals to see how he distinguishes between choice and autonomy. Kant claims that animals are a means to an end, they are instruments, and we do not have to respect them as ends in themselves. We have duties to animals but these duties are really 'indirect duties towards humanity' rather than direct duties to animals. He claims that if we treat animals harshly, we are failing in our duty, not for the animals sake but because we damage the humanity in ourselves. Cruelty generates more cruelty, so if we treat animals with cruelty we are failing to cultivate duties which we owe to the rest of humanity. As an example, Kant argues that a dog who has served his master long and faithfully must be taken care of till the end, even if it can serve no longer:

> If a man has his dog shot, because it can no longer earn a living for him, he is by no means in breach of any duty to the dog . . . but he thereby damages the

kindly and humane qualities in himself, which he ought to exercise in virtue of his duties to mankind.[55]

For Kant, choices made by animals do not warrant respect. Animals can make choices such as when they choose food but this is 'brute' or a 'merely sensitive power of choice' in which they are 'determined by stimuli alone.'[56] This kind of choice is not free because the impulse which determines action can be overcome by involuntary impulses that are stronger still.[57] Because the choices of animals are not free in a Kantian sense animals are not ends in themselves. This suggests we can have choice without autonomy. For Kant, animals have the capacity to choose but the thing that prevents them from being autonomous and worthy of respect is that the choices they make are 'necessitated by incentives and stimuli.'[58] He claims:

> All animals have the capacity to use their powers according to choice. Yet this choice is not free. . . . If all creatures had such a choice, tied to sensory drives, the world would have no value. But the inner worth of the world, the *summun bonum,* is freedom according to a choice that is not necessitated to act.[59]

For Kant, respect applies, therefore, only to persons or rational beings, but not to things. Things 'can awaken inclinations, and even love if they are animals (horses, dogs, etc.), or fear, as do the sea, a volcano, or a beast of prey; but they never arouse respect.'[60] People are very special and it seems to be something to do with the fact that they are ends in themselves and this is because they are rational beings.

Choice can be both free and necessitated and is free to the extent that it is determined by reason.[61] Choice which is determined only by inclination is 'animal choice' and not worthy of respect because it is caused by outside forces. According to Kant, there is a kind of free choice which is made independently from sensuous impulse, but it is not necessarily autonomy. It means only that we are 'not necessitated to act by any sensuous determining ground.'[62] It is merely 'freedom *from* something' and is 'arbitrary and lawless in itself.'[63] It is simply to choose between alternatives. The mere exclusion of feeling and desire is not enough to warrant respect. What is more, Kant does not exclude feeling and desire. He requires more in the sense that reason needs to be in control. Kant associates a positive concept of freedom with autonomy. It is something that is self-imposed. Reason is autonomous to the extent that it 'cares for its own interest to the exclusion of all else' rather than being a 'mere guardian of the inclinations.'[64]

THE CATEGORICAL IMPERATIVE

For Kant, rational beings are autonomous and can act in ways that are regarded as free. When we are free and we act according to the moral law, our actions have a certain consistency that is not in any way dependent on desires or inclinations. Kant's categorical imperative is a kind of test that we apply to our maxims and when we obey the categorical imperative it shows that we are not entirely determined by our sensuous nature and the physical world.

The categorical imperative tests whether an act is autonomous or heteronomous. It shows whether an act has moral worth and whether it is permissible. In order for our actions to have moral worth Kant claims we 'must be able to will' that a maxim, which is the subjective principle on which we *act*, 'should become a universal law'[65]—something that is valid for both myself and others in all situations. This means that the activity of our will represents an action as 'objectively necessary' *in itself* and not *as a means* to other goals or ends.[66] The categorical imperative is a principle on which we *ought* to act and the moral worth of our action is in the willing (acting for the sake of the law), not the ends of the action.

As rational beings we have a power to act on ideas and reasons and we can *choose* a course of action rather than allowing ourselves to be passively determined by outside forces. The categorical imperative tests whether we are free and self-legislating in this sense. It is also the expression of a law based in reason. This kind of command is opposed to a hypothetical imperative which commands an action *if* we seek a particular end. A hypothetical imperative is a conditioned response and it is characterized by an 'if.' Conditioned or hypothetical imperatives 'rest on an artistry employed for a purpose.' They depend on my desires and therefore, they only tell me what I should do '*if I will* this or that.'[67] They merely counsel or advise: 'I ought not to lie if I want to maintain my reputation.' The categorical imperative, on the other hand, is directed at rational beings in general rather than someone in a specific situation with a particular desire. The categorical imperative is something that we *ought* to obey. The emphasis is on the 'ought': 'I ought not to lie even if so doing were to bring me not the slightest disgrace.'[68]

Kant gives several formulations of the categorical imperative. Each sets forth the rules of a good will:

> Act only on that maxim through which you can at the same time will that it should become a universal law.[69]

> Act in such a way that you always treat humanity, whether in your own person or in the person of any other, never simply as a means, but always at the same time as an end.[70]
>
> Every rational being must so act as if he were through his maxims always a law-making member in the universal kingdom of ends.[71]

Kant specifically calls one formulation of the categorical imperative 'the principle of autonomy.' It is the 'Idea of the will of every rational being as a will which makes universal law.'[72] In the form of a command he states it in this way:

> Never . . . choose except in such a way that in the same volition the maxims of your choice are also present as universal law.[73]

Kant maintains that these formulations are equivalent and amount to the 'strictest method' which is: 'act on the maxim which can at the same time be made a universal law.'[74]

According to Kant, we can know we are autonomous when we act from the moral law of reason but the moral law does not tell us specifically what we should do in particular situations. For Kant, moral action amounts to testing our maxims, so while the categorical imperative is in one sense a command, it is primarily a test that we apply to our maxims. The test, however, is more than a tool for measuring autonomy. We shall see that the activity involved in doing the test is, in itself, meaningful.

The categorical imperative is not just an appeal to some version of the golden rule. Kant claims that while the idea of not doing to others what you don't want done to yourself, subject to certain qualifications, may be derived from the categorical imperative, it cannot be a universal law: 'for many a man would readily agree that others should not help him if only he could be dispensed from affording help to them.'[75] The categorical imperative is more than an appeal to our desires or even our needs as beings in the physical world. It *tests* the moral acceptability of what we plan to do and is independent of and even contrary to our needs and desires. It does not look at the results of action and it is not meant to give rise to a plan of action.[76]

The categorical imperative is a test and a command and as such, it seems to be for the use of agents rather than observers. It commands us to impose a certain consistency or rationality on our actions by asking that we act according to a maxim which we can, 'at the same time will that it should become a universal law.'[77] Kant uses promise keeping as an example on which to try out the categorical imperative. When confronted with a choice of action an agent can subject his maxims to the test of the categorical imperative to find whether it is 'unlawful and contrary to duty.'[78] If a man promises to pay back money in order to get a loan, while knowing that he will not be able to repay it, his maxim runs like this: 'Whenever I believe myself short of money, I will borrow money and promise to pay it back, though I know that this will never be done.' The principle of action here is 'self-love or personal advantage' and Kant asks: 'How would things stand if my maxim became a universal law?' His answer is that 'this maxim can never rank as a universal law of nature and be self-consistent, but must necessarily contradict itself.'[79] If breaking promises was to become a universal law, if everyone acted in this way when it suited them, no one could place confidence in promises: 'promising would abolish itself.' There is a contradiction in the sense that if the maxim were made into a rule it would be untenable: 'no one would believe he was being promised anything, but would laugh at utterances of this kind as empty shams.'[80] Although we could decide to keep promises because it is the prudent thing to do, that will not pass the test of the categorical imperative: 'To tell the truth for the sake of duty is something entirely different from doing so out of concern for inconvenient results.'[81] The categorical imperative serves as a rule on which we test our maxims and the prudential maxim fails on that test:

> could I really say to myself that every one may make a false promise if he finds himself in a difficulty from which he can extricate himself in no other way? I then become aware at once that I can indeed will to lie, but I can by no means will a universal law of lying.[82]

All imperatives of duty can be derived from a single categorical imperative. When our maxim is made into universal law and is not in conflict with itself, it is our duty. The content of our maxims is not important. According to Kant, maxims undeniably have content and this comes from an object of our desires. It is not the presence of the desire or empirical condition that matters, but that it should not be the 'determining ground and condition of the maxim.' Kant maintains: 'If it were, the maxim could not be presented as giving universal law.'[83] The moral law has no content and the pure form of the moral law needs no content: 'let the consequences be what they may.'[84] This leaves us with the idea of universal law; a moral law which is empty of content. Kant's concern is solely with the 'form' and the 'principle' of an action. He claims that 'what is essentially good in the action consists in the mental disposition.' The activity (the use of reason) involved in applying the categorical imperative, is itself meaningful. He calls the imperative which commands absolutely (not hypothetically) the 'imperative of morality.'[85] From this notion of the categorical imperative the ideas of autonomy and human or free choice acquire value:

> In the moral imperative the end is quite undetermined, nor is the action determined by the end, for it relates only to free choice, be the end what it may. Hence the moral imperative commands absolutely, without looking to the end. Our free acting and refraining has an inner goodness, and thus gives man an immediate inner absolute worth or morality.[86]

SELF-LEGISLATION

For Kant, self-legislation is a self-enforced constraint on lawless freedom. It is morality which we impose on ourselves. Self-legislation is an idea that was foreshadowed by Rousseau who saw an 'essential connection between law and freedom' in politics.[87] Rousseau's concern was in finding a form of association that protected and defended people while allowing each to retain their freedom. He found a difficulty in securing the collective strength of the people without restricting their individual freedom. Kant's interest is in determining a law that the will can obey, that 'limits freedom and renders it lawful,' without taking away the freedom of the will. The difficulty here is that submission to law seems contrary to freedom. Kant develops Rousseau's connection between law and freedom (or duty and freedom) into a 'moral and metaphysical' concept of autonomy.[88] Kant's concept of autonomy as self-legislation or self-directed action is inextricably bound up with freedom and duty: 'to the Idea of freedom there is inseparably attached the concept of *autonomy*, and to this in turn the universal principle of morality—a principle which in Idea forms the ground for all the actions of *rational* beings.'[89]

As already mentioned, self-legislation (obedience to a self-imposed law) is an alternative to the idea that morality is something imposed on us by an outside authority. Self-legislation is an expression of our reason—reason in the sense of going beyond mere things such as offered by sensibility. Self-legislation is more than using reason to simply choose between premises which are desires. It is choosing to act according to the *idea* of law:

> What I recognize immediately as law for me, I recognize with reverence, which means merely consciousness of the *subordination* of my will to a law

> without the mediation of external influences on my senses. Immediate determination of the will by the law and consciousness of this determination is called '*reverence*' . . . the *object* of reverence is the *law* alone—that law which we impose on *ourselves* but yet as necessary in itself.[90]

Kant maintains that although reverence could be called a feeling it is one that is 'self-produced by a rational concept' and is distinct from feelings '*received* through outside influence.'[91] For Kant, there is a dignity in our rational nature and our reverence for a mere idea: '...it is just this freedom from dependence on interested motives which constitutes the sublimity of a maxim and the worthiness of every rational subject.'[92]

RESPECT FOR PERSONS AS ENDS

Kant appeals to the idea that rational beings have unconditional and absolute value. This is his often quoted idea of treating persons as ends rather than means which he expresses as a constraint on action: 'Act in such a way that you always treat humanity, whether in your own person or in the person of any other, never simply as a means, but always at the same time as an end.'[93] Respect for persons in Kant's sense, however, goes beyond the idea of a constraint on action. It also amounts to more than acknowledging and sharing other peoples' ends. Central to the notion of respect for persons are the ideas of a systematic union of rational beings under common laws, moral agents as simultaneously making the law and being subject to the law, the fitness of the maxims we act on and reverence for an 'idea.'

For Kant, the value of a person as an end derives from the fact that, as a rational being, persons are moral agents and capable of acting autonomously. The respect owed to persons, according to Kant, is owed not only because we do our duty, but because we are also the makers of moral law to which we, at the same time, subject ourselves.

We are worthy of respect by way of our part in making the moral law and this is something we share with all rational beings. According to Kant, it 'unquestionably follows' from the respect for persons version of the categorical imperative that we must always choose our maxims not only from our own point of view but also that of every other rational being 'as a maker of law.'[94] This means that we enter into a relationship with other rational beings and become a member of a union under common laws which Kant calls the 'kingdom of ends.' This is an ideal rather than something that really exists. We cannot count on every other person to always follow the categorical imperative but in acting as if all other rational beings will act in accordance with the law or moral feeling and do the same, we bring moral worth to our actions. Our dignity consists in *acting* in view of the *idea* of a 'kingdom of ends.'

A kingdom of ends would eventuate if we all acted on maxims that could be universally followed and for Kant it is enough that we act on the *idea* that every rational being, ourselves and others, 'may at the same time count in [our] maxim as an end in himself':[95] 'morality lies in the relation of actions to the autonomy of the will—that is, to a possible making of universal law by means of its maxims.'[96] This means that when we act in relation to another person we ought to take into account that he can make laws for himself. The idea of a kingdom of ends is central to the idea of respect for autonomy or respect for persons as ends because it prevents us from viewing and treating another person as merely a thing that is acted upon. It requires us to regard others as also making universal law (we assume the fitness of that person's maxims). When we do this we treat that person as an end.

To be an end in himself, a rational being 'must always be regarded as making universal law.'[97] The 'sole condition' under which anything can be an end in itself and in which it has intrinsic value or dignity is the 'morally good attitude of mind' which affords a rational being a 'share' in the 'making of universal law.' It enables him to be a member in a possible kingdom of ends.[98] In other words, freedom of the will or autonomy is the basis of the dignity of a rational being.[99]

Kant's idea of respect for persons as ends is not separable from his 'kingdom of ends' formulation of the categorical imperative. It is through the idea of a kingdom of ends that we assume and assure the fitness of another person's maxims. Without this we could only respect other peoples' ends on the basis of experience and the empirical world and that is something that Kant explicitly rejects. The 'reverence for a mere Idea' which the kingdom of ends version of the categorical imperative commands is, according to Kant, connected with both our dignity and our rational nature.

In order to treat persons as ends we have to *act as if* we are through our maxims 'always a law-making member in the universal kingdom of ends.'[100] In other words we act as if what is merely possible actually exists: 'All maxims as proceeding from our own making of law ought to harmonize with a possible kingdom of ends as a kingdom of nature.'[101] This is not a conditional or hypothetical imperative. According to Kant, it is a self-imposed rule that is without any end or advantage, and is free from interested motives. It assures the fitness of our maxims and constitutes the 'worthiness of every rational subject to be a law-making member in a kingdom of ends; for otherwise he would have to be regarded as subject only to the law of nature—the law of his own needs.'[102] Acting in view of the idea of a kingdom of ends distinguishes us from nonrational beings: 'Everything in nature works in accordance with laws. Only a rational being has the power to act *in accordance with his idea* of laws—that is, in accordance with principles.'[103] In other words reason moves us to act in the sense that it derives actions from laws.

The notion of a kingdom of ends which is 'reverence for a mere Idea' lifts us out of the purely physical realm. Reason becomes practical when we obey the kingdom of ends formulation of the categorical imperative. When we act on this version of the categorical imperative, we act on an idea to bring something about. Reason has a power such that when we act as though a kingdom of ends is possible, we 'bring into existence what does not exist but can be made actual by our conduct.'[104] There is a theoretical possibility that the kingdom of ends will become actual if we act in accordance with the categorical imperative. This is autonomy—we are not determined by the laws of nature. In contrast to acting in accordance with our 'idea of a law' which is possible only through freedom of the will, all other imperatives are conditioned and classed under heteronomy.[105]

It would be a mistake to think that it would be a desirable goal to make the kingdom of ends a kingdom of nature, in other words, for a 'mere Idea' to achieve any reality at all. Kant argues that this would not add any intrinsic worth: 'it would still be necessary to conceive the unique and absolute lawgiver himself as judging the worth of rational beings solely by the disinterested behaviour they prescribed to themselves in virtue of this Idea alone.'[106] Again, it is the 'form' of the principle, not the end results that are important for Kant. Respect for persons, therefore, involves more than instrumental value and it cannot be simply equated with acknowledging or sharing another person's ends.

Kant is not supporting or defending the content of people's goals. His concern is only with the 'form of a kingdom of ends' made up of persons 'capable of willing personal ends' which are 'in conformity with universal law.'[107] The command to respect persons as ends concerns the conduct of the agent. According to Kant, when we agree negatively with 'humanity as an end in itself' we refrain from deliberately impairing their happiness. When we agree positively with 'humanity as an end in itself,' it is not another person's particular ends that we seek to promote but our own attitude of mind which assumes the fitness of their maxims: 'For the ends of a subject who is an end in himself must, if this conception is to have its *full* effect in me, be also, as far as possible, *my ends*.'[108] It is significant that Kant refers to the effect in the agent rather than the result. According to Kant, my own and other peoples happiness is not an end which is also my duty: 'to maintain the integrity of my morality, that is my end and also my duty.'[109]

Respect for persons in Kant's sense entails not interfering with other people's goals or choices but this is not an endorsement of their ends and it is not concerned with bad consequences or possible harm. The concept of a kingdom of ends means that when we respect persons as ends, the critical aspect is the abstract idea that we, as moral agents, form in assuming the fitness of other peoples' maxims. This is a 'speculative use of reason' which assures the fitness of their maxims as well as our own. In doing this, we respect their ends regardless of content. This is respect for logic or respect for the like status of others as lawmaking members in a kingdom of ends.

Without the idea of universal law and without the kingdom of ends formulation of the categorical imperative, a principle of respect for persons is no more than an appeal to good consequences. According to Kant, we have to act from duty and discount the details of particular ends, such as happiness, well being, or even the promotion of autonomous action by others. Otherwise our will is only 'relatively good' and merely a means rather than an end. The various formulations of Kant's categorical imperative are equivalent but also, in a sense, parts of a whole which cannot be appealed to in isolation. Any defense of autonomy based on Kant's ideas has to include the ideal of a kingdom of ends and of acting on universal laws. Otherwise it is not grounded in Kantian arguments.

NOTES

1. J. J. Rousseau, *The Social Contract,* in *The Essential Rousseau*, translated by Lowell Bair (New York: A Mentor Book, 1974).
2. Rousseau, *The Social Contract*, 17.
3. Rousseau, *The Social Contract*, 20–21.
4. Rousseau, *The Social Contract*, 20.
5. Rousseau, *The Social Contract*, 20.
6. Rousseau, *The Social Contract*, 20–21.
7. Rousseau, *The Social Contract*, 13.
8. J. B. Schneewind, "Autonomy, Obligation, and Virtue: An Overview of Kant's Moral Philosophy" in *The Cambridge Companion to Kant*, ed. Paul Guyer (Cambridge: Cambridge University Press, 1992), 309–41, 314.
9. Rousseau, *The Social Contract*, 18–19.
10. Rousseau, *The Social Contract*, 27.
11. Rousseau, *The Social Contract*, 19–20.

12. Rousseau, *The Social Contract*, 11.

13. Rousseau, *The Social Contract*, 20–21.

14. Isaiah Berlin, "Two Concepts of Liberty" in *Four Essays on Liberty*, (London: Oxford University Press, 1969), 145.

15. Onora O'Neill, "Kantian Ethics," in *A Companion to Ethics*, ed. Peter Singer (Oxford: Blackwell, 1993), 179.

16. Rousseau, *The Social Contract*, 20.

17. See O'Neill, "Kantian Ethics," 183–34. e.g., O'Neill refers to a 'Kantian ethics' which is the image of Kant's ethics often used in modern debates and in which the 'specific understanding of Kantian ethics varies very much from context to context.' She also refers to John Rawls' 'Kantian ethics' which has features that are clearly Kantian but 'assumes a quite different account of rationality from Kant's.'

18. J. B. Schneewind, *The Invention of Autonomy: A History of Modern Moral Philosophy*, Cambridge University Press, 1998, p. 485. According to Schneewind, Kant had arrived at this view by 1765.

19. Schneewind, *The Invention of Autonomy*, 485 referring to Kant's, *Observations on the Feeling of the Beautiful and the Sublime*, 1763.

20. Schneewind, *The Invention of Autonomy*, 485.

21. Immanuel Kant, *Critique of Practical Reason and Other Writings in Moral Philosophy*, Translated and Edited with an Introduction by Lewis White Beck, (Chicago: University of Chicago Press, 1949), 6.

22. Rousseau, *The Social Contract*, 21.

23. Immanuel Kant, *Groundwork of the Metaphysic of Morals*, in *The Moral Law*, H. J. Paton, (Hutchinson Of London, 3rd. ed., 1956), 123 (Berlin page no. 455). Berlin page numbers will be enclosed in brackets.

24. Kant, *Groundwork*, 117 (449).

25. Kant, *Groundwork*, 118 (451).

26. Kant, *Groundwork*, 130 (462).

27. Kant, *Groundwork*, 120–21 (107–108).

28. Kant, *Groundwork*, 131 (463).

29. Kant, *Groundwork*, 119 (451).

30. Kant, *Groundwork*, 120 (452).

31. Kant, *Groundwork*, 80, (412).

32. Kant, *Groundwork*, 108 (440).

33. Kant, *Groundwork*, 80 (412).

34. Kant, *Groundwork*, 64 (396).

35. Kant, *Groundwork*, 65 (397).

36. Kant, *Groundwork*, 57 (389).

37. Kant, *Critique of Practical Reason*, 180.

38. Kant, *Groundwork*, 66 (398).

39. Kant *Critique of Practical Reason*, 180.

40. Kant, *Groundwork,* 66 (398).
41. Kant, *Groundwork,* 103 (436).
42. Kant, *Groundwork,* 61 (393).
43. Kant, *Groundwork,* 63 (394).
44. Kant, *Groundwork,* 63 (395).
45. Kant, *Groundwork,* 69 (401) f.n.
46. Immanuel Kant, in *Immanuel Kant, Lectures on Ethics*, eds. Peter Heath and J.B. Schneewind (Cambridge: Cambridge University Press, 1997), 125 (27:344).
47. Kant, *Groundwork,* 120 (452).
48. Kant, *Groundwork,* 69 (401).
49. Kant, *Groundwork,* 92 (425).
50. Kant, *Groundwork,* 68 (400).
51. Kant, *Groundwork,* 93 (425).
52. Kant, *Groundwork,* 69 (401) f.n.
53. Kant, *Groundwork,* 71 (403).
54. The fact that we are autonomous when we act from reasons rather than inclination, and that there is moral worth in acting from duty alone, should be distinguished from claims that Kant is advocating rule fetishism. See Barbara Herman, "Rules, Motives, and Helping Actions" *Philosophical Studies*, 45, (1984): 370, 372–73. Kant's idea of the moral worth of acting from duty should be distinguished from the idea that the object of an action is duty or that 'acting from the motive of duty is acting from concern for moral principle.' As we have seen, Kant suggests that when confronted with a choice of action there is an option that has a certain irresistibility or compulsion for a being with reason and Kant calls this option our duty. This does not mean that Kant is advocating a form of rule worship.
55. Kant, *Lectures on Ethics*, 212.
56. Immanuel Kant, *Lectures on Metaphysics*, translated and edited by Karl Ameriks and Steve Naragon, (Cambridge: Cambridge University Press, 1997) 484.
57. Kant, *Lectures on Ethics*, 234.
58. Kant, *Lectures on Ethics*, 125.
59. Kant, *Lectures on Ethics*, 125.
60. Kant, *Critique of Practical Reason,* 184.
61. Kant, *Critique of Practical Reason,* 30 (Intro).
62. Immanuel Kant, *The Doctrine of Virtue, Part II of The Metaphysic of Morals,* Trans. by Mary J. Gregor, (New York: Harper Torchbooks Harper and Row, 1964), 10, 26.
63. Kant, *Critique of Practical Reason,* 30 (Intro).
64. Kant, *Critique of Practical Reason,* 222 (V,118).
65. Kant, *Groundwork,* 91 (424), 88 (421 fn).
66. Kant, *Groundwork,* 82 (414).
67. Kant, *Lectures on Ethics*, 260 (27:491).

68. Kant, *Groundwork,* 108 (89).
69. Kant, *Groundwork,* 88 (421).
70. Kant, *Groundwork,* 96 (429).
71. Kant, *Groundwork,* 106 (438).
72. Kant, *Groundwork,* 98 (431).
73. Kant, *Groundwork,* 108 (440).
74. Kant, *Groundwork,* 104 (436–37).
75. Kant, *Groundwork,* 97 (430fn).
76. Onora O'Neill, *Constructions of Reason: Explorations of Kant's Practical Philosophy,* (Cambridge: Cambridge University Press, 1989), 83–84.
77. Kant, *Groundwork,* 88 (421).
78. Kant, *Groundwork,* 89–90 (422).
79. Kant, *Groundwork,* 90, (422).
80. Kant, *Lectures on Ethics*, 232 (29:608); Kant, *Groundwork,* 90 (422).
81. Kant, *Groundwork,* 70 (402).
82. Kant, *Groundwork,* 71 (403).
83. Kant, *Critique of Practical Reason,* 144–45 (V, 33–34).
84. Kant, *Groundwork,* 84 (416).
85. Kant, *Groundwork,* 84–85 (416).
86. Kant, *Lectures on Ethics*, 44.
87. Lewis White Beck, *A Commentary on Kant's Critique of Practical Reason,* (Chicago: The University of Chicago Press, 1960), 196–200, 179. For the idea of lawless or unrestricted freedom see also Kant, *Lectures on Ethics,* 125.
88. Beck, *A Commentary*, 196–200.
89. Kant, *Groundwork,* 120 (452–53).
90. Kant, *Groundwork,* 69 (401fn).
91. Kant, *Groundwork,* 69 (401fn).
92. Kant, *Groundwork,* 106 (439).
93. Kant, *Groundwork,* 96 (429).
94. Kant, *Groundwork,* 105–106 (438).
95. Kant, *Groundwork,* 105 (437).
96. Kant, *Groundwork,* 107 (439).
97. Kant, *Groundwork,* 102 (434).
98. Kant, *Groundwork,* 102–103 (435).
99. Kant, *Groundwork,* 103 (436).
100. Kant, *Groundwork,* 106 (438).
101. Kant, *Groundwork,* 104 (436).
102. Kant, *Groundwork,* 106 (439).
103. Kant, *Groundwork,* 80 (412).
104. Kant, *Groundwork,* 104 (fn436).
105. Kant, *Groundwork,* 100–101 (433–34).
106. Kant, *Groundwork,* 107 (439).

107. Kant, *Groundwork,* 141 [fn74 n.1. from 101 (433)].
108. Kant, *Groundwork,* 98 (430).
109. Kant, *The Metaphysics of Morals* in *Immanuel Kant: Critique of Practical Reason and Other Writings in Moral Philosophy,* Translated and edited by Lewis White Beck (Chicago: The University of Chicago Press, 1949), 357 (VI, 388).

2

MILLIAN IDEAS IN CONTEMPORARY INTERPRETATIONS OF AUTONOMY

ETHICAL FOUNDATIONS

In contrast to Kant, Mill's concern is with the consequences or ends of action. He argues for liberty and that argument involves the idea that we should be able to pursue our various ends without interference. For Mill 'all action is for the sake of some end.'[1] He claims that we begin with an idea of that which we are pursuing and our actions need to be justified in terms of that end: 'rules of action, it seems natural to suppose, must take their whole character and color from the end to which they are subservient.'[2] Mill's utilitarianism is grounded in the idea that pleasure and freedom from pain are basic desirable ends and things are desirable for the pleasure inherent in them or as means to the promotion of pleasure and the prevention of pain.'[3] The promotion of happiness, however, is not the end of all actions. According to Mill the utilitarian end of human action is also the standard of morality for human conduct: 'I regard utility as the ultimate appeal on all ethical questions; but it must be utility in the largest sense, grounded on the permanent interests of a man as a progressive being.'[4]

Utility or the greatest happiness principle, according to Mill, is an ethical standard. He claims there is 'nothing embarrassing' to those who view utility as the 'ultimate sanction' of all morality. Because of his concern with the consequences of our actions, Mill is also concerned with the agent and his character. Utility, for Mill, is a 'subjective feeling' in our minds and its basis and its force is the 'conscientious feelings of mankind.' This is an empirical thing—a fact of human nature. Mill differs from Kant who avoids altogether any appeal to anything empirical such as human nature. In contrast to Kant who maintains actions have moral worth when done from duty alone, Mill values a sympathetic temperament. This is evident in his discussion of whether the feeling of duty is innate in us. Although Mill does not believe this to be true (Mill claims moral feelings are acquired), he claims the principle of utility is the natural response of a sympathetic temperament: 'If there be anything innate in the matter, I see no reason why the feeling which is innate should not be that of regard to the pleasures and pains of others. If there is any principle of morals which is intuitively obligatory, I should say it must be that.'[5] According to Mill: 'few but those whose mind is a moral blank could bear to lay out their course of life on the plan of paying no regard to others except so far as their own private interest compels.'[6] This is part of the 'basis of powerful natural sentiment' which is the 'strength of utilitarian morality.' Its binding force is the sympathy individuals have for all others or 'the deeply rooted conception' individuals have of themselves as social beings:

> the desire to be in unity with our fellow creatures. . . . The social state is at once so natural, so necessary, and so habitual to man, that except in some unusual circumstances or by an effort of voluntary abstraction, he never conceives himself otherwise than as a member of a body. . . . Any condition, therefore, which is essential to a state of society becomes more and more an inseparable part of every person's conception of the state of things which he is born into, and which is the destiny of a human being . . . people grow up unable to conceive as possible to them a state of total disregard of other people's interests.[7]

Although Mill discusses the question of whether a feeling of duty is innate in us, he is not concerned with any notion of duty irrespective of the consequences. For Mill, the 'justification' for all ends is utility or the promotion of happiness. Action in which happiness is sacrificed can only be justified in terms of the promotion of happiness where it can be shown that 'on the whole more happiness' will come about. While utilitarian morality does recognize the sacrifice of our own greatest good for the good of others it does not view the sacrifice as a good in itself.[8]

THE ARGUMENT FOR LIBERTY: THE LINK WITH AUTONOMY

Several things in Mill's argument about liberty link into current debates about autonomy. First of all there is the question of the legitimate bounds of government interference with the individual. This fits in with the idea that noninterference with an individual's autonomous action is good and the idea that paternalism is the antithesis of, or a competing value with autonomy. In a famous passage from *On Liberty*, Mill argues that we should not interfere with the actions of other individuals simply because we dislike or disapprove of the actions they choose:

> the only purpose for which power can be rightfully exercised over any member of a civilized community, against his will, is to prevent harm to others. His own good, either physical or moral, is not a sufficient warrant. He cannot rightfully be compelled to do or forbear because it will be better for him to do so, because it will make him happier, because, in the opinions of others, to do so would be wise, or even right. These are good reasons for remonstrating with him, or reasoning with him, or persuading him, or entreating him, but not for compelling him, or visiting him with any evil in case he do otherwise. To justify that, the conduct from which it is desired to deter him, must be calculated to produce evil to some one else. The only part of the conduct of any one, for which he is amenable to society, is that which concerns others. In the part which merely concerns himself, his independence is, of right, absolute. Over himself, over his own body and mind, the individual is sovereign.[9]

In this passage Mill defends liberty of action and discusses the sole condition which allows or justifies intervention by the state. According to Mill, however, the prevention of harm to others, although a reason for state intervention, is not a sufficient condition for intervention. Sometimes we can cause pain or loss to others in a legitimate way. For instance, in overcrowded professions, competitive exams, and in contests where there is an object which more that one person desires, it is inevitable that there will be 'disappointed competitors.' Society admits no right to immunity from this kind of suffering.[10] 'At most,' claims Mill, 'harm to others is a necessary condition for intervention.'[11] Despite the fact that there may be ambiguities and difficulties with Mill's concept of harm,[12] and this causes problems with the justification for intervention, it is clear what, for Mill, constitutes *insufficient* grounds. He regards the fact that the agent may bring harm to self and that others may not approve of the action as insufficient grounds for intervention. Even though others think an agent's actions are foolish or wrong and not in his or her own best interests, this does not justify interference or force. Mill defends the choices an individual makes even when they come into conflict with the majority view: 'All errors which he is likely to commit against advice and warning are far outweighed by the evil of allowing others to constrain him to what they deem his good.'[13]

For Mill, where questions of conduct are concerned, the 'likings and dislikings' of society are not the ultimate appeal:

> There are many who consider as an injury to themselves any conduct which they have a distaste for, and resent it as an outrage to their feelings. . . . But there is no parity between the feeling of a person for his own opinion, and the feeling of another who is offended at his holding it; no more than between the desire of a thief to take a purse, and the desire of the right owner to keep it.[14]

Mill argues that until there is a definite risk of harm to another individual or to society, we may use persuasion or reason but not compulsion to change another's mind. Our opinion that an individual's actions are wrong is not sufficient justification for intervention. When no 'specific duty' to the public is violated or obvious harm is done to any 'assignable individual' other than the agent: 'the inconvenience is one which society can afford to bear, for the sake of the greater good of human freedom.'[15] As we shall see, it is from Mill that we get the idea of respect for autonomy as respect for choice.

INDIVIDUALITY

Another aspect of Mill's argument for liberty that links into current debates about autonomy is his argument for the value of individuality which involves the idea of 'character.' Even though he does not use the term 'autonomy,' Mill's argument about individuality as one of the elements of well-being can, without difficulty, be interpreted as an argument for why we should respect or value autonomy.

Despite a concern with both our desire to be in unity with others and with our social conscience in which we have joint or collective interests, it is individual human nature that Mill is mostly concerned with. Mill deals with the struggle between liberty and authority in *On Liberty*. He advocates individual independence and argues for a limit on social control. The social control he wants to restrict is 'the tyranny of the majority' or 'social tyranny' in the sense of the 'prevailing opinion and feeling' of society which fetters the development of individuals 'not in harmony with its ways'; which 'compels all characters to fashion themselves upon the model of its own.'[16] This kind of collective Mill refers to in a derogatory way as 'masses' or 'collective mediocrity.'[17] 'All wise or noble things' he argues, 'must come from individuals; generally at first from some one individual.'[18] The idea of society as a type of association in the sense of Rousseau's general will or Kant's kingdom of ends is not an idea that would appeal to Mill. For Mill, the whole which is society or a collective, is not in some way greater than the sum of its parts:

> The laws of the phenomena of society are, and can be, nothing but the laws of the actions and passions of human beings united together in the social state. Men, however, in a state of society, are still men; their actions and passions are obedient to the laws of individual human nature. Men are not, when brought together, converted into another kind of substance, with different properties; as hydrogen and oxygen are different from water. . . . Human beings in society have no properties but those which are derived from, and may be resolved into, the laws of the nature of individual man.[19]

For Mill, although the principle of utility is the ultimate appeal on all ethical questions, he also claims that the elevation of character or free development of individuality is something which is valuable in itself. This does not conflict with the principle of utility. Mill claims that the promotion of happiness is not itself the end of all actions or rules of action. Instead, it is 'the justification, and ought to be the controller, of all ends.'[20] The development of individual character can therefore be a goal to be pursued for itself:

> The character itself should be, to the individual, a paramount end, simply because the existence of this ideal nobleness of character, or of a near approach to it, in any abundance, would go further than all things else towards making human life happy; both in the comparatively humble sense, of pleasure and freedom from pain, and in the higher meaning, of rendering life . . . such as human beings with highly developed faculties can care to have.[21]

Individuality, according to Mill, 'is the privilege and proper condition of a human being, arrived at the maturity of his faculties, to use and interpret experience in his own way.'[22] A person who develops individuality has a character, whereas the person 'whose desires and impulses are not his own, has no character, no more than a steam engine has a character.'[23] Although the emphasis is on the development of individuality in conditions of freedom, Mill's ideas about individuality and character as required by the liberty principle are a recognizable influence on many contemporary accounts of the autonomous person. Even though Mill is discussing liberty, he could easily be describing the idea of the autonomous person in some contemporary discussions:

> the principle requires liberty of tastes and pursuits; of framing the plan of our life to suit our own character; of doing as we like subject to such consequences as may follow: without impediment from our fellow creatures, so long as what

> we do does not harm them, even though they should think our conduct foolish, perverse, or wrong . . . the only freedom which deserves the name, is that of pursuing our own good in our own way. . . . Each is the proper guardian of his own health, whether bodily, *or* mental and spiritual.[24]

CHOICE

The idea of choice is of importance in Mill's argument for the assertion of individuality. He claims that we express our individuality and our humanity when we make choices. Qualities such as 'perception, judgement, discriminative feeling, mental activity, and even moral preference' are, according to Mill, the 'distinctive endowment of a human being' and are exercised and developed only in the making of choices.[25] The value is not in the choice, however, but in our individuality which involves the idea of fully developing our capacities. The emphasis and the value is in the idea of character or self-development:

> He who lets the world, or his own portion of it, choose his plan of life for him, has no need of any other faculty than the ape-like one of imitation. He who chooses his plan for himself, employs all his faculties.[26]

In addition to the distinctive human qualities mentioned, Mill argues that once we have used these faculties to decide, we need 'firmness and self-control' to hold to our 'deliberate' decisions. We get practice in discerning or desiring what is best when we make choices and it is 'only in making a choice' that we develop our distinctive human qualities.[27] Mill seems to be giving a special role to choice and this may play a part in the fact that the notion of choice has become the focus of some contemporary accounts of autonomy.

C. L. Ten claims that Mill is often misunderstood as holding the view that all choices are good or valuable. This is not what Mill's argument is about. It is the importance of freedom and individuality that Mill is concerned with and it is in terms of the agent and his character that he argues for this. As mentioned earlier, for Mill, the development of character is for individuals a 'paramount end.' Mill emphasizes choice because it develops a person's capacities. He is not suggesting that a freely chosen act is necessarily a moral one, nor does he deny that good consequences may come out of a coerced or unfree act.[28]

Mill claims he is not arguing for one way of life or a particular ideal of character. He likens attempts to force human beings into a uniform way of life to being cramped and dwarfed or maimed by compression: 'like a Chinese lady's foot.'[29] From Mill's arguments we get a sense of what it is to be an autonomous person. What is more, the idea of the autonomous individual, derived from Mill's arguments, gives rise to a psychological sense of autonomy. Characteristics such as self-development, firmness, self-control, and the idea of choosing a plan of life are defended in the notion of autonomy associated with Mill.

Mill's view contrasts sharply with that of Kant whose concern is with the question of whether we are directed by our intellect as opposed to outside forces or the physical world. When Kant distinguished us from animals, it was to show that we express our humanity when we act from reason. When Mill distinguishes us from animals he refers to the 'ape-like' faculty of imitation, and contrasts this with the human individual whose desires or impulses are his own (who has a character). Mill seems to have a positive attitude to impulses and desires as long as they are our own. He claims that there is a tendency to view desires and impulses as a 'peril and a snare' but argues that 'desires and impulses are as much a part of a perfect human being as beliefs and restraints.'[30] According to Mill, it is not our desires or the strength of our desires that leads to bad actions, but that our 'consciences are weak,' that we 'act ill.'[31] Mill views desires and impulses as 'the raw material of human nature' which may be turned to bad use but certainly also to good. He favors intellectual activity and the possession of strong impulses and desires to a nature that is 'indolent and impassive.' Mill disputes the desirability of those who merely ask 'what is suitable to my position?' rather than 'what do I prefer? or, what would suit my character and disposition?'[32] Mill describes the condition of those who have no inclination other than custom as follows:

> the mind itself is bowed to the yoke: even in what people do for pleasure, conformity is the first thing thought of; they like in crowds; they exercise choice only among things commonly done; peculiarity of taste, eccentricity of conduct, are shunned equally with crimes: until by dint of not following their own nature they have no nature to follow: their human capacities are withered and starved: they become incapable of any strong wishes or native pleasures, and are generally without either opinions or feelings of home growth, or properly their own.[33]

It is not really clear what Mill means when he says that our desires and impulses must be our own. From his claim that a person's desires and impulses 'are the expression of his own nature, as it has been developed and modified by his own culture' with the additional claim that desires and impulses need to be balanced and 'under the government of a strong will,' we get the impression that for Mill, reason also has a role.[34] A role for reason suggests some convergence in ideas—but there is still a significant difference between Mill and Kant.

THE ROLE OF REASON IN ACTION

The differences between Kant and Mill on the role of reason in autonomous action stem from their different views on the role of reason in action. Mill seems to be a Humean about practical reason. That is, although he discusses the need for desires and impulses to be under the control of a strong will he is not giving reason a dominant role. He claims that it is absurd to say that 'my conscience prevails over my desires' because conscience itself is a desire—'the desire to do right.'[35] Mill calls into question the view that represents this kind of struggle as a contest between the individual and 'some foreign power' which the individual conquers or is overcome by. He describes a 'struggle between passions' in which the agent suffers a 'conflict of feelings' in this way:

> it is obvious that "I" am both parties in the contest; the conflict is between me and myself; between (for instance) me desiring a pleasure, and me dreading self-reproach. What causes Me, or, if you please, my Will, to be identified with one side rather than with the other, is that one of the Me's represents a more permanent state of my feelings than the other does. After the temptation has been yielded to, the desiring "I" will come to an end, but the conscience stricken "I" may endure to the end of life.[36]

The difference between a good man and a bad man, according to Mill, is that the desire to do right and the aversion to doing wrong in the good man are strong enough to overcome other desires. He claims that this is what makes humans capable of 'moral government.'[37] Mill is a Humean in the sense that he claims it is desires that motivate us to act. Kant takes the opposite view on this point. For Kant, reason motivates us while desires and passions distract us from the path of moral integrity.

IMPARTIALITY

For Kant, when we act on a maxim which can at the same time be made a universal law, our actions have moral worth and achieve a sort of consistency. This is more than the *desire* to be consistent or to do right. Moral worth, in the Kantian sense, in not an idea to be found in Mill.

Mill's view could be termed 'universalist' in the sense that he holds actions to be right in proportion to the happiness promoted, not just of the agent but of all concerned in the action.[38] The universal aspect in Mill is the idea that we go beyond our own personal view and take into account the view or interests of all who will be affected by an action. Taking this universal or impartial view does not depend on obedience to reason or to a universal moral law and it is not something which is good in itself.

MILL'S DETERMINISM

Mill is a determinist, but one who gives a role to choice and to responsibility. He believes that if we know a person thoroughly and if we know all of the influences such as desires, aversions, habits, and dispositions which they are subject to, we can, with certainty, predict that persons conduct in the same way we can predict physical events: 'given the motives which are present to an individual's mind, and given likewise the character and disposition of the individual, the manner in which he will act may be unerringly inferred.'[39] Determinism in Mill's sense, however, does not mean that things are so irrevocably fixed that we cannot or should not try to change them. The sense in which our actions are inevitable does not detract in any way from our feeling of freedom: 'We do not feel ourselves the less free, because those to whom we are intimately known are well assured how we shall will to act in a particular case.'[40]

Mill argues against the view that our actions do not depend on our desires and also the view that our character is innate or fixed and we are not responsible for it. He calls himself a 'moral causationist' which means he believes that the improvement of the character is possible and that the only 'needful condition' for that is desire.'[41] Mill holds that 'the vital truth in moral psychology' is that we can 'improve our character.' His argument for how we can improve our character shows that, although he is a determinist he also thinks we have a kind of freedom:

> we can, by employing the proper means, improve our character; and . . . if our character is such that while it remains what it is, it necessitates us to do wrong, it will be just to apply motives which will necessitate us to strive for its improvement, and so emancipate ourselves from the other necessity. We shall not indeed do so unless we desire our improvement, and desire it more than we dislike the means which must be employed for the purpose.[42]

It is not difficult to see how the idea of character and the role of desires derived from Mill's arguments find a place in contemporary ideas of autonomy. According to Mill, by way of our desires we are self-determining and we are responsible for our actions:

> A person feels morally free who feels that his habits or his temptations are not his masters, but he theirs: who even in yielding to them knows that he could resist; that were he desirous of altogether throwing them off, there would not be required for that purpose a stronger desire than he knows himself to be capable of feeling.[43]

On the other hand we are not autonomous when our desires are thwarted or unfulfilled: 'if we have wished and not attained, we have, to that extent, no power over our own character, we are not free.'[44]

Mill does not use the word 'autonomy' but his arguments for individual liberty can be interpreted as providing reasons for respecting other people's autonomy. From Mill we get the idea that autonomy is noninterference and because he refers to certain character traits that seem to define an autonomous person we also get the idea that autonomy is a psychological state.

Quite separate notions of autonomy are derived from Mill and Kant. Kant is defending an ethics based on reason and for Kant reason is much more than a guardian of the senses. Reason determines its own end and choice is only free when it is determined by reason alone. When choice originates in feelings or desires, it is somehow not *our* choice and therefore not autonomous. For Mill, on the other hand, autonomy is not negated by choice that originates in our feelings and desires. Furthermore, Mill's concern is with political civil liberty whereas Kant's concern is with autonomy as a fundamental moral principle. As we are about to see, these very different, incompatible, views are the source of confusion in some contemporary accounts of autonomy.

NOTES

1. J. S. Mill, *Utilitarianism* in *Mill: Utilitarianism*, ed. Samuel Gorovitz (Indianapolis: The Bobbs-Merrill Company, Inc., 1971), 14.
2. Mill, *Utilitarianism*, 14.
3. Mill, *Utilitarianism*, 18.
4. Mill, *Utilitarianism*, 21; J. S. Mill *On Liberty*, in *On Liberty and Considerations on Representative Government*, ed. R. B. McCallum (Oxford: Basil Blackwell, 1948), 9.

5. Mill, *Utilitarianism*, 32–33.
6. Mill, *Utilitarianism*, 36.
7. Mill, *Utilitarianism*, 34–35.
8. Mill, *Utilitarianism*, 24.
9. Mill, *On Liberty*, 8–9.
10. Mill, *On Liberty*, 84–85.
11. C. L. Ten, *Mill on Liberty* (Oxford: Clarendon Press, 1980), 66–67.
12. John Gray, *Mill on Liberty: A Defence* (London: Routledge & Kegan Paul, 1983), 49.
13. Mill, *On Liberty*, 69.
14. Mill, *On Liberty*, 75.
15. Mill, *On Liberty* 73.
16. Mill, *On Liberty*, 4.
17. Mill, *On Liberty*, 58.
18. Mill, *On Liberty*, 59.
19. J. S. Mill, *System of Logic: Ratiocinative and Inductive*, vol. II, 7th ed. (London: Longmans, Green, Reader, and Dyer, 1971), 466.
20. Mill, *System of Logic*, 554.
21. Mill, *System of Logic*, 554.
22. Mill, *On Liberty*, 51.
23. Mill, *On Liberty*, 53.
24. Mill, *On Liberty*, 11.
25. Mill, *On Liberty* , 51.
26. Mill, *On Liberty*, 51–52. Mill may have been unfair to apes here as there is evidence that they are not limited to imitation. See Jane Goodall, 'Chimpanzees—Bridging the Gap'; Toshisada Nishida, ' Chimpanzees Are Always New to Me'; Adriaan Kortlandt, 'Spirits Dressed in Furs?'; and Roger S. Fouts and Deborah H. Fouts, 'Chimpanzees' Use of Sign Language,' in *The Great Ape Project: Equality beyond Humanity*, eds P. Cavalieri and P. Singer (London: Fourth Estate, 1993).
27. Mill, *On Liberty*, 51.
28. Ten, *Mill on Liberty*, 79–80.
29. Mill, *On Liberty*, 55, 62.
30. Mill, *On Liberty*, 53.
31. Mill, *On Liberty*, 53.
32. Mill, *On Liberty*, 54.
33. Mill, *On Liberty*, 54.
34. Mill, *On Liberty*, 53.
35. J. S. Mill, *An Examination of Sir William Hamilton's Philosophy and of the Principal Philosophical Questions Discussed in His Writings* (Toronto: University of Toronto Press, 1979), 451.
36. Mill, *An Examination*, 452.
37. Mill, *An Examination*, 453.

38. J. O. Urmson and Jonathan Ree, *The Concise Encyclopedia of Western Philosophy and Philosophers*, (London: Unwin Hyman, London, 1991), 210.

39. Mill, *System of Logic*, 418; H. J. McCloskey, *John Stuart Mill: A Critical Study* (London: Macmillan, 1971), 91.

40. Mill, *System of Logic*, 418.

41. Mill, *An Examination*, 465–66.

42. Mill, *An Examination*, 466.

43. Mill, *System of Logic*, 423.

44. Mill, *System of Logic*, 423.

3

THE DEVELOPMENT OF THE CONTEMPORARY IDEA OF AUTONOMY

THE BELMONT REPORT

Having looked at the historical development of autonomy, we have seen that both Mill and Kant have influenced current concepts of autonomy. Now we will turn to the twentieth century to see why and how the idea of autonomy became so dominant in contemporary bioethics. I will also trace the influence of Mill and Kant through *The Belmont Report* and *Principles of Biomedical Ethics*—key documents in contemporary thinking about autonomy.

The Belmont Report is a set of guidelines issued by a United States National Commission, created in 1973 to identify basic ethical principles that should underlie the conduct of research involving humans. Respect for persons was one of the principles identified. This principle was transformed into the contemporary idea of autonomy by Beauchamp and Childress, who have been very influential in the development of bioethics, particularly in the discussion of autonomy. Their book, *Principles of Biomedical Ethics,* has become a central bioethical text and they have produced five editions with major changes. In view of the influence of *The Belmont Report* and the wide influence of *Principles of Biomedical Ethics,* it is worth looking at both in more detail. It is worth looking at the selection of the principle of respect for persons in *The Belmont Report* and tracing in detail the changes to the chapter on autonomy through the five editions of the Beauchamp and

Childress text. This will show us how many others in the field have seen the concept of autonomy.

In contemporary bioethical discussions various senses of autonomy are often run together and Beauchamp and Childress have been cited as being 'to some extent' to blame for for mixing the different senses of autonomy.[1] One of the ideas being referred to in contemporary discussions is a psychological view of autonomy which is seen as the ability to make choices based on an individual's own values and preferences. This sense of autonomy describes a state of affairs, and is not itself evaluative, although from some well-known ethical viewpoints this state of affairs is a desirable one. Then there is Kant's view in which to act autonomously is to act with reason alone as the determining ground of the will, and thus is to act from duty or from respect for the moral law. For Kant, these actions alone have moral worth. We will see how these different senses of autonomy are often mixed together in contemporary discussions.

Principles of Biomedical Ethics, which is 'close to a canonical text' in medical ethics, has lead to the widespread common idea that autonomy construed as a psychological state is a moral value 'independent of the utilitarian value of beneficence.'[2] In later editions of the text we will see how Beauchamp and Childress's approach changes to a procedural one where the focus is on gaining informed consent and resolving conflict without force. This idea of autonomy, even though it is an approach more than an idea, still contains many psychological assumptions. And this approach is still not a Kantian one.

Beauchamp and Childress attribute the work of the National Commission for the Protection of Human Subjects with having an influence on the writing of their book.[3] *Principles of Biomedical Ethics* and *The Belmont Report* were 'written simultaneously, the one inevitably influencing the other' during the period in which Beauchamp was a staff member of the National Commission for the Protection of Human Subjects of Biomedical and Behavioral Research.[4] Beauchamp had the task of writing 'The Belmont Paper,' later called '*The Belmont Report*' and claims that the two projects—one focused 'largely on issues in clinical ethics and health policy' and the other focused solely on 'research ethics'—had 'many points of intersecting interest.'[5]

According to Beauchamp, *The Belmont Report* had an 'enormous impact on the development of U.S. bioethics,' and until about 1983, had a 'much wider impact on the field' than the book he and James Childress published.[6] The impact of the National Commission and *The Belmont Report* was in part due to the influence it had on the emerging field of bioethics. Over the four years of its existence, the National Commission enlisted various people to contribute papers on specific topics. This served to actively involve many scholars in the emerging field and it promoted the study of bioethics.[7]

The Belmont Report is a key document in contemporary thinking about autonomy and even now, the influence of *The Belmont Report* continues.[8] The report was issued by a commission concerned with the regulation of human experimentation that was created by the U.S. Congress in 1973 with the official name; the National Commission for the Protection of Human Subjects of Biomedical and Behavioral Research. This commission was a response to a combination of things which I outline below.

In 1966 Henry Beecher, a Harvard Medical School professor, published an article in the *New England Journal of Medicine* containing details of twenty-two experiments in which researchers had risked the life or the health of human subjects. For instance a number of human subjects (hospitalized patients) were injected with live cancer cells. In this study of immunity to cancer, the subjects were told only that they were receiving 'some cells.' The word cancer was not mentioned to them at all. In other studies, known effective treatments were withheld without the subjects being informed. This was done without their consent or even their awareness that they were involved in an experiment. Another experiment involved a group of investigators who recognized an effective treatment for typhoid fever in an earlier study and then conducted a further study to determine relapse rates. Of four hundred and eight charity (impoverished) patients, two hundred and fifty-one received the known effective treatment while it was withheld from the other one hundred and fifty-seven. The death rates were 7.97 percent and 22.9 percent respectively. According to this data, twenty-three patients died for the sake of the study.[9] Beecher concluded that widespread disregard for human subjects existed and that unethical or questionable practice was not uncommon.[10] There was a conflict between the interests of researchers and the interests of patients. Patient well being was being treated as less important than research.

Part of the background to these revelations were the Nazi war experiments. Arthur Caplan argues that 'bioethics was born from the ashes of the holocaust' and the holocaust made it clear to society that medicine was incapable of, and should not be left to set its own ethical standards.[11] The Beecher cases reawakened this concern.

The censure of recurring abuses in human experimentation played a significant part in the establishment of the commission that had as its primary concern the protection of human subjects. Its mandate, however, went further than preventing particular abuses. Ethical issues arising from the use of vulnerable subjects was also a focus. In the aftermath of the abortion decision in *Roe vs Wade* and reports in the press about experiments on fetuses and exploitative or coercive research on special populations, the commission was required to consider vulnerable subjects such as young children, prisoners, the mentally disabled, and also human fetuses.[12] In *Strangers at the Bedside: A History of How Law and Bioethics Transformed Medical Decision Making*, David Rothman argues that it was circumstances such as the ones just mentioned that brought outsiders, people outside the medical profession, into the group of people interested in the practice of medicine.[13]

Additionally, there were certain developments occurring in society at that time which are likely to have contributed to the establishment of the commission. The civil rights movement, the growth of consumer groups, and an increasingly politically active disabilities community, added to the numbers of those interested in medical ethics and medical decision making. Also, according to David Rothman, author of the first formal history of bioethics, there was an enormous amount of conflict and tension in the development of bioethics and in those early days the ideology of the movement 'had a quite heroic quality about it.' The ideology of the movement had to do with civil rights which meant that the patient was 'understood as a member of a minority.' This gave the movement an 'extraordinary power' and ideas of autonomy and issues of consent were built onto that.[14] These developments all coincided with a general distrust of authority and institutions.[15] One of the topics the commission was instructed to deliberate on was the ethical requirements for psychosurgery. It has even been suggested that the misgivings and unease generated by Ken Kesey's critique of frontal lobotomy in mental institutions in *One Flew Over the Cuckoo's Nest* had some effect.[16]

Increasingly those outside the medical profession saw no reason to believe that the profession was capable of self-regulation, and they agreed on one thing, 'the need to reduce physicians' discretion and enhance patients' autonomy.'[17] It seems that the need for a commission, bioethics in general, and the demand for patient autonomy, has to some extent, developed as a reaction to medical paternalism. Over and above that, however, was the fact that doctors were seen not to be acting in a genuinely paternalistic manner—they were acting in ways that were *not* in the best interests of their patients.

The National Commission for the Protection of Human Subjects of Biomedical and Behavioral Research was charged with identifying 'basic ethical principles that should underlie the conduct of research involving human subjects' and with developing 'guidelines to assure that such principles

[were] followed.' These instructions are contained in the commission's mandate under Public Law 93–348.[18] From 1974 to 1978 the commission issued ten reports. One of those was *The Belmont Report*. Belmont was the Conference Center of the Smithsonian Institution, where a four-day period of intensive discussions took place in February 1976.[19] Part of the recommendation of the report was that its principles and guidelines be adopted as a statement of departmental policy on the conduct of research involving human subjects for use by federal employees, members of institutional review boards, and researchers.[20]

The Belmont Report is a document for the public rather than a philosophical analysis of concepts. The report identifies three 'basic ethical principles' which it offers as an 'analytical framework' to 'guide the resolution of ethical problems arising from research involving human subjects.'[21] The three principles are respect for persons, beneficence, and justice.

While *The Belmont Report* has three principles, *Principles of Biomedical Ethics* contains four principles: respect for autonomy, nonmaleficence, beneficence, and justice. The principle of respect for autonomy in *Principles of Biomedical Ethics* corresponds to the principle of respect for persons identified in *The Belmont Report*. *The Belmont Report* states that: 'Respect for persons incorporates at least two basic ethical convictions.' These are: 'individuals should be treated as autonomous agents' and 'persons with diminished autonomy are entitled to protection.'[22] According to the report, 'the principle of respect for persons thus divides into two separate moral requirements: the requirement to acknowledge autonomy and the requirement to protect those with diminished autonomy.'[23]

In *The Belmont Report* an 'autonomous person' is described as 'an individual capable of deliberation about personal goals and of acting under the direction of such deliberation.' It also says that 'respect' for autonomy is 'to give weight to autonomous persons' considered opinions and choice' and that also means refraining from 'obstructing their actions unless they are clearly detrimental to others.' A 'lack of respect' for an autonomous person is 'to repudiate that person's 'considered judgements, to deny an individual the freedom to act on those considered judgements, or to withhold information necessary to make a considered judgement, when there are no compelling reasons to do so.'[24]

Essentially this is all *The Belmont Report* has to say about the principle of respect for persons. Albert Jonsen, one of the commissioners, who was intimately involved in writing *The Belmont Report* says: 'I can attest that relatively little philosophical profundity went into it (although some philosophically profound people worked on it).' He says 'we were trying to capture the general idea of Nuremberg's voluntary consent and lift it to a plane of wider generalization.' Although at Belmont itself, the subcommittee which was considering the principles used the term 'respect for self-determination of human beings' the full commission preferred respect for persons.[25]

In *The Belmont Report* and bioethics discussions in general, 'respect for persons,' 'respect for autonomy,' and 'respect for self-determination' are often used interchangeably.[26] They may or may not be describing the same thing. An example of how these terms are interchanged occurs in an article about the use of principles in bioethics by Raymond J. Devettere. He claims that the three basic principles identified on page four of *The Belmont Report* were 'autonomy, beneficence, and justice.'[27]

George Annas, who argues that American bioethics 'is rooted in and dominated by American law,' also does not distinguish between these terms. He suggests that the values and ideals of American law, as expressed in the Declaration of Independence and the Constitution, dominate ethical discourse and that the first and third ethical principles of *The Belmont Report* center on 'fundamental American legal principles: autonomy (liberty), beneficence, and justice.'[28]

These examples reveal a looseness in the terminology which could be attributed to the settling down of the terminology. In other words, the various terms may be describing the same things. I will argue, however, that these terms are not always describing the same things. Sometimes respect for persons and respect for autonomy signify different things and using the terms interchangeably invites confusion. We may claim that we are appealing to the value of autonomy but what we are really appealing to may be something different. For instance we may invoke the idea of respect for autonomy as it is construed in *The Belmont Report* (as freedom to follow one's considered judgments), but incorporate the idea of respect for persons or respect for autonomy as a value in itself.

HOW RESPECT FOR PERSONS GOT INTO *THE BELMONT REPORT*

Jonsen believes that it was he who suggested the term 'respect for persons.'[29] Although the principle 'variously called "respect for persons" or "respect for autonomy"' came to dominate in bioethics and the idea of autonomy played a role in Western philosophy for some centuries before that, Jonsen notes that modern moral philosophy gave little attention to the phrase 'respect for persons' or 'respect for autonomy.' Neither term appeared in the indices of the most influential textbooks.[30]

Jonsen says that, at the time of the National Commission, he thought 'respect for persons' was a 'suitably general ethical principle which could include both acknowledgment of autonomy and protection of those lacking autonomy.' He remembers that 'it seemed efficient' to link these ideas together and adds that *The Belmont Report* was a document for the public rather than for philosophers. He states that the reason he suggested the term was that he had recently read R.S. Downie and Elizabeth Telfer's *Respect for Persons*, which he describes as a fairly straightforward interpretation of Kantian autonomy. He also claims: 'the title seemed to me a good one to express our ideas.' The commission also had a paper written by H. Tristram Engelhardt which named 'respect for persons' as one of the basic moral values.[31] It is worth looking at these influences on the selection of the principle of respect for persons in *The Belmont Report* to see how the idea of autonomy in contemporary bioethics originated and developed.

As already mentioned, Jonsen claims that the National Commission for the Protection of Human Subjects of Biomedical and Behavioral Research was trying to 'capture the general idea of Nuremberg's voluntary consent.' The Nuremberg Code has an instrumental value in the sense that it was a device to make sure that atrocities like the Nazi experiments could never happen again. The notion of respect for autonomy is made clearly evident by the standard of conduct set out in the Nuremberg Code. The code emphasizes and insists on the voluntary informed consent of human subjects:

> The voluntary consent of the human subject is absolutely essential. This means that the person involved should have legal capacity to give consent; should be so situated as to be able to exercise free power of choice, without the intervention of any element of force, fraud, deceit, duress, overreaching, or other ulterior form of constraint or coercion; and should have sufficient knowledge and comprehension of the elements of the subject matter involved as to enable him to make an understanding and enlightened decision.[32]

The Nuremberg Code also states the conditions necessary for a subject to reach this kind of autonomous choice:

> before the acceptance of an affirmative decision by the experimental subject there should be made known to him the nature, duration and purpose of the experiment; the method and means by which it is to be conducted; all inconveniences and hazards reasonably to be expected; and the effects upon his health or person which may possibly come from his participation in the experiment.[33]

Obviously the Nazis would never have been able to obtain voluntary informed consent from the subjects of their experiments. The standards set out in the code are a strategy to prevent any reoccurrence of abuse of human subjects.

As well as respect for autonomy, there are aspects of the Nuremberg Code that are indicative of respect for persons. The opening statement of the code suggests that, even though they may benefit a lot of people, results produced by experiments are not the only moral consideration. It rejects the idea of people being used merely as a means and introduces the idea that this involves acting on principles rather than seeking a particular end:

> The great weight of the evidence before us is to the effect that certain types of medical experiments on human beings, when kept within reasonably well-defined bounds, conform to the ethics of the medical profession generally. The protagonists of the practice of human experimentation justify their views on the basis that such experiments yield results for the good of society that are unprocurable by other methods or means of study. All agree, however, that certain basic principles must be observed in order to satisfy moral, ethical and legal concepts.[34]

It seems that both ideas, respect for autonomy and respect for persons, are in the Nuremberg Code. They are not clearly distinguished and it is not clear whether it was one or both of these ideas that had an influence on *The Belmont Report*.

According to Jonsen, R. S. Downie and Elizabeth Telfer's *Respect for Persons* had some influence in bringing respect for persons and then respect for autonomy into American bioethics via Jonsen and via *The Belmont Report*. In their book Downie and Telfer adopt and defend 'respect for persons as ends' as a 'supreme regulative principle.'[35] The idea of the individual having 'supreme worth' is, they say, 'fundamental to the moral, political and religious ideals of our society.' They claim that it has been given a 'central place' in philosophical writings such as Kant's *Groundwork of the Metaphysic of Morals* and J. S. Mill's *On Liberty*. In fact, despite the linking of their notion of respect for persons to Kant, Downie and Telfer's version actually moves away from Kant.

Downie and Telfer claim that respect for persons as ends is a way of regarding people that gives rise to ways of treating them. The sense of 'to respect' that is relevant to their notion of 'respect for persons' is 'to value' or 'to esteem.'[36] What is of value in persons, according to Downie and Telfer, 'can be characterized roughly as the exercise of rational will, taking that concept in a broad sense which does not exclude the concomitant presence of feeling and desire.'[37] This is not incompatible with Kant. Kant emphasises reason but he does not exclude the presence of feelings and desires. Downie and Telfer, however, go further. They want to include feelings and desires as things that move us to action and they want to make that a necessary part of respecting persons as ends.

The 'possession of a rational will' according to Downie and Telfer, is the 'distinctive endowment' of the human person. They also claim that when we accept the concept of a rational will, we must accept the view that reason is practical as well as theoretical. This practical sense of reason involves 'the ability to choose for oneself, and, more extensively, to formulate purposes, plans and policies of one's own.'[38] It is, they claim, this ability to exercise the rational will that gives human personality its intrinsic value and it is something that is 'cognitive, conative and affective.'[39] In other words, the ability to feel and express certain things is characteristically human and the perception and discrimination needed for that involves the rational will. Downie and Telfer argue that the distinction Kant makes between feeling and reason may be artificial. They include feelings and emotions as a motivating force for action. Active sympathy, they claim, is practical concern for others and a necessary component of the attitude of respect:

> Our claim is that active sympathy is one form of 'creative emotional response,' and that it is a response to the conception of persons as self-determining agents pursuing ends of inclination.[40]

According to Downie and Telfer, we respect other persons by 'showing active sympathy with them.' They claim the equivalent 'in Kant's language' is 'we make their ends our own.'[41] A second necessary component of the attitude of respect, is 'a readiness to at least consider the applicability of other men's rules both to them and to ourselves.' Downie and Telfer claim that these two components are 'independently necessary and jointly sufficient to constitute the attitude of respect which it is fitting to direct at persons conceived as rational wills.'[42]

For Kant, the idea of respecting persons as ends has more to do with the fact that we are rational beings than it has with acknowledging and sharing another person's ends. It is something we are owed because of the dignity and worth we possess insofar as we are capable of morality. When Downie and Telfer invoke Kant and the language of people as ends to legitimize the inclusion of inclinations and desires they seem to be using (or at least not distinguishing between) different senses of 'ends.' They attribute to Kant the idea that 'we should treat the ends of others, their ends of inclination, or what they pursue in the exercise of their self-determination, as if they were our own.'[43] Contrary to Kant, this could be interpreted as an undiscriminating respect for whatever ends, including desires, that people happen to have, rather than respect for persons as ends. For Kant, not all ends are duties. Downie and Telfer do not distinguish between what motivates respect (our intellect) and the goals people have which may belong entirely to the physical world. They include the pursuit of objects of inclination as ends in their interpretation of the exercise of self-determination. This is significantly different to Kant. According to Kant, in order for a rational being 'to be conceived as *an end in himself*' the will 'must always be regarded as *making universal law*' and this is 'in no way based on feelings, impulses, and inclinations.'[44] We conceive another person as an end because of our part in making universal law and our recognition that this is something we share with all rational beings. It means we choose our maxims from the point of view of ourselves 'and also of every other rational being.'[45] This is not the same thing as the wholesale promotion of other people's ends.

Downie and Telfer invoke Kant but then depart from him again in their discussion of the rational will. They name two distinctive features of human beings or the rational will. There is the ability to be self-determining, and secondly, the ability to 'govern one's conduct by rules' and to make rules which are valid for all rational beings. This second feature Kant calls 'autonomy of the will' and, in his view, is something which distinguishes us from animals. According to Downie and Telfer, it is a feature much stressed by Kant.[46] Having invoked Kant, however, Downie and Telfer do not want to adhere to Kant. They do not want to embrace his idea of autonomy of the will. Instead, they aim to cast doubt on his notion of self-validating moral legislation and take from Kant 'the weaker thesis' that as well as being self-determining we also formulate and follow rules, some of which (such as moral rules)' we hold as 'binding on others' as well as ourselves.[47] Downie and Telfer's notion of respect for persons differs from Kant in the sense that it does not capture the Kantian idea that this respect is due to persons in so far as they are able to act according to moral law. Perhaps Downie and Telfer would claim that they capture the Kantian idea of respect in the positive concern they prescribe for others as self-determining agents and in the act of making their ends our ends. For Kant, however, we have a capacity to legislate universal moral law and a corresponding duty to respect the moral law. It involves the subjugation of our inclinations to the moral law. To the extent that Downie and Telfer were influential in bringing the idea of 'respect for persons' into modern bioethics, they did so in a way that is a significant departure from the original Kantian conception of autonomy, despite what Jonsen says and what their terminology seems to imply.

Another influence on the selection of 'respect for persons,' according to Jonsen, was an article written by Tristram Engelhardt. Engelhardt was one of the scholars nominated by the National Commission to prepare a statement on the ethical principles that should govern human subject research. He names respect for persons as a basic moral value and argues that there are two central but separate concerns at issue when considering experimentation involving human subjects. There are deontological concerns (involving rights and duties) and teleological concerns (involving goals and goods):

1. questions bearing on respect for persons as moral agents, and
2. questions bearing on the achievement of goods and values which humans in general esteem.[48]

According to Engelhardt the literature concerning human experimentation focuses on three principles or 'cardinal ethical issues.' These are:

- respect for human subjects as free agents,
- concern to foster the best interests of human subjects, and
- concern to maximize the benefits accruable to society.[49]

The first principle is a deontological principle: 'an appeal to respect for the freedom of persons whether or not such respect would in the long run contribute to the benefit of society.' The other two principles involve goals and goods.[50] Engelhardt's notion of respect for persons is in some ways tied to a notion of freedom. The idea that freedom is a necessary condition of morality is attributed by Engelhardt to Kant and freedom is presupposed in much of what Engelhardt says about respect for persons. It seems doubtful, however, whether Engelhardt is confining himself to a Kantian idea of freedom.

> This analysis of basic ethical principles concerning experimentation with human subjects begins with the presupposition that there is a sense of moral responsibility, and that this sense has meaning only if persons think of each other as being free.[51]

Kant's idea of freedom is more than freedom *from* something. Nevertheless, Engelhardt invokes Kant and uses Kantian terminology. He invokes Kant's distinction between the dignity of persons and the value of things and claims that the notion of respect is also connected to the 'dignity of a free agent.' By this, he means that 'a person has the right to be treated not merely as an object, but also as self-determining—an entity who can be used only with his or her consent.'[52] This does not quite capture the Kantian idea of dignity or the idea that a free will is a will under moral laws.

To see why Engelhardt's view is not Kant's we need to look more closely at what he says about respect for persons. Although Engelhardt differentiates between the concern to respect persons as moral agents and our interest in autonomy which we express in the requirement for informed consent, he also runs these different ideas together. The first standard of the Nuremberg Code is a demand for informed consent which, according to Engelhardt, stresses the significance of the notion of respect for persons: 'The voluntary consent of the human subject is absolutely essential.' Engelhardt claims that this appeals to the principle of respect for human subjects as free agents.[53] He also claims that the notion of informed consent can serve more than one purpose because other values can be pursued simultaneously. Informed consent serves as a focal point for the central concerns at issue in experimentation involving human subjects and, according to Engelhardt, the various principles are located in this one concept:

> Respect for human subjects as persons requires gaining their free and informed consent in order to use them, not as mere objects, but as collaborating persons in an experiment. . . . And, again, the other roles of consent must be emphasized: to encourage autonomy as a general social value, and to ensure that the best interests of the subject are secured.[54]

Engelhardt distinguishes between concerns such as duties and rights on the one hand and goals and goods on the other and he views all of these concerns as central and necessary within the notion of informed consent. He claims his view of freedom and morality is one that 'draws heavily' on Kant,[55] but it is doubtful whether it really is Kant's. A point to note is that he is invoking Kant and appealing to Kant together with ideas such as the best interests of the subject. The ideas Engelhardt refers to are non-Kantian ideas more often associated with Mill.[56]

According to Engelhardt, in matters relating to human experimentation, appeals to freedom in the concepts of free and informed consent are important. Persons need to be 'free to choose good reasons over bad.'[57] He reformulates his three basic principles as procedural maxims to secure ethical conduct in experimentation. Gaining free and informed consent is a way to ensure respect for persons and also a way to pursue other values. For instance, we value a society where individuals live without fear of being used in experiments without their consent.[58] Basically, Engelhardt's four procedural principles are:

- obtaining free and informed consent,
- obtaining proxy consent where individuals are unable to consent,
- avoiding coercion, and
- the weighing of benefits and risks.[59]

With this reformulation, he provides us with a procedural approach rather than a substantive concept of autonomy or persons. It is a view about why we should respect autonomy rather than why we should respect persons or what it is for a person to be autonomous.

Although Engelhardt names respect for persons as a basic value, in the context of the conduct of biomedical and behavioral research, his focus becomes general principles of moral conduct, which enjoy general assent and which can function as a regulative ideal.[60] He invokes and appeals to Kantian notions to some extent, but he also moves away from Kant. His notion of freedom seems more Millian than Kantian, and for Engelhardt, rationality does not have a central role in ensuring respect for persons:

> One cannot try (nor should one) to force subjects who can be rational free agents to use that rationality and freedom to its fullest. . . . The concept of informed consent thus functions to guarantee that researchers will not act in disregard of their subjects as persons. It cannot, however, function to guarantee that subjects will be ideal moral agents who will act on their choices in a fully free and informed fashion. It is only that the deficiency in their choice should not be attributable to the investigator.[61]

THE LAW'S INFLUENCE

George Annas claims that American bioethics is 'rooted in and dominated by American law' and he attributes this dominance, in part, to the involvement of the legal profession. The National Commission for the Protection of Human Subjects of Biomedical and Behavioral Research had eleven commissioners, and three of them belonged to the legal profession. There was a professor of law, an associate professor of law, and an attorney. The director of the Commission Staff was also a lawyer. In addition to the makeup of the commission, law was central in other ways. A main primary source document (the Nuremberg Code) used by the commission to develop federal regulations was a legal document. The National Commission was also charged with producing a legal document—i.e., with producing federal regulations or legal rules to guide clinical research (*The Belmont Report*).[62]

Legal scholars and lawyers have been prominent and more deeply involved than a lot of others in the developing field of American bioethics. Many physicians and scientists are interested in and versed in bioethics but, according to Daniel Callahan, apart from notable exceptions, it is mainly those with a legal, philosophical or theological background who have devoted themselves to scholarly work in bioethics.[63]

The involvement and role of law and lawyers means that bioethical debates are often partly shaped by American law, particularly constitutional law. The Declaration of Independence is a foundational document of the American experience, and because of this, bioethical discourse is often framed in terms of rights. The essence of the Declaration of Independence is the belief that all citizens have certain inalienable rights including the rights to 'life, liberty and the pursuit of happiness.'[64] Annas claims that the influence of law on bioethics is inevitable because American law is the ethos that holds the American people together. He refers to mythologist Joseph Campbell's claim that 'there is no other ethos' and suggests that there is 'no other bioethics either. Law becomes, of necessity, our lowest common denominator ethics.'[65]

The dominance of legal concerns over ethics and medical practice is evident in the language of certain ethical debates. The debate about physician-assisted suicide is often reduced to concerns such as legal prohibition or the provision of legal immunity for physicians who actively assist. The abortion debate has been argued in terms of a woman's constitutional right to privacy and end of life questions in terms of a constitutional right to liberty to refuse medical intervention. Although the language of the law helps us to express ethical issues and to argue for certain values, talk of rights can also cause confusion. There is a tendency to conflate moral values or rights with statutory rights and constitutional rights.

Annas notes a tendency to defer to the law and an 'insistence on legal immunity' that 'pervades and often dominates ethical discourse in medicine.' He also claims that rather than being a 'self-imposed ethical principle' the most important ethical requirement in medicine had to come to us through the courts. He is referring to the requirement for informed consent and says: 'It is remarkable that information sharing had to be imposed by law, and that many in the medical profession still view information sharing with patients as either optional or inappropriate.'[66]

Jay Katz also argues that the impetus for the requirement of informed consent came from law rather than medicine.[67] Better disclosure practices and communication between doctors and patients came about only in order for physicians to escape legal liability. He claims that even though judges base informed consent on patient self-determination or autonomy, the doctrine was not designed in response to medical considerations or patients' interests. The impact of law, according to Katz, is that while the medical profession may bow to the doctrine of informed consent, that does not mean that they accept it. He argues that in order to show a real commitment to the value of patient autonomy, '[u]ltimately, medicine and not law must formulate a doctrine of informed consent.'[68]

We can see the impact of the law's influence on the developing notion of autonomy in the landmark case *Canterbury vs Spence* (1972). This case is not exactly about autonomy but it involves a crucial decision about informed consent and the two are closely related in the sense that autonomy is the justification if asked why the law requires informed consent. In *Canterbury vs Spence* a patient suffered major paralysis after a fall from a hospital bed following a medical procedure for severe back pain. The patient had not been warned about the danger of paralysis from an event such as falling out of bed. An appeals court held that the patient should have been informed of the risk of possible paralysis and the judge's opinion focused on autonomy:

> The root premise is the concept, fundamental in American jurisprudence, that 'every human being of adult years and sound mind has a right to determine what shall be done with his own body.'[69]

In regard to the sufficiency of information, the court held that:

> The patient's right of self-decision shapes the boundaries of the duty to reveal. That right can be effectively exercised only if the patient possesses enough information to enable an intelligent choice.[70]

This case marks a shift from a beneficence-based standard of disclosure to an autonomy-based standard. It is a rejection of the professional practice standard of disclosure (determined by the traditional practice of physicians or what is 'customary') for a patient based standard of disclosure.[71] The decision in *Canterbury vs Spence* was a shock to the medical community and met with opposition from some who saw the requirements for informed consent as an impossible goal and an imposition on physicians.[72]

To the extent that law has an influence on American bioethics in general and on the selection of the principle of respect for persons by the National Commission in particular, it has added to the conflation of different senses of autonomy. The influence of law has served to confuse moral values with legal values.

PRINCIPLES OF BIOMEDICAL ETHICS, BY BEAUCHAMP AND CHILDRESS

Beauchamp and Childress have had a wide influence on the emerging field of bioethics. They have been particularly influential at the level of people who are dealing with practical bioethical questions. According to one commentator, the Beauchamp and Childress approach to medical ethics became '*the* standard approach heard on hospital rounds, read in prestigious medical journals, and found in policy reports.'[73]

From the first edition of *Principles of Biomedical Ethics* to the fifth edition, Beauchamp and Childress make a lot of changes to the chapter on autonomy. As the influence of their book grew, the authors produced new editions and in each, they acknowledge immense changes to the field of bioethics and major changes to their text. These changes are worth tracing in some detail because in view of the wide influence of their book, we can see the how the concept of autonomy has been seen by many others in the field.

Dworkin's Influence

Gerald Dworkin's writings on autonomy, which have been generally influential in their own right, also had an influence on Beauchamp and Childress. In the first edition of *Principles of Biomedical Ethics*, Beauchamp and Childress state that parts of their treatment of autonomy were 'heavily influenced' by an unpublished manuscript written by Gerald Dworkin.[74] This has since been published as the chapter called 'Moral Autonomy' in Dworkin's *The Theory and Practice of Autonomy*.[75]

Dworkin's influence is noticeable in Beauchamp and Childress's interpretation of Kantian self-legislation as critical reflection. They draw attention to the notion of 'acceptance by the agent' and equate it with an understanding of Kant that means 'each individual must *will the acceptance* of his principles.' They include rationality but they reject an 'extreme interpretation' of Kant which holds that each person 'must *make* (author or originate) his own moral principles.'[76] Dworkin's influence is most apparent in the idea of autonomy as critical reflection and the concession to outside influences. Dworkin claims that autonomy as critical reflection is a worthy conception of autonomy because it is consistent with objectivity in the sense that it aims at what is good and it is not incompatible with 'the recognition of a notion of (limited) authority. It can accept the relevance (if not the conclusiveness) of tradition in moral life.'[77] Likewise, Beauchamp and Childress find no compelling inconsistency between autonomy and authority. They claim that autonomy is 'more closely linked to the notion of reflective individual choice or acceptance of a view than it is to the rejection of authority and traditional views.'[78]

Dworkin's conception of autonomy is sometimes termed a hierarchical or higher-order theory of autonomy. It involves the notion of first-order and second-order desires. The interest for Beauchamp and Childress, however, seems to be in the idea that the critical reflection somehow confers rationality or autonomy.

The Influence of the National Commission and *The Belmont Report*

According to Tom Beauchamp who, with James Childress, wrote *Principles of Biomedical Ethics*, there was a 'reciprocity in the drafting' of *The Belmont Report* and *Principles of Biomedical Ethics*. Beauchamp describes this 'bilateral influence' thus:

> I was often sumultaneeously drafting material on the same principle or topic for both the commission and Childress; and Childress was at the same time writing material for me to inspect. I would routinely write parts of *The Belmont Report* during the day at commission headquarters . . . then go to my office at Georgetown in the evening and draft parts of chapters for Childress to review. He would critique my work in the next few days and suggest changes. Our work on the book thus influenced how I drafted the Belmont document, and the converse.[79]

Beauchamp also reports that the Belmont document was 'contracted over time' and a lot of the material he wrote on the principles including respect for persons was eliminated but he would 'scoop up the reject pile' and use it for their book:

> One might say that various late-written chunks of this book were fashioned from the more philosophical, but abjured parts of what I wrote for the commission, the parts that never found the light of day.[80]

There were some aspects of the commission's report however, that he and Childress were not in agreement with:

> In a nutshell, I thought then and still do that the commission was mistaken in the way it delineated the principle of respect for persons. I thought it was mixing together two independent principles: a principle of respect for autonomy and a principle of protection and avoidance of harm to incompetent persons.[81]

Instead of the three principles named in *The Belmont Report*, Beauchamp and Childress have four main principles. They choose the principle of respect for autonomy rather than the principle of respect for persons and they add the principle of nonmaleficence to the principles of beneficence and justice.

Changes in the Chapter on Autonomy in Successive Editions of *Principles of Biomedical Ethics*

Beauchamp and Childress start out in the first edition with a view of autonomy that is Kantian to some extent. There are significant references to Kant and his influence seems to be quite pervasive. At the same time, despite the prominence given to Kant's ideas, there are some instances where it seems that Beauchamp and Childress may only be paying lip service to Kant.

According to Beauchamp and Childress in the first edition of their book, Kant can be credited with having 'shaped our understanding of autonomy' as 'freedom of the will.' They also credit Mill with shaping our understanding of autonomy, but in the sense of 'freedom of action.'[82] The 'most general idea of autonomy' they claim is 'that of being one's own person, without constraints either by another's action or by psychological or physical limitation.' This mixes together Kantian freedom of the will and Millian freedom of action and it involves quite a lot of assumptions about what autonomy means.

Beauchamp and Childress refer to Kant's contrast of autonomy with heteronomy (being directed by outside forces—either external or internal). They cite Kant's view that persons acting 'out of desire, rather than reason' are not acting autonomously, and that while coerced actions are obviously heteronomous, Kant regarded actions which are the result of 'desire, impulse and habit' in the same way.[83] Beauchamp and Childress do not specifically endorse this view but neither do they challenge it. The fact that it is quoted in connection with their claim that Kant was one of the figures who shaped our understanding of autonomy can be taken as tacit acceptance of the view that reason or rationality has a dominant role in the concept of autonomy.

There is more evidence of the dominant role given to rationality in Beauchamp and Childress's suggestion that Kant's contribution to a theory of autonomy is the idea of critical reflection. This is what they say:

> For our purposes, Kant's main contribution to a theory of autonomy is his discussion of self-legislation: the reasons for actions for autonomous persons are their own reasons, and they are principled rather than arbitrary reasons. This notion of self-directed action based on a rational principle accepted by the agent is the central ingredient in "autonomy" in the remainder of this chapter.[84]

Beauchamp and Childress state that there is an 'extreme interpretation' of Kant but that is not the view which they hold. The 'extreme interpretation' is a view in which persons must '*make* (author or originate [their] own moral principles.' According to Beauchamp and Childress this interpretation 'denies much of what we know about the moral life.' They interpret Kant to mean that 'each individual must *will the acceptance* of his principles.' Beauchamp and Childress emphasise 'acceptance by the agent.'[85] In this discussion they do not criticize the importance of rationality or the notion of self-legislation itself. What is more, they do not disassociate themselves from the view that in order for our actions to count as autonomous we need to act from reason rather than desire.

Beauchamp and Childress link the role of reason as critical reflection or reflective choice to autonomy. Reasons are important and have weight, they claim. Even though the idea that autonomy is radically inconsistent with authority is a common one and seems to follow from the philosophies of both Mill and Kant, there is 'no fundamental inconsistency,' according to Beauchamp and Childress, because the 'provision of reasons' which 'justify commands' is what gives authority some legitimacy. Beauchamp and Childress argue that 'autonomy is perfectly compatible with authority, as long as the authority is autonomously accepted' and they maintain that 'reflective individual choice' constitutes autonomous acceptance.[86]

Reason and rationality are also appealed to as that which makes persons worthy of respect. Beauchamp and Childress adopt Kant's notion of respect for persons and use his language of persons as ends rather than means in order to determine what it means to 'be *respected* as an autonomous agent and to respect the autonomy of others.'[87] According to Beauchamp and Childress one aspect of the principle of autonomy (called the principle of respect for autonomy in later editions) is the principle of respect for persons. In judging the self-regarding actions of others, they claim: 'we ought to respect them as persons with the same right to their judgments as we have to our own.' This is a demand for respect simply because the other person is a 'rational determiner of his or her own destiny.' It is not they claim, for reasons of utility.[88]

Mill provides the other aspect of Beauchamp and Childress's principle of autonomy. From Mill they add a 'moral demand of noninterference.' This means that as long as we do not infringe the autonomous actions of others, we should be free to do what we wish, even if that involves serious risk for ourselves and even though others may think our action foolish.[89]

Beauchamp and Childress claim, in the first edition of *Principles of Biomedical Ethics*, that the views of autonomy presented by Mill and Kant, 'two very different philosophers' are 'both acceptable and in no major respects incompatible.'[90] While Beauchamp and Childress find some middle ground between the two views, the compromise this involves seems to undermine, in particular, the Kantian ideas which are invoked and appealed to.

The following examples suggest that although, in the first edition, Beauchamp and Childress are using Kantian terminology, the content is not really Kantian. Beauchamp and Childress invoke Kant's idea of persons as ends in themselves (together with Mill's views on individualism) as a basis for respecting autonomy:

> To respect autonomy for Kant is bound up with conceiving the other person as having unconditional worth, solely because persons are ends in themselves determining their own destiny and are not to be treated merely as means.[91]

Kant's notion of respect for persons and the idea of them being ends in themselves is more to do with the fact that they are rational beings and involves more than acknowledging or sharing other people's ends. The unconditional worth of persons is also tied in with our being rational beings and our 'reverence for a mere Idea.' It is not simply an irreducible value that belongs to human beings. Beauchamp and Childress do not address the role of or the importance of rationality in their formulation of respect for autonomy. They formulate respect for autonomy in a way that is more Millian than Kantian:

> To respect autonomous agents is to recognize with due appreciation their own considered value judgments and outlooks even when it is believed that their judgments are mistaken.[92]

Beauchamp and Childress also define violations of autonomy in Kant's language of means and ends, but then interpret that (a violation of autonomy) in a way that is not Kantian. They interpret it as a lack of respect. Earlier on, Beauchamp and Childress had linked respect to the Kantian idea of rational beings. 'Lack of respect,' however, is not defined in terms of rational beings. It seems to be a Millian notion rather than a Kantian one:

> To treat a person merely as a means always involves a violation of autonomy. . . . To show a lack of respect for an autonomous agent, then, is either to reject that person's considered judgments or to deny him the freedom to act on those considered judgements.[93]

Here we also see the closeness to *The Belmont Report.* Some of this is almost word for word from *The Belmont Report,* where respect for autonomy is defined as giving weight to the 'considered opinions and choices' of autonomous persons 'while refraining from obstructing their actions unless they are clearly detrimental to others.'[94] This is not based on Kant at all.

Despite the role given to reason in the first edition of *Principles of Biomedical Ethics,* Beauchamp and Childress reject the idea of moral autonomy. They claim that it does not follow that an action is morally acceptable or morally principled just because it is autonomous.[95] This is contrary to Kant's view of autonomy. For Kant, an action that is autonomous is necessarily in accordance with the moral law. It is morally required and therefore right.

From starting out in the first edition with a view that is Kantian in terminology and to some extent in substance, in later editions Beauchamp and Childress increasingly bring in more Millian ideas. With this comes a move from the question 'what is autonomy?' to the question 'why should we respect or value autonomy?' This shift can be seen in Beauchamp and Childress's reference to the influence of Mill and Kant. In the first edition they are introduced as 'two figures in the history of philosophy who have shaped our understanding of autonomy.' By the fourth edition and the fifth edition they are credited with having 'influenced contemporary interpretations of respect for autonomy.'[96] While Kant did help shape our understanding of autonomy in terms of a system of reason and choice, Mill did not really do that. Mill produced arguments for individual liberty which could be interpreted as giving reasons why we should respect the autonomy of others. From the first edition onward, there is also a shift from rationality to choice. By the fourth edition, even though Beauchamp and Childress still use Kantian terminology, the substance of their notion of autonomy is no longer Kantian.

There is more reference to Mill in the second edition than in the first. In the second edition, Mill's name features with Kant as one of the figures in philosophy who 'have held that morality requires autonomous persons.'[97] In this edition Beauchamp and Childress expand on Mill's part in shaping our understanding of autonomy—what he referred to as 'the individuality—of *action* and *thought*.'[98] They contrast this with Kant's concern with '*moral* autonomy—the idea of giving oneself the moral law, or self-determination in accordance with morally valid principles.' Mill's interest, they claim, was in the concept of '*individual* autonomy or self-determination from a personal point of view.' Characteristics such as 'firmness and self-control' and the idea of 'choosing a plan of life' are associated with Mill. Although Kant's ideas also contribute to Beauchamp and Childress's notion of autonomy, Mill's ideas are ones that are readily understood in relation to autonomous persons or why we should value autonomy. They are more accessible to the reader and more attainable in a practical sense than the Kantian idea of moral autonomy or self-legislation. As noted, Beauchamp and Childress abandon some of Kant's ideas about self-legislation in the second edition and retain only the idea that 'each individual must *will the acceptance* of his or her principles.' This means that reasons for action are 'principled rather than arbitrary' but action is based on a 'principle freely accepted by the agent.' This is central to Beauchamp and Childress's notion of autonomy in the second edition of their text. Principled action is self-directed action and it does not have to be based on a 'valid universal principle.'[99]

While the second edition is similar in many ways to the first edition, Beauchamp and Childress begin omitting reference to rationality. 'Action based on a rational principle' becomes 'action based on a principle freely accepted.'[100] 'A rational determiner of his or her own destiny' becomes just a 'determiner.'[101] The latter omission is especially significant because the Kantian notion of respect for persons gains its significance from the fact that persons are rational beings. Therefore, when Beauchamp and Childress describe persons merely as determiners rather than rational determiners of their destiny, they lose the grounds for respect for persons—in Kant's sense. Respect for persons is reduced to acknowledging or sharing other people's ends: 'In evaluating the autonomous actions of others we ought to respect them as persons with the same right to their choices and actions as we have to our own.'[102] Kant claims that we are required to view other rational beings as also making universal law. In doing that we assume the fitness of that person's maxims and we treat that person as an end. To be an end in him/herself, a rational being must always be regarded as making universal law. Beauchamp and Childress are certainly diluting, if not abandoning the connection with rationality, and appeals to Kant's notion of respect for persons seems to be a misappropriation. For Kant, the ability to make choices is not a sufficient basis for respect. We saw that, for Kant, the fact that animals may be able to choose is not enough to warrant respect.

After the second edition of *Principles of Biomedical Ethics*, even though there is an increasing shift toward Mill's ideas there is less direct reference to either Mill or Kant. This suggests that as well as a move away from Kant there is less concern with the history or the origins of the idea of autonomy. This indicates a shift in focus from autonomy for individuals to autonomy as a procedural notion. As we shall see, in a pluralistic society, the principle of respect for autonomy becomes a framework on which everyone can agree.

Beauchamp and Childress write with public policy in mind. They are driven by the search for agreement in a pluralistic society, and this approach puts heavy weight on autonomy. We may not be able to agree on the question of what autonomy is or what an autonomous person is like, but we can agree to respect each other's autonomy.[103] 'At a minimum,' this involves acknowledging a person's 'right to hold views, to make choices, and to take actions based on personal values and beliefs.' Beauchamp and Childress's account of respect involves respectful action as well as a respectful attitude. In addition to a need for nonintervention, they include 'obligations to maintain capacities for autonomous choice.'[104] Their procedural approach is therefore often viewed as a defense of autonomy rather than a method for bioethics.[105] This procedural sense of autonomy, as something on which we can all agree, leads to a rather thin concept of what it means to be a person. To be a person on this view amounts to no more than having the capacity to make choices. A more substantive view would not do because it may contain ideas and meanings that people do not share. This increases the opportunity for disagreement. I will discuss the procedural approach to autonomy in more detail in a later chapter.

Beginning in the third edition, the principle of respect for autonomy has become the main focus. Theories or formulations of autonomy are virtually immaterial. Instead it is context that counts. Beauchamp and Childress's concern is with ordinary people or normal choosers. By the fourth and the fifth editions they talk in terms of 'respect for the autonomous choices' of persons and they claim that little agreement exists about the 'nature, scope or strength' of the principle.[106] They focus on the notion of respect for choice rather than autonomous persons, because their interest is in decision making and in the fourth edition they claim 'being autonomous is not the same as being respected as an autonomous agent.'[107] This suggests a move away from a substantive psychological view of the person. They say their concern is with '*autonomous* choice' rather than 'capacity for governance' because people who are qualified to act autonomously sometimes fail to do so and people who are generally not autonomous can sometimes make autonomous choices. For this reason they do not focus on traits or capacities such as 'understanding, reasoning, deliberating, and independent choosing.'[108]

By the fourth edition, in moving away from any connection with rationality, Beauchamp and Childress no longer include the idea of critical reflection or reflective choice. They criticize higher-order theories of autonomy on the grounds that critical reflection that results in the acceptance or repudiation of a desire may be caused by 'an overriding desire that is simply *stronger*, not more *rational* or *autonomous*.' [109] Theories of autonomy which require individuals to be 'exceptionally authentic, self-possessed, consistent, independent, in command, resistant to control by authorities, and the original source of personal values, beliefs, and life plans,' are too exacting they claim.[110]

Beauchamp and Childress want a way for 'ordinary' people to 'qualify as deserving respect for their autonomy.'[111] These people may not have reflected on their preferences and may not meet the rigorous standards required by some theories of autonomy. An 'aspirational ideal of autonomy' is, according to Beauchamp and Childress 'beyond the reach of normal choosers' and this means that 'few choosers' and 'few choices' would be deemed autonomous.[112] This is an important point in which context (the medical context) and practical concerns are given more weight than what it means to be autonomous. It shows Beauchamp and Childress's commitment to achieving consensus and their move toward a procedural approach. They claim that they 'vigorously defend rights of autonomy in biomedical ethics' and they acknowledge that the obligation to respect autonomy does not extend to persons who cannot act in an autonomous manner, but, they want more rather than fewer choices to be worthy of respect.[113] This leads to a dilution of the role of reason. And the dilution of reason makes it more difficult to see why respect for autonomy is important.

Beauchamp and Childress argue that in the health-care setting, 'meaningful decision making' is a more practical goal than completely autonomous decision making, and substantially autonomous rather than fully autonomous decisions are achievable and sufficient for that purpose. They argue that 'to limit adequate decision making by patients to the ideal of fully or completely autonomous decision making strips these acts of any meaningful place in the practical world.' Requirements for decision making in the context of health care are comparable to other kinds of decisions they claim, such as 'making a financial investment, hiring a new employee, buying a new house, or selecting a university.' Beauchamp and Childress want us to respect patients' decisions about participation in research or medical interventions in the same way that we respect these other kinds of decisions.[114]

In the fourth and fifth editions of the text there is much less reference to Kant and the role of reason is diluted further. From the first through to the third editions, the autonomous acceptance of authority has centered on the idea that the provision of justifying reasons legitimates authority. In the fourth edition, however, it changes. Beauchamp and Childress say there is 'no fundamental inconsistency' between autonomy, authority and community 'because individuals can exercise their autonomy in choosing to accept and submit to the authoritative demands of an institution, tradition, or community that they view as a legitimate source of direction.'[115] The autonomous acceptance of authority becomes 'choosing to accept and submit to' whatever individuals view as a 'legitimate source of direction.'[116] In the fifth edition they add that '[r]ules or codes of professional ethics are also not an individual's invention, and they, too, are compatible with the exercise of autonomy.'[117] Concern with what constitutes an autonomous choice seems to have switched to a concern with exercising autonomy.

The only substantial reference to Kant by the fourth edition is in relation to the wrongness of violating autonomy, or to what is described as 'respectful treatment of persons as ends rather than merely as means.' Although there seems to be a move away from Kant starting with the second edition and increasingly clear by the fourth edition, Kant's language is reserved for and employed in the idea of autonomy violations. From the third to the fourth edition, the terminology becomes more consistently Kantian in that area.

In the third edition the description of autonomy violations is a mixture of Kantian and Millian ideas:

> To violate a person's autonomy is to treat that person merely as a means, to treat that person in accordance with one's own goals and without regard to that person's goals. To reject that person's goals and considered judgments or to restrict his or her freedom to act on those goals and judgments is to fail to respect autonomy.[118]

The first sentence appeals to the Kantian idea of treating persons as ends but the second sentence is more Millian than Kantian. In the fourth edition the notion of the autonomy violations is couched almost entirely in Kantian terms:

> To violate a person's autonomy is to treat that person merely as a means, that is, in accordance with others' goals without regard to that person's own goals. Such treatment is a fundamental moral violation because autonomous persons are ends in themselves capable of determining their destinies.[119]

In the fifth edition they drop the second sentence but reemphasize the idea of persons as ends in themselves. They remind us that Kant's contribution, which supports the principle of respect for autonomy, is the 'moral imperative of respectful treatment of persons as ends in themselves.'[120]

Beauchamp and Childress appeal to Kant's idea about persons as ends as though it is something which is almost indisputable. However, they do not show the connection with autonomy. The idea of treating persons as ends is something that most people would agree is a good thing. It gets our approval without the need for any notion of autonomy or respect for autonomy. Beauchamp and Childress' use of Kant is really a misappropriation because, although they appeal to Kant and use his language, they reject his ideas about autonomy and the role of reason.

Beauchamp and Childress fluctuate between a procedural approach and a psychological concept of autonomy. Neither of these approaches is a genuine appeal to a Kantian notion of autonomy. They appropriate the value Kant gives autonomy but attribute it to something else such as a kind of psychological ideal—but don't acknowledge this. Beauchamp and Childress are an example of modern theorists who appeal to Kant but reject crucial aspects of his metaphysics, sometimes without even realizing they are doing so.

NOTES

1. Howard Klepper, Medical College of Wisconsin Bioethics Discussion, February 21, 1997, and personal communication.
2. Klepper, MCW Bioethics Discussion and personal communication.
3. Tom L. Beauchamp and James F. Childress, *Principles of Biomedical Ethics* (New York: Oxford University Press, 1st edition 1979), xiii. Beauchamp and Childress also name another hidden source which "heavily influenced" their treatment of autonomy. They refer to an unpublished manuscript by Gerald Dworkin which has since been published as "Moral Autonomy" in H. Tristram Engelhardt, Jr., and Daniel Callahan, ed., *Morals, Science, and Sociality* (Hastings-on-Hudson, N.Y.:

Hastings Center, 1978), 156–71. This has also become the third chapter of Gerald Dworkins *The Theory and Practice of Autonomy* (Cambridge: Cambridge Universtiy Press, 1988), 34–47.

4. Tom L. Beauchamp, "The Origins, Goals, and Core Commitments of *The Belmont Report* and *Principles of Biomedical Ethics*," in *The Story of Bioethics*, ed. Jennifer K. Walter and Eran P. Klein (Washington, D.C.: Georgetown University Press, 2003), 17–46.

5. Beauchamp "The Origins, Goals, and Core Commitments," 17 and 20.

6. Tom L. Beauchamp, "The Principles Approach," Special Supplement "The Birth of Bioethics" *Hastings Center Report* 23, (6 suppl), (November–December, 1993), S9.

7. Ruth Ellen Bulger, Elizabeth Meyer Bobby, and Harvey V. Fineberg, ed., *Society's Choices: Social and Ethical Decision Making in Biomedicine* (Washington D.C.: National Academy Press, 1995), 70, 91.

8. Nancy M. P. King, Gail E. Henderson, and Jane Stein, ed., in *Beyond Regulations: Ethics in Human Subject Research* (Chapel Hill: University of North Carolina Press, 1999), 12. The influential sets of guidelines for epidemiological research and for biomedical research produced by the Council for International Organizations of Medical Sciences (CIOMS) adopt the approach and reflect the basic premises of *The Belmont Report*. *The Belmont Report* and the three ethical principles (respect for persons, beneficence, and justice) are also invoked in the *National Statement on Ethical Conduct in Research Involving Humans*, issued by the National Health and Medical Research Council (NHMRC) (Canberra: Commonwealth of Australia, 1999), 4, 11–12.

9. Henry K. Beecher, "Ethics and Clinical Research," *New England Journal of Medicine* 274, no.24 (June 1966): 1,354–60.

10. David J. Rothman, *Strangers at the Bedside: A History of How Law and Bioethics Transformed Medical Decision Making* (New York: Basic Books, 1991), 15–16.

11. George J. Annas "The Dominance of American Law (and Market Values) over American Bioethics," in *Meta Medical Ethics: The Philosophical Foundations of Bioethis*, ed. Michael A Grodin (Dordrecht: Kluwer Academic Publishers, 1995), 83–96. Quoting Arthur Caplan, p. 85.

12. Albert R. Jonsen and Stephen Toulmin, *The Abuse of Casuistry: A History of Moral Reasoning* (Berkley: University of California Press, 1988), 16–17.

13. Rothman, *Strangers at the Bedside*, 4.

14. David J. Rothman, "Three Views of History," Special Supplement "The Birth of Bioethics" *Hastings Centre Report*, ed. Albert R. Jonsen (November–December 1993), S11–S12. Rothman argues that the "extraordinary power" of "this sense of patient as minority" is something that is overlooked by critics of the bioethics movement, e.g., Renee Fox and Judith Swazey who took the movement seriously and understood it, but complained that bioethics elevated individual rights above all other rights.

15. Michael A; Grodin, ed., *Meta Medical Ethics: The Philosophical Foundations of Bioethics* (Dordrecht: Kluwer Academic Publishers, 1995), 4.

16. Stephen Toulmin "The National Commission on Human Experimentation: Procedures and Outcomes," in *Scientific Controversies: Case Studies in the Resolution and Closure of Disputes in Science and Technology*, ed. H. Tristram Engelhardt, Jr., and Arthur L. Caplan (Cambridge: Cambridge University Press, 1987), 599.

17. Rothman, *Strangers at the Bedside*, 5.

18. The National Commission for the Protection of Human Subjects of Biomedical and Behavioral Research, *The Belmont Report: Ethical Principles and Guidelines for the Protection of Human Subjects Research* (DHEW Publication No (OS) 78-0012, 1978) (Letter to the President from the Chairman, Kenneth J. Ryan, M.D.).

19. Beauchamp, "The Origins, Goals, and Core Commitments," 17. According to Tom Beauchamp, this is where the 'idea for the Belmont paper originate.'

20. The National Commission (Letter to the President).

21. The National Commission (Letter to the President).

22. *The Belmont Report*, 4.

23. *The Belmont Report*, 5.

24. *The Belmont Report*, 5.

25. Albert R. Jonsen, personal communication.

26. See Albert R. Jonsen, *The Birth of Bioethics* (New York: Oxford University Press, 1998), 348n29. Jonsen argues that phrases such as 'respect for persons,' 'respect for autonomy' and 'respect for personal autonomy' are not synonomous but are carelessly interchanged in contemporary bioethics discussions. He adds that 'respect for persons seems a much wider concept than respect for autonomy.'

27. Raymond J. Devettere, "The Principled Approach: Principles, Rules, and Actions," in *Meta-Medical Ethics: The Philosophical Foundations of Bioethics*, ed. Michael A. Grodin (Dordrecht: Kluwer Academic Publishers, 1995), 39.

28. Annas, "The Dominance of American Law," 86.

29. Albert R. Jonsen, personal communication.

30. Jonsen, *The Birth of Bioethics*, 334 and 348. The phrase 'respect for persons' (or 'respect for autonomy') does not appear in the indices of philosophy textbooks by 'luminaries' such as William Frankena in his *Ethics* 2nd ed. (Englewood Cliffs, Prentice Hall, 1973) or Richard Brandt in *Ethical Theory*. 'Nor are the terms found in the *Encyclopedia of Philosophy* or even in the 1978 *Encyclopedia of Bioethics*!' It is philosophers Downie and Telfer, in their book *Respect for Persons* (London, Allen and Unwin 1969) who saw the need for a 'sustained examination of the idea [of the individual person as of supreme worth] in the language of contemporary analytical philosophy.' It was this book which put the phrase 'respect for persons' into Jonsen's 'moral vocabulary.'

31. Jonsen, personal communication and *The Birth of Bioethics*, 334.

32. *Nuremberg Code*, ohsr.od.nih.gov/guidelines/nuremberg.html (accessed 22 August 2004).

33. *Nuremberg Code.*
34. *Nuremberg Code.*
35. R. S. Downie and Elizabeth Telfer, *Respect for Persons* (London: George Allen and Unwin Ltd., 1969), 15.
36. Downie and Telfer, *Respect for Persons,* 18
37. Downie and Telfer, *Respect for Persons,* 23. The authors say they will 'assume' this 'for the present' and the 'gaps in the detailed argument required to establish the practical force of reason will be supplied later' in chapter 5.
38. Downie and Telfer, *Respect for Persons,* 20.
39. Downie and Telfer, *Respect for Persons,* 22.
40. Downie and Telfer, *Respect for Persons,* 27.
41. Downie and Telfer, *Respect for Persons,* 28.
42. Downie and Telfer, *Respect for Persons,* 29.
43. Downie and Telfer, *Respect for Persons,* 24.
44. Kant *Groundwork,* 102 (76).
45. Kant *Groundwork,* 102 (434).
46. Downie and Telfer, *Respect for Persons,* 21.
47. Downie and Telfer, *Respect for Persons,* 21.
48. H. Tristram Engelhardt, Jr., "Basic Ethical Principles in the Conduct of Biomedical and Behavioral Research Involving Human Subjects," in *Appendix: Vol. 1, Belmont Report,* National Commission for the Protection of Human Subjects of Biomedical and Behavioral Research, 2.
49. Engelhardt, "Basic Ethical Principles in the Conduct," 5, 39.
50. Engelhardt, "Basic Ethical Principles in the Conduct," 6–7.
51. Engelhardt, "Basic Ethical Principles in the Conduct," 3.
52. Engelhardt, "Basic Ethical Principles in the Conduct," 41n7.
53. Engelhardt, "Basic Ethical Principles in the Conduct," 8–9, 13.
54. Engelhardt, "Basic Ethical Principles in the Conduct," 28.
55. Engelhardt, "Basic Ethical Principles in the Conduct," 40n3.
56. For example, Mill's idea that each person is the best judge and guardian of his own interests. See Mill, *On Liberty,* 8–9.
57. Engelhardt, "Basic Ethical Principles in the Conduct," 2.
58. Engelhardt, "Basic Ethical Principles in the Conduct," 13.
59. Engelhardt, "Basic Ethical Principles in the Conduct," 13–14.
60. Engelhardt, "Basic Ethical Principles in the Conduct," 1.
61. Engelhardt, "Basic Ethical Principles in the Conduct," 22.
62. Annas, "The Dominance of American Law," 85–86.
63. Albert R. Jonsen and Andrew Jameton, "Medical Ethics, History of: The Americas," in *Encyclopedia of Bioethics,* vol. 3. Revised ed., ed. Warren Thomas Reich (New York: Simon & Schuster Macmillan, 1995), 1,616–32.
64. Annas, "The Dominance of American Law," 83–84.
65. Annas, "The Dominance of American Law," 87.
66. Annas, "The Dominance of American Law," 86–87.

67. Jay Katz, "Informed Consent: Must It Remain a Fairy Tale?" *Journal of Contemporary Health Law and Polic* 10, (Spring, 1994): 69–91.

68. Katz, "Informed Consent: Must It Remain a Fairy Tale?" 71.

69. *Canterbury vs Spence*, 464F.2d 786, quoting *Schloendorff vs Society of New York Hospitals* in Tom L. Beauchamp and Lauranec B. McCullough, "The Management of Medical Information: Legal and Moral Requirements of Informed Consent," in *Bioethics: A Collection of Readings*, ed. Edwards and Graber (San Diego: Hacourt Brace Jovanovich, 1988), 130–41.

70. *Canterbury vs Spence*, 786 in Beauchamp and McCullough, "The Management of Medical Information," 133.

71. Beauchamp and McCullough, "The Management of Medical Information," 133–35. Even though there was a shift to a patient based standard, the court favoured the 'objective reasonable person' standard in which the physician must disclose 'all information relevant to a decision, as judged by what a hypothetical reasonable person would want to know.' *Canterbury* rejected the subjective standard of disclosure (the requirement to meet the informational needs of individual patients) because physicians would be vulnerable to the 'vindictive hindsight' of patients. It seems that the most appropriate standard of disclosure from a legal point of view may be quite different from the best standard in the moral sense. The standard required by law is not necessarily the best standard in terms of the doctor-patient relationship. Even though autonomy may be invoked as the justification, informed consent in the legal context is not strictly about respect for autonomy or promoting autonomous decision making.

72. Beauchamp and McCullough, "The Management of Medical Information," 133.

73. Ezekiel J. Emanuel, "The Beginning of the End of Principilism," *Hastings Center Report* 25, no. 4 (July–August 1995): 37–38.

74. Beauchamp and Childress, *Principles of Biomedical Ethics*, 1979, 1st ed., xii.

75. Gerald Dworkin, *The Theory and Practice of Autonomy* (Cambridge: Cambridge University Press, 1988), 34–47.

76. Beauchamp and Childress, *Principles of Biomedical Ethics*, 1979, 1st ed., 58.

77. Dworkin, *The Theory and Practice of Autonomy*, 47.

78. Beauchamp and Childress, *Principles of Biomedical Ethics*, 1979, 1st ed., 62.

79. Beauchamp, "The Origins, Goals, and Core Commitments," 27.

80. Beauchamp, "The Origins, Goals, and Core Commitments," 22.

81. Tom L. Beauchamp, "The Principles Approach," P.S9; Beauchamp, "The Origins, Goals, and Core Commitments," 23.

82. Beauchamp and Childress, *Principles of Biomedical Ethics*, 1979, 1st ed., 57.

83. Beauchamp and Childress, *Principles of Biomedical Ethics*, 1979, 1st ed., 57.

84. Beauchamp and Childress, *Principles of Biomedical Ethics*, 1979, 1st ed., 58.

85. Beauchamp and Childress, *Principles of Biomedical Ethics*, 1979, 1st ed., 58.

86. Beauchamp and Childress, *Principles of Biomedical Ethics*, 1979, 1st ed., 60–62.

87. Beauchamp and Childress, *Principles of Biomedical Ethics*, 1979, 1st ed., 58.
88. Beauchamp and Childress, *Principles of Biomedical Ethics*, 1979, 1st ed., 59.
89. Beauchamp and Childress, *Principles of Biomedical Ethics*, 1979, 1st ed., 59.
90. Beauchamp and Childress, *Principles of Biomedical Ethics*, 1979, 1st ed., 58.
91. Beauchamp and Childress, *Principles of Biomedical Ethics*,1979, 1st ed., 58–59.
92. Beauchamp and Childress, *Principles of Biomedical Ethics*, 1979, 1st ed., 58.
93. Beauchamp and Childress, *Principles of Biomedical Ethics*, 1979, 1st ed., 59.
94. *The Belmont Report*, 5.
95. Beauchamp and Childress, *Principles of Biomedical Ethics*, 1979, 1st ed., 61.
96. Beauchamp and Childress, *Principles of Biomedical Ethics*, 1994, 4th ed., 125; and Beauchamp and Childress, *Principles of Biomedical Ethics*, 2001, 5th ed., 63.
97. Beauchamp and Childress, *Principles of Biomedical Ethics*, 1883, 2nd ed., 59.
98. Beauchamp and Childress, *Principles of Biomedical Ethics*, 1883, 2nd ed., 60.
99. Beauchamp and Childress, *Principles of Biomedical Ethics*, 1883, 2nd ed., 61
100. Beauchamp and Childress, *Principles of Biomedical Ethics*, 1979, 1st ed., 61.
101. Beauchamp and Childress, *Principles of Biomedical Ethics*, 1979, 1st ed., 63.
102. Beauchamp and Childress, *Principles of Biomedical Ethics*, 1883, 2nd ed., 63.
103. Gilbert C. Meilaender, *Body, Soul, and Bioethics* (Notre Dame: University of Nortre Dame Press, 1995), 18–19.
104. Beauchamp and Childress, *Principles of Biomedical Ethics*, 1994, 4th ed., 125.
105. Meilaender, *Body, Soul, and Bioethics*, 18.
106. Beauchamp and Childress, *Principles of Biomedical Ethics*, 1994, 4th ed., 20; and Beauchamp and Childress, *Principles of Biomedical Ethics*, 2001, 5th ed., 57.
107. Beauchamp and Childress, *Principles of Biomedical Ethics*, 1994, 4th ed., 125.
108. Beauchamp and Childress, *Principles of Biomedical Ethics*, 1994, 4th ed., 121; and Beauchamp and Childress, *Principles of Biomedical Ethics*, 2001, 5th ed., 58.
109. Beauchamp and Childress, *Principles of Biomedical Ethics*, 1994, 4th ed., 122; and Beauchamp and Childress, *Principles of Biomedical Ethics*, 2001, 5th ed., 59.
110. Beauchamp and Childress, *Principles of Biomedical Ethics*, 1994, 4th ed., 123.
111. Beauchamp and Childress, *Principles of Biomedical Ethics*, 1994, 4th ed., 122–23; and Beauchamp and Childress, *Principles of Biomedical Ethics*, 2001, 5th ed., 59.
112. Beauchamp and Childress, *Principles of Biomedical Ethics*, 1994, 4th ed., 122; and Beauchamp and Childress, *Principles of Biomedical Ethics*, 2001, 5th ed., 59.

113. Beauchamp and Childress, *Principles of Biomedical Ethics*, 1994, 4th ed., 127; and Beauchamp and Childress, *Principles of Biomedical Ethics*, 2001, 5th ed., 65.

114. Beauchamp and Childress, *Principles of Biomedical Ethics*, 1994, 4th ed., 123; and Beauchamp and Childress, *Principles of Biomedical Ethics*, 2001, 5th ed., 59–60.

115. Beauchamp and Childress, *Principles of Biomedical Ethics*, 1994, 4th ed., 124.

116. Beauchamp and Childress, *Principles of Biomedical Ethics*, 1994, 4th ed., 124.

117. Beauchamp and Childress, *Principles of Biomedical Ethics*, 2001, 5th ed., 60.

118. Beauchamp and Childress, *Principles of Biomedical Ethics*,1883, 3rd ed., 71–72.

119. Beauchamp and Childress, *Principles of Biomedical Ethics*, 1994, 4th ed., 125.

120. Beauchamp and Childress, *Principles of Biomedical Ethics*, 2001, 5th ed., 64.

II

DIFFERENT NOTIONS OF AUTONOMY

4

DIFFERENT NOTIONS OF AUTONOMY IDENTIFIED

As we have seen, there are historically quite distinct strands of the idea of autonomy. There is a Kantian and a Millian conception of autonomy and we will see that there is a psychological and a procedural approach to making sense of autonomy as it is applied in the clinical setting or to the doctor/patient relationship. In some instances autonomy is viewed as an ideal of character while in others it is task related. Disentangling these strands is an essential preliminary to any clear and coherent discussion about autonomy and its role in the clinical context.

Additionally, it is possible that part of the confusion is due to the approach that is adopted when autonomy is discussed in a particular context. This is quite apart from its historical roots. There are four broad categories into which the various notions of autonomy can be classified. Autonomy can be a psychological, an evaluative, a procedural, or a metaphysical idea. Some overlap occurs where a particular strand divides and can fit more than one category. For instance, we shall see that we can view the notion of autonomy derived from Mill as a psychological state or as a procedural concept. As well as disentangling the different strands of the idea of autonomy it will also be instructive to see the differences when autonomy is construed as a metaphysical, a psychological, a procedural, or an evaluative concept.

In this chapter I am identifying and defining these distinct notions/approaches to autonomy. The critical analysis will follow this chapter.

AUTONOMY AS A METAPHYSICAL CONCEPT

I have discussed Kant's idea of autonomy in some detail in an earlier chapter so in this section I will refer only to those aspects which distinguish it as a metaphysical account of autonomy and I will discuss ways in which others have appropriated some of its features. We shall see that one of the ways in which modern theorists appropriate and confuse Kant's ideas is by using a metaphysical concept as something different.

Kant's idea of autonomy is a metaphysical one. It is a worked out view with a certain philosophical coherence about it. In short, his notion of autonomy depends on a specific metaphysics about the nature of the world and the kind of beings humans are. We have seen that Kant makes a distinction between the sensible (phenomenal) world and the intellectual (noumenal) world. He claims that as rational beings we belong to both worlds and we therefore can be considered subject to two standpoints. We are simultaneously under the laws of nature (heteronomy) and under laws which 'are not empirical'; which have their ground in 'reason alone.'[1] According to Kant, these characteristics are quite compatible. As members of the intelligible world we are free but we are also determined by the sensible world. We are subject to desires and impulses, but, because we are intelligent beings, we do not have to indulge or give in to our desires.[2] This is not simply about wanting to eradicate sensibility. It is because we are subject to the influence of sensuous desires that we are led to the notion of moral obligation:

> when we think of ourselves as free, we transfer ourselves into the intelligible world . . . whereas when we think of ourselves as under obligation, we look upon ourselves as belonging to the sensible world and yet to the intelligible world at the same time. . . . The moral 'I ought' is thus an 'I will' for a man as a member of the intelligible world; and it is conceived by him as an 'I ought' only in so far as he considers himself at the same time to be a member of the sensible world.[3]

Only because we are beings who belong to both worlds is morality an issue. If we were solely members of the intelligible world and perfect in the sense that we were not subject to desires and inclinations, obligation or the *need* for morality would not exist. Similarly, if we belonged only to the sensible world morality would be unrealizable. We would be driven simply by our appetites and there would be nothing on which to base the moral 'I ought.' Therefore, when Kant claims that our actions have moral worth, when we act from reason alone, he does not mean that we must shun the world of sense or that we belong only to the intelligible world. He means that reason alone determines what we do but in the sense that we are 'necessarily' subject to the laws of nature at the same time that we are members of the intelligible world.[4] This metaphysical picture of the world and of human action is an essential part of Kant's ethics, which cannot be understood without it.

Kant's concept of autonomy is metaphysical and it follows from what has just been said that it is not a psychological state to be derived from observation and experience. Kant is not concerned with observable human behaviour or 'whether this or that has happened' but with actions 'of which the world has perhaps hitherto given no example.'[5] Those who rely entirely on experience to demonstrate and confirm the existence of things, he claims, may doubt the reality of these kinds of actions. The actions he is concerned with are the actions which 'reason by itself' commands 'ought to happen.' For instance, 'pure loyalty in friendship' is something (an idea) that can exist even though 'up to now there may have existed no loyal friend.'[6] In other words, there are things such as duties which exist in the sense that they are 'commanded unrelentingly by reason' even though they may not eventuate.

Although Kant's idea of autonomy is a metaphysical one it often becomes transformed into a kind of psychological ideal. Various notions such as rationality, dignity, moral worth, freedom, making universal law, duty, intellect, principles, a good will, good in itself, and value, are all involved in Kant's conception of autonomy. Given the nature of some of these ideas, it is understandable that an ideal or noble image of an autonomous person is often assumed. This psychological ideal is not, however, an idea that is true to Kant. It is no longer a metaphysical concept. Onora O'Neill refers us to a 'misplaced' view of an autonomous person often attributed to Kant. She claims that no one describes this 'antithesis' of Kant's idea of autonomy more vividly than Iris Murdoch:

> Stripped of the exiguous metaphysical background which Kant was prepared to allow him, this man is with us still, free, independent, lonely, powerful, rational responsible, brave, the hero of so many novels and books of moral philosophy. . . . He is the ideal citizen of the liberal state, a warning held up to tyrants. He has the virtue which the age requires and admires, courage.[7]

This is autonomy construed as a psychological state. It is descriptive (which will be explained more fully in the next section) rather than metaphysical and quite different to Kant's concept of autonomy which is the property of any rational being and a 'property of particular acts' rather than the 'special achievement of the most independent.'[8] Kant's concern is with what we *ought* to do rather than what we *in fact* do. He repeatedly stresses his disdain for the idea that morality derives from experience or the empirical world:

> We cannot do morality a worse service than by seeking to derive it from examples. . . . What it turns out is a disgusting hotchpotch of second-hand observations and semirational principles on which the empty headed regale themselves, because this is something that can be used in the chit chat of daily life. Men of insight, on the other hand, feel confused by it and avert their eyes.[9]

According to Kant, the use of examples does have a role and can be justified as a way of giving philosophy a popular character, of 'winning acceptance,' but not as a first enquiry. This must wait till later. Moral philosophy must be first grounded on metaphysics.[10]

Kant's idea of autonomy is both revered and reviled. According to Onora O'Neill, Kant is 'revered' for his concern with human freedom, his idea of respect for persons, and for his 'insistence that reason can guide action.'[11] In discussions about autonomy, it is the kudos of these ideas that modern theorists are after when they appeal to Kant. At the same time that Kant is invoked by modern theorists, he is also reviled for his analysis of the connection between freedom and morality. The emphasis he places on duty and his neglect of the value of acting from motives such as fellow feeling, loyalty, or sympathy are the subject of much criticism. For many, there is something objectionable about insisting that we have moral worth only when we act from duty. According to O'Neill, 'many contemporary proponents of "Kantian" ethics want the nicer bits of his ethical conclusions without the metaphysical troubles. They hope to base a "Kantian" account of justice and of rights on broadly empiricist conceptions of self, freedom and action.'[12] The same applies for accounts of autonomy.[13]

Kant's notion of autonomy is a metaphysical concept and like other key notions in Kant's ethics, such as acting from duty and also respect for persons, is often popularly misunderstood and treated in a nonmetaphysical way. The distinctive thing about Kant's concept of autonomy is that autonomy is related to freedom and yet it is something that is required of us. We are autonomous only when we act on the basis of reason which is to act in accordance with the moral law or universal law or from duty. Theories of action or accounts of autonomy that involve desires, wants, or preferences are really theories of 'heteronomy' in Kant's sense of that term.

Rousseau's ideas about freedom and reason also fit into the metaphysical category. According to Rousseau, who foreshadows Kant, when we choose obedience to a self-imposed law, we demonstrate that we are intelligent beings who use reason. This distinguishes us from 'stupid short-sighted' animals.[14] We are free in the sense that we become our 'own master,' whereas those who are driven by appetite and determined by outside forces are not free. Rousseau claims that to renounce one's freedom is to renounce one's humanity.

These connections of freedom with duty and Rousseau's notion of the general will depend on a metaphysical view. Surrendering to the general will is not the same thing as an act of prudence.[15] It is not something that can be described in terms of an individual's psychological state or a person's particular will, or the will of the majority, or even as a common element of the actual wills of all members of the community. The idea of the general will, of listening to the voice of reason, is not a way to achieve some end. It is a metaphysical explanation of abstract concepts.

Kant's metaphysics has a political aspect as well. Recalling his kingdom of ends formulation of the categorical imperative (Every rational being must so act as if he were through his maxims always a law-making member in the universal kingdom of ends'),[16] we find a relationship between morality and politics. It suggests a 'plurality of free and rational agents' who act in ways that do not prevent others from doing likewise.[17] Some of Kant's political writings show us just how much like Rousseau's ideas his ideas are and how very far Kant's idea of autonomy is from modern ideas about autonomy. Like Rousseau, Kant saw a kind of conflict between individuals and society. Kant claims that at the same time that man has an inclination to come together in society he also has a 'great tendency to live as an individual.'[18] In society he feels more able to develop but as an individual, he encounters the 'unsocial characteristic of wanting to direct everything in accordance with his own ideas.'[19] Like Rousseau, Kant recognizes the paradox of political freedom in which we must submit to coercion or law in order to preserve our freedom. For Rousseau, we are 'forced to be free'[20] and for Kant we have to remain our own law giver:

> And this is indeed the most stringent of all forms of necessity, for it is imposed by men upon themselves, in that their inclinations make it impossible for them to exist side by side for long in a state of wild freedom. But once enclosed within a precinct like that of civil union, the same inclinations have the most

beneficial effect. In the same way, trees in a forest, by seeking to deprive each other of air and sunlight, compel each other to find these by upward growth, so that they grow beautiful and straight—whereas those which put out branches at will, in freedom and in isolation from others, grow stunted, bent and twisted.[21]

Kant's ideas about the paradox of freedom reinforce for us the idea that his notion of autonomy cannot be detached from his metaphysics. It emphasizes the fact that action takes place in relation to other people and that autonomy is bound up with the ideas of a kingdom of ends, self-legislation, and universal law. Kant claims that 'man is an animal who needs a master':

For he certainly abuses his freedom in relation to others of his own kind. And even although, as a rational creature, he desires a law to impose limits on the freedom of all, he is still misled by his self-seeking animal inclinations into exempting himself from the law where he can. He thus requires *a master* to break his self-will and force him to obey a universally valid will under which everyone can be free. But where is he to find such a master? Nowhere else but in the human species. But his master will also be an animal who needs a master.[22]

On the one hand, we get from Kant the idea that no individual is in a privileged position where he or she can say what another must or must not do, but, on the other hand it seems that Kant may be prepared to justify political authoritarianism. We have seen that Kant asserts the independence of the individual in the face of authority or outside forces. Further to this, because of a similarity between the spirit of Kant's ideas and those of the French Revolution, according to Hans Reiss, Kant 'has rightly been called the philosopher of the French Revolution.'[23] It is paradoxical then, that despite his sympathy for the French Revolution, Kant does not endorse the idea of revolution. In fact, in his political writings he argues for the prohibition of revolution:

It thus follows that all resistance against the supreme legislative power, all incitement of the subject to violent expressions of discontent, all defiance which breaks out into rebellion, is the greatest and most punishable crime in a commonwealth, for it destroys its very foundations. This prohibition is *absolute*.[24]

By exploring this apparent inconsistency in Kant's moral and political thinking we are reminded that Kant's view is a metaphysical one. Kant's argument against the right of revolution can be understood in the sense that revolution means a 'return to nature.'[25] L. W. Beck argues that Kant cannot and does not appeal to a utilitarian justification for a revolution—to do so would be inconsistent with his moral principles.[26] Kant claims that those who plead on behalf of the people to oppose the sovereign are making the mistake of allowing the principle of happiness to influence their judgment and they have also 'assumed the idea of an original contract (a basic postulate of reason) is something which must have taken place *in reality*, even where there is no document.'[27] According to Kant, the principle of happiness which he claims is 'not in fact a definite principle,' is misused in the political sense just as it is in morality, despite the good intentions of those who promote it.[28]

These last points show that it is wrong to assume that politically Kant is opposed to paternalistic political authority, or that Kant is a defender of liberty in the small "l" liberal sense. Furthermore, Kant's political ideas dramatize and sharpen the contrast between the metaphysical view and the way in which Kant's notion of autonomy is invoked today.

According to Beck, Kant's formalism and the ideal of the social contract in which 'sovereignty is indivisible' explain Kant's opposition to revolution.[29] These are metaphysical notions. Kant argues that the maxim on which revolution is based is not a legitimate principle of action because it cannot be made into universal law: 'such resistance would be dictated by a maxim which, if it became general, would destroy the whole civil constitution and put an end to the only state in which men can possess rights.'[30] For Kant, following Rousseau, revolution is a return to nature because (in Rousseau's terms), anything less than the general will is only an individual will and individual wills tend toward partiality and impulsion by appetite.[31]

The idea that 'sovereignty is indivisible' emphasises further the disparity between Kant's metaphysical view of autonomy and many contemporary ideas of autonomy. According to Andrew Levine, Kant appropriates Rousseau's idea that since autonomy is maintained only if the general interest is willed, 'autonomous agents cannot be at odds.' Kant develops this into the doctrine that rationality 'establishes a strong consensus on ends, a "harmony of rational wills."'[32] This is quite different from the idea of autonomy that makes negative liberty worth having. On that view, individuals have particular ends and there is no reason why they should not find themselves 'at odds' with each other. Their wills are independent of one another's.[33] Unlike those who argue the right of individuals to pursue and express diverse views and for the promotion of negative liberty, Kant's concern is with the form and the principle of action: 'let the consequences be what they may.'[34]

AUTONOMY AS A DESCRIPTIVE PSYCHOLOGICAL CONCEPT

Autonomy is sometimes construed as a kind of psychological ideal. Sometimes it is used to describe persons and at other times choices. As mentioned earlier, it is often viewed as a 'special achievement of the most independent' and this is the antithesis of Kant's idea.[35] Thomas Hill claims that, particularly in practical contexts, autonomy has come apart from its Kantian roots and has come to be viewed as a 'sort of psychological maturity.' He describes autonomy construed in this way as something which people have, or do not have, in varying degrees and as something we attribute on the basis of empirical evidence:

> An autonomous person, in this sense, has a kind of independence of judgment which young children and unthinking conformists lack. One shows a deficiency of autonomy when one blindly follows parental wishes, peer pressures, traditional norms, church authorities, or local fads, fashions, or folk heroes. Impulsive rebellion against custom and authority, however, does not mark one out as autonomous, for autonomy is typically associated with a high degree of rational self-control. Compulsive gamblers and drug addicts, for example, are common paradigms of the nonautonomous.[36]

Kant's metaphysical concept does not admit degrees of autonomy. Kant thought that we are all autonomous. Rather than the achievement of some, he thought that autonomy is a fate we cannot escape. This point marks a notable difference between the metaphysical and the psychological concept. However, the idea that autonomy is a psychological state, but, nevertheless derived from Kant seems to be one that is prevalent in contemporary discussions. Instead of understanding that these are very different kinds of concepts, autonomy as a psychological concept is sometimes viewed as an improvement on or even a refinement of Kant's idea. David Richards makes the startling claim that: 'Understandably, Rousseau's and Kant's articulation of the notion of autonomy is limited by the undeveloped state of the psychology and social theory of the period.'[37] Richard's claim is on the wrong track because, as we saw earlier, Kant is not concerned with observable human behavior and his concept of autonomy is not a psychological state to be derived from observation and experience.[38]

The arguments of John Stuart Mill present us with a conception of autonomy as a psychological state. Mill's argument for liberty involves the agent and his character and Mill discusses the development of individuality in conditions of freedom. From this we get the idea that autonomy involves characteristics such as self-development, firmness, self-control, and the ability to choose a plan of life. The development of individuality and character are important for Mill in the sense that 'nobleness of character' is one of the things that makes life happy.[39] In contemporary accounts of autonomy, the idea of individuality is linked to and sometimes equated with autonomy.

Fundamental to the idea of autonomy in a context such as the medical one is the assumption that agents can choose and act, and are competent or not competent in certain ways. This accounts for an explication of autonomy that is, at least partly, in psychological terms.[40] This is evident in *The Belmont Report* where an autonomous person is described as one who is 'capable of deliberation about personal goals and of acting under the direction of such deliberation.' Autonomous persons are also described as making choices and as having considered opinions.[41]

Beginning in the first edition of *Principles of Biomedical Ethics*, Beauchamp and Childress present a largely psychological account of autonomy:

> Autonomy is a form of personal liberty of action where the individual determines his or her own course of action in accordance with a plan chosen by himself or herself. The autonomous person is one who not only deliberates about and chooses such plans but who is capable of acting on the basis of such deliberations, just as a truly independent government has autonomous control of its territories and policies. A person's autonomy is his or her independence, self-reliance, and self-contained ability to decide. . . . The most general idea of autonomy is that of being one's own person, without constraints either by another's action or by a psychological or physical limitation.[42]

By the fourth and fifth editions, Beauchamp and Childress state that their interest is in decision making which leads them to focus on 'autonomous choice' rather than the autonomous person and their capacities for self-government.[43] They do not want to depict autonomy as an ideal so they set out in the fourth edition to tie their analysis to 'the assumptions of autonomy underlying moral requirements of "respect for autonomy"'[44] and in the fifth edition to the 'nonideal moral requirements of "respect for autonomy."'[45] It is not really clear what this means but it seems they do not want to give content to the word 'autonomy.' Nevertheless, they say that they analyze 'autonomous action in terms of normal choosers who act (1) intentionally, (2) with understanding, and (3) without controlling influences that determine their action.'[46] This approach still involves many psychological assumptions and relies on a description of the psychology of the person choosing. For instance, in the third edition when Beauchamp and Childress introduce these ideas, they state that intentional action as a condition is a 'matter of planning.'[47] In the fourth and fifth editions they merely claim that intentional action is not a matter of degree and drop reference to 'planning.'[48] Intentional action, nevertheless, requires the idea of an agent who deliberates and who has certain capacities.

Beauchamp and Childress have a negative formulation and a positive aspect to the principle of respect for autonomy in the medical context. The negative part is to do with negative or political freedom: 'Autonomous actions should not be subjected to controlling constraints by others.'[49] The 'affirmative demands' or the positive aspect of the principle includes disclosing information and 'fostering autonomous decision making.'[50] They claim that it sometimes involves an obligation by physicians to help equip patients 'overcome their sense of dependence and achieve as much control as possible or as they desire.'[51] These are practical matters which involve attention to psychological detail. Beauchamp and Childress are unable to disentangle themselves from the idea of autonomy as a psychological state, even though they want to focus on 'autonomous choice' rather than 'autonomous persons' and the 'capacity for governance.' They do not want autonomy to be conceived as a psychological state because people, who are not generally autonomous in the psychological sense, even some who are declared legally incompetent, can 'at times make autonomous choices'[52] and these are choices that Beauchamp and Childress want protection for.[53]

Many other contemporary theorists do not try to disassociate themselves from the idea of autonomy construed as a psychological state. In fact many embrace the idea of autonomy as a psychological concept and as we shall see the idea of autonomy seems to lend itself most readily and particularly well to psychological descriptions.

I am now going to outline the major descriptive psychological accounts of autonomy. There are important differences in these accounts and by putting them into the same category (the descriptive psychological account of autonomy) I am not denying that there are important differences between them.

Robert Young's well-developed account of autonomy is a descriptive account explicated in psychological terms. It tells us what autonomy involves and it gives us a detailed picture of what an autonomous person is like. Young argues for a notion of autonomy that is broader than the idea of negative liberty. He claims that autonomy is more than 'freedom from' something and is more appropriately construed in a positive way as self-government or self-determination.[54] Autonomy 'has to be worked at.' He likens this to the idea that a woman is not made autonomous by the repeal of laws prohibiting abortion even though antiabortion laws can interfere with a woman's liberty and thereby her autonomy.[55] Autonomy is to do with persons and actions and autonomous persons are those whose actions are self-directed or self-determined.[56]

Young claims that an autonomous person makes choices and acts in ways expressive of their preferences, and an autonomous person can be described as 'his own man or her own woman.' Yet beyond this, he claims, there is an even 'richer sense' of autonomy. Young emphasizes long-term planning by making what he claims is a 'more comprehensive or dispositional claim' that relates to the 'overall course of a person's life.' He claims that '[*l*]*ives* are the primary referents in talk of autonomy'[57] and that it is the dispositional or comprehensive notion of autonomy which 'enables an individual to enjoy a life that is unified, orderly, and free from self-defeating conflict over fundamentals.' It involves the possession of positive qualities such as rationality, strength of will, and self-knowledge. Young describes this kind of self-directed life thus: 'in the main, it is ordered according to a plan or conception which fully expresses one's own will.' He relates it to things like career, life style, and what he calls 'dominant pursuits' and claims that it is the 'following through' on this plan or conception that unifies the various pursuits and that this is the basis of judgments about autonomy.[58]

Gerald Dworkin states that his concern is with 'what it means to be an autonomous person'—not with the notion of 'autonomous acts.'[59] Autonomy, he claims, is 'a feature of persons.'[60] His concern, therefore, is with a certain capacity persons have and with its exercise. It is a 'second-order' capacity to 'reflect critically' upon 'first-order preferences, desires, wishes, and so forth.' It involves the ability to 'accept or attempt to change' preferences, desires and wishes in light of 'higher-order preferences or values.' According to Dworkin, when a person exercises this capacity they 'define their nature, give meaning and coherence to their lives, and take responsibility for the kind of person they are.' That is what it means to be autonomous.[61] Dworkin warns that this capacity is not a 'fully articulated, and explicit process' in the sense that only certain kinds of people such as philosophy professors could qualify as autonomous. He argues that even isolated and relatively uneducated people can be autonomous. What makes such a person autonomous is the way that they shape and mold their life 'according to reflective procedures.' And this is empirically discernible: 'This will be shown not by what [a person] says about his thoughts, but in what he tries to change in his life, what he criticizes about others, the satisfaction he manifests (or fails to) in his work, family, and community.'[62] Further to this, the 'condition of being a chooser' is integral to being an autonomous person.[63] And, like Young, he claims that 'intuitively' autonomy seems to be a 'global' rather than a 'local' concept in the sense that it is about a 'whole way of living one's life.' It needs to be assessed over 'extended portions of a person's life.'[64]

Richard Lindley also provides us with a descriptive psychological account of autonomy. He claims that in order for a person to be autonomous 'freedom from external constraints' is required. This means that an autonomous person 'has a will of her or his own, and is able to act in pursuit of self-chosen goals.' He claims that this is one aspect of being autonomous, but that the notion of 'a developed self' is the first requirement. In other words, we need the idea of an agent together with a description of the psychology of the agent in order to explicate the idea of autonomy. The underlying idea, according to Lindley, is that of self-mastery.[65] He argues that autonomy is a matter of degree and that it is more helpful to delineate the ways in which a person may be heteronomous than to give a definition of perfect or complete autonomy.[66] This still amounts to a psychological account of autonomy. It is one which requires some capacity for reasoning in order for an agent to avoid the label of heteronomy.

Lindley rejects the idea that autonomy requires rationality of the kind that means persons must desire specific ends which conform to a stringent criterion of rationality. We still get a picture of what an autonomous person is like through his claim that autonomy requires that a person 'not act irrationally.' This means that autonomy entails some conception of rationality and Lindley claims that that can be expressed loosely as 'do as well as you can.' According to Lindley, the autonomous person's psychology is such that the person has some capacity for 'critical rational enquiry' and is autonomous to the extent that he or she acts in accordance with what he or she 'judges to be best.'[67]

Preferences and desires are central to psychological accounts of autonomy. Autonomy is sometimes tied in with the idea that critical reflection of a person's first-order desires and preferences by higher-order desires and preferences signifies autonomy. Harry Frankfurt is best known for this view which is presented in his influential paper titled 'Freedom of the Will and the Concept of a Person.'[68] Frankfurt claims that the philosophical interest in the word 'person' is to do with capturing 'those attributes which are the subject of our most humane concern with ourselves and the source of what we regard as most important and most problematical in our lives.'[69] Although he does not use the word 'autonomy,' he is referring to the 'capacity for reflective self-evaluation that is manifested in the formation of second-order desires'[70]and a preference that one of the desires 'be paramount over the other.'[71] Frankfurt's description of what it takes to have freedom of the will fits the conception of autonomy construed as a psychological state.

For Frankfurt, it is an agent's concern with 'his own free will' that is essential to being a 'person' and he distinguishes being a 'person' from being a 'wanton.' A wanton does not care about which desire wins out or about his will. Freedom of the will is not an issue for a wanton. Some adult humans, all very young children, and all nonhuman animals can be included in the class of wantons.[72] According to Frankfurt: 'The concept of a person is not only, then, the concept of a type of entity that has both first-order desires and volitions of the second order. It can also be construed as the concept of a type of entity for whom the freedom of its will may be a problem.'[73] In other words, in the same way that many accounts of autonomy need to include the concept of a person, Frankfurt is saying that the concept of a person necessarily involves the issue of freedom of the will or autonomy. Because Frankfurt's concept of a person is a psychological one, autonomy will be conceived and described as a psychological concept.

Based on Frankfurt's ideas, autonomy means more than just doing what we want. We can be characterized as autonomous when we are doing what we want to want.[74] An extension of this is the idea of authenticity as a possible condition for autonomy. Diana T. Meyers claims that an autonomous person is one who lives in harmony with his or her authentic self. According to Meyers, there is more to this than just desire satisfaction. What one 'really wants' is something that originates in the true self.[75] Distinguishing between 'real and apparent desires' is what concerns Meyers because she is arguing in the context of socialization and she argues that reclaiming this distinction is the 'chief task of a theory of autonomy.'[76] For Meyers this involves personal identity considerations and she articulates and makes explicit the idea of a 'true self.' She claims that 'really wanting' something is a 'qualitative distinction' we make with regard to our desires but it does not just mean that one desire is stronger. It means that one desire is 'more integral to our identity.'[77]

According to Meyers, the 'major accounts' of personal autonomy presented by Dworkin, Frankfurt, and Young,[78] construe autonomy as a 'special case of free will.' She claims autonomy is unintelligible on that kind of account because agents are required to 'elude socialization'; any notion of a true self amounts to a 'socialization-transcending agent.'[79] Therefore, according to Meyers, free will accounts are 'fatalistic' and 'incomplete.' They must rely on the idea of 'innate attributes' to explain a self 'untainted by socialization.'[80] In order to avoid this kind of 'static' conception of a self, she introduces the idea of a dynamic process.[81] She claims it is the 'spirit' in which a person lives and 'the way in which' a person makes their decisions that determines whether they are autonomous. This involves 'active engagement' in 'shaping' one's self and an 'intimate knowledge' of one's self.[82] Life plans are important and necessary for Meyers' because they 'facilitate the harmony autonomy requires.' She questions whether anyone can be autonomous without a life plan and claims that the alternative requires consulting one's self 'at length with regard to each and every personal decision.' Life plans constitute 'preaffirmed dispositions' and 'preestablished policies.' Our self-concepts are in 'reciprocal relation' to our life plans, so in order to have a self-concept that is not untested or tenuous we need a life plan. What this amount to is that persons must be equipped and disposed to pose and answer this question: 'What do I really want, need, care about, value, etcetera?' Meyers argues that the ability to 'act on the answer' and to make corrections when wrong are skills which constitute what she calls 'autonomy competency.'[83]

Meyers is trying to improve on and give a more sophisticated picture of the autonomous person than the accounts given by Young, Dworkin, and Frankfurt.[84] Ultimately, however, although she provides more detail about the autonomous person, her account fits into the same category. It is a descriptive psychological account of autonomy spelt out in terms of the psychology of an agent. Preferences and desires, notions of the self, life plans, and rationality have a central role.

IN SUMMARY

Descriptive psychological accounts of autonomy give us a substantive account of what an autonomous person is and the more developed the account the better the picture and the measure of what it is to be autonomous. This view of autonomy is easily understood; autonomy is more than an abstract notion. Even though an idea such as authenticity may not be easy to measure, autonomy is empirically definable and therefore discernible to some extent. In other words, it seems that if we have the description right we will be able to know and identify autonomy. It is then a separate question as to whether we should respect or value autonomy highly. Those who do value it will adopt the principle of respect for autonomy which will be construed as respect for beings who exhibit certain psychological characteristics.

A PROCEDURAL APPROACH TO AUTONOMY[85]

Procedures are important in situations where autonomy is viewed as a competing value with paternalism. Many modern theorists seem to be concerned with the agent whose actions require protection from interference. Procedures to respect persons and their autonomy are given importance and appeals to autonomy act as a limit to the authority of others to interfere.

It is from Mill that we get the idea of autonomy as being in tension with paternalism. Mill's argument for individual liberty in which he asserts 'one very simple principle' about the state or society not encroaching on or interfering with the individual, is a classic example of a procedural principle of *liberty*. I have already discussed Mill's ideas but we can see the procedural notion of liberty at work in his principle of liberty:

> That principle is, that the sole end for which mankind are warranted, individually or collectively, in interfering with the liberty of action of any of their number, is self-protection. . . . His own good, either physical or moral, is not a sufficient warrant. . . . The only part of the conduct of any one, for which he is amenable to society, is that which concerns others. In the part which merely concerns himself, his independence is, of right, absolute. Over himself, over his own body and mind, the individual is sovereign.[86]

These ideas are closely related to procedural ideas of autonomy and Mill's antipaternalistic principle can be applied to the doctor-patient relationship. Autonomy can act as a constraint on moral authority and respect for autonomy becomes the procedure that limits intervention by others.

Some kind of limit or check on interventions is particularly relevant in biomedical research, an area in which abuses have occurred. The creation of regulatory standards in relation to human subject experimentation establishes autonomy as a procedural concept. Both the autonomy and the well being of the patient/subject is the moral basis of these kinds of regulations. Autonomy, in particular, is appealed to as the underlying value of informed consent.

In the article he prepared for the National Commission for the Protection of Human Subjects of Biomedical and Behavioral Research, Engelhardt takes a procedural approach to autonomy. He appeals to two ideas. There is the idea of respect for persons which he claims is a basic moral value and there is the idea that there is value in self-determination. In other words, he is making a disctinction between an intrinsic value and an instrumental value for autonomy and then runs both ideas together in the concept of informed consent. For Engelhardt, the notion of informed consent takes into account two things at stake in the issue of human experimentation. Gaining free and informed consent ensures respect for persons and it gives consideration to goals and values such as the best interests of the subject and the benefits for society.[87] This approach does not demand anything special in terms of the choice made by the research subject. There is no requirement that the decision to consent must meet. The function of informed consent, according to Engelhardt, is to ensure that any 'deficiency' in a person's choice 'should not be attributable to the investigator.'[88] For Engelhardt, there is no special role for the rationality of the subject because his procedural approach functions to guarantee that researchers do not disregard their subjects as persons.[89]

Autonomy is also a procedural concept in Engelhardt's *The Foundations of Bioethics* (1986). Autonomy is a condition for morality in the sense that it generates mutual respect out of the interest in resolving disputes without force.[90] According to Engelhardt, autonomy reaches across moral communities and creates a 'morality of mutual respect'[91] whereas the pursuit of particular values or ranking of goods blocks the condition necessary for the possibility of mutual respect.[92] Engelhardt suggests that what he terms the 'principle of autonomy' is inescapable on account of the fact that it is required for the very coherence of the notion of morality.[93] The 'principle of beneficence' on the other hand he claims, is less basic. In the medical context the principle of beneficence has content; there are particular goods to which medicine ought to be directed but there are competing rankings of these goods and ethical disagreement results. Consensus is a problem, he claims, because the principle of beneficence is specified 'within the terms of a *particular* moral community.' Autonomy, however, is an appeal to mutual respect and it is 'the necessary condition for the possibility of resolving moral disputes without force and for sustaining a minimum ethical language of praise and blame.'[94]

According to Engelhardt, the principle of autonomy 'provides the empty process for generating moral authority' through 'mutual agreement' in a pluralist society where neither religion or reason has been able to establish a concrete account of the good life.[95] Engelhardt uses the term 'moral strangers' to describe the relationship between people who do not share a concrete moral vision. Without a common moral framework there is a difficulty in resolving disputes. Sometimes there may be enough shared in common to decide right and wrong and to establish public policy, but, often a lack of commonly shared moral premises means that moral strangers regard other people's views as morally misguided or even offensive.[96] The principle of autonomy or mutual respect is the way to resolve controversies. It is a form of peaceable negotiation or a constraint which is integral to the resolution of disputes. According to Engelhardt, this constraint is 'not grounded in a value given to autonomy, liberty or persons' but is a way to 'ground a common moral world for moral strangers without arbitrarily endorsing a particular ranking of values.'[97] The principle of autonomy can be relied on to resolve disputes without having to give a definitive answer of right or wrong to a content-full moral question:

> It can show that abortion, contraception, and suicide may not be forbidden with moral authority, but it cannot show that it is good to pay for abortion and contraception for the indigent or to assist rational individuals seeking to commit suicide who need aid.[98]

Engelhardt argues that the principle of autonomy is more fundamental than the principle of beneficence because an individual who violates the principle of autonomy violates moral authority and places him or herself 'outside the peaceable community.' This is a 'full rejection' of the moral life whereas a failure of beneficence merely impoverishes the moral life.[99] According to Engelhardt beneficence and autonomy together are two major moral principles in bioethics. The two are usually intertwined and 'express the fact that the moral point of view is one of beneficence within constraints of respect for persons.'[100] The morality of mutual respect or autonomy is more central in the sense that the nature of public policy is not discoverable by the principle of beneficence alone. It is created by common agreement. Mutual respect or the principle of autonomy is the basis for public policy or programs of beneficence.[101]

In the health care setting, in the absence of particular religious or moral premises, an interest in legitimating conduct and resolving disputes puts the focus on free and informed consent. It provides a common moral framework for moral strangers:

> Even if people cannot agree about when treatment should terminate, about whether they should practice euthanasia, or about whether and under what circumstances it would be appropriate to seek an abortion, they can at least agree that they will not subject persons to medical treatment, euthanasia, or abortion without their consent, and will not stop those who competently choose to make use of such modalities.[102]

According to Engelhardt, the principle of autonomy, even though it is quite neutral indicates the need for free and informed consent. Authority for actions involving others is derived from consent and in a secular pluralist society morality is 'the practice of doing the good within the bounds of moral authority.'[103] Engelhardt justifies the principle of autonomy by the fact that it expresses the agreement of participants in a dispute:

> Therefore, consent is the origin of authority, and respect of the right of participants to consent is the necessary condition for the possibility of a moral community. The principle of autonomy provides the minimum grammar for moral language. It is as inescapable as the interest of persons in blaming and praising with justification and resolving issues with authority.[104]

Consensus can be achieved and authority is derived from the principle of autonomy, but the procedural concept of autonomy has nothing to say about matters such as the moral status of persons, the value of liberty or the grounds for respecting persons.[105]

In a later edition of *The Foundations of Bioethics* Engelhardt renames the principle of autonomy as 'the principle of permission.' This, he claims, is to show that 'what is at stake is not some value possessed by autonomy or liberty' and it is the 'recognition' that moral authority is not derived from God or from reason, but from the 'permission of individuals.'[106] In other words moral authority comes from agreement among individuals, not as a response to some characteristic of the decision. Engelhardt's idea of autonomy has had an important part in the history of the development of the idea of autonomy in contemporary bioethics. He has had an influence through *The Foundations of Bioethics* and we have seen that his ideas were also influenctial in *The Belmont Report*. Even though Engelhardt no longer wants to use the label autonomy, his notion of autonomy as a procedural concept still has influence in terms of other people's acceptance of his ideas.

Gilbert Meilaender refers to ways in which autonomy seems to be a procedural concept. He claims that because consensus or public policy has become our aim, bioethics has become a procedure: 'lacking substantive agreement there remains only the search for ways to honor everyone's autonomy.'[107] He also claims that autonomy has been incorporated into our understanding of what it means to be a person with the result that modern bioethics has become a defense of autonomy.[108] Meilaender, who prefers religious concerns and ideas of human dignity as the basis of a substantive view of persons, laments the circumstances in which respect for persons has come to be 'grounded in autonomy alone.'[109] As an example of the modern defense of autonomy, he refers us to *Principles of Biomedical Ethics* which he acknowledges is popular and influential.[110] He claims that the approach used by Beauchamp and Childress is a procedural one and their idea of being a person has no substantive content. To be a person is about being an 'autonomous chooser.'[111]

The principle of respect for autonomy that Beauchamp and Childress use in *Principles of Biomedical Ethic,* from the third edition onward, is at times, but not consistently, a public policy or procedural approach to autonomy. A public policy approach is a view about why we should respect autonomy rather than what constitutes autonomy and it is an approach that seeks to build a framework for a pluralistic society where people do not share the same ideas about a whole range of substantive moral questions. Autonomy becomes something on which everyone can agree.

Beauchamp and Childress want ways of allowing more choices and 'ordinary' or 'normal choosers' to qualify as worthy of respect. They use the words 'ordinary' and 'normal' in the sense that they oppose an aspirational ideal of autonomy 'beyond the reach of normal choosers.'[112] Because the development of 'general moral action guides' for use in a biomedical context is one of their main concerns, some kind of shared consensus is required.[113] In a pluralistic society, Beauchamp and Childress are committed to this kind of procedural approach and respect for autonomy is the obvious procedure because everyone can agree to the extent that they all agree to respect each other's autonomy. It is important to note, however, that Beauchamp and Childress claim they are not making respect for autonomy a 'trump moral principle'[114] even though some of their conclusions support professional conduct that exceeds current legal and regulatory requirements. For instance, with regard to public policy they argue that the demands of justice sometimes clearly outweigh the demands of respect for autonomy.[115] Their interest, therefore, seems to be more with finding *a procedure* to generate moral authority and resolve disputes than with promoting autonomy itself as a principle. Nevertheless, although public policy requires procedures rather than particular moral principles, the principle of respect for autonomy seems to be the obvious contender. With an emphasis on *respect*, it adapts readily into a procedure. Where consensus or public policy is a particular concern, Meilaender's argument (about a lack of substantive agreement resulting in a search for ways to honor everyone's autonomy) is a reasonable one.

In circumstances where the principle of respect for autonomy is the best procedure to resolve disagreements or to generate authority, the content of a person's choice is not the important issue. Likewise, the question of what it means to be autonomous is not important—that may contain ideas and meanings that people disagree on. In the clinical context the emphasis on 'respectful action' and a 'respectful attitude' is related to the conduct of health care professionals and public policy rather than what constitutes an autonomous person or choice. For Beauchamp and Childress, like Engelhardt, consent is the thing that legitimates forms of authority and conduct. In fact, Beauchamp and Childress claim that consent is the 'basic paradigm of autonomy in health care, research, politics, and other contexts.'[116] Beauchamp and Childress refine the idea somewhat and claim that it is '*express* consent' that is important. Other forms of consent such as tacit or implied consent can occur under conditions that render consent invalid and presumed consent based on a theory of human goods or a theory of rationality is problematic.[117] In the fourth edition of their text they argue that they accept and want to 'give depth' to the premise that the 'primary function and justification of informed consent is to enable and protect individual autonomous choice.'[118] Since Beauchamp and Childress are disinclined to give a clear account of what an autonomous choice is, it is hard to see that the word 'autonomous' (as it is added into the previous sentence) can be anything other than some kind of evaluative term.[119]

AUTONOMY AS AN EVALUATIVE CONCEPT

What does it mean to say that autonomy is an evaluative concept? When we use autonomy in this way it means we are making a judgment rather than describing something. An evaluative term expresses a value judgment which may be a moral judgment. Alternatively it could be expressing some nonmoral value as in an aesthetic judgment. Statements in which a term is used descriptively are factual statements; they can be true or false, whereas a statement which uses the same term evaluatively is arguably quite different. Statements involving an evaluative term can be affirmed by one person and denied by another without it necessarily being the case that one of them is right and the other wrong. Evaluative terms depend on a certain standard which in turn is seen by some as depending on what the speaker approves or disapproves of.[120] When a term such as 'autonomy' is used evaluatively we are 'explaining or conveying or setting forth the standard' of autonomous persons or choices rather than describing some characteristic of the action or person.[121]

We can see the difference between a descriptive and an evaluative concept in the debate about abortion and infanticide. Michael Tooley distinguishes between a descriptive and an evaluative use of the term 'person.'

When the term functions in a purely descriptive way the only thing we can establish is that the entity has certain characteristics. No ethical conclusions are implied by the fact that something is a 'person.' It can tell us things such as, this entity has the capacity for thought, it is self-conscious, and it has rationality.[122] When 'person' is an evaluative concept, an entirely different approach is taken. This occurs at the level of formulating the concept and in the implications we draw from the term. With an evaluative approach, we would begin from the idea that some entities have a right to life and we want to understand the term 'person' in a way that applies to those beings only. This gives moral content to the term 'person.' 'Person' is an evaluative concept in the sense that to say that something is a person entails that it has a right to life.[123] In a similar way, in discussions about autonomy, we can detect in some authors a shift from a descriptive account of autonomy in which autonomy has certain characteristics and it remains an open question whether or not we ought to respect it, to an account in which it follows by definition that an autonomous decision ought to be respected. This has moral content but no descriptive content. When autonomy is an evaluative concept, what counts as an autonomous decision is left open and depends on people's evaluations.

When we use autonomy as an evaluative concept it implies that someone or something is deserving of respect rather than indicating anything about what it means to be autonomous. This contrasts with the descriptive use of the term in which saying that someone is autonomous means something like—this person is independent, has self-control and acts in accordance with his or her stable values. When we use the term evaluatively it is a way of saying that this person qualifies as deserving of respect. It implies that this person should not be interfered with, has a right to autonomy, or that interference is a violation of autonomy.

If we begin with the idea that it is prima facie wrong to violate a person's autonomy, the descriptive sense of autonomy drops away and the term shifts to an evaluative one in the sense that the thing foremost in our mind is the idea that there are particular choices that deserve protection and should not be overridden paternalistically. The idea of autonomy underlying Beauchamp and Childress's principle of respect for autonomy seems, at times, to be an evaluative concept. Nevertheless, it is important not to confuse autonomy as an evaluative concept with giving an excessive amount of value to autonomy. For Beauchamp and Childress, respect for autonomy has prima facie standing and they insist that they do not want to overvalue it by making it a 'trump moral principle.' It is 'one principle in a framework of prima facie principles.'[124]

In the third edition of *Principles of Biomedical Ethics*, Beauchamp and Childress's argument focuses in large part on whether it is good or bad to protect a patient's choices. They claim that: 'For an action to be autonomous we should only require a substantial degree of understanding and freedom from constraint, not a full understanding or a complete absence of influence.'[125] From the fourth edition, they declare that their interest is in decision making[126] and their particular concern is with what they call 'meaningful decision making' in the 'practical world.'[127] They argue that if it is only an ideal of 'fully or completely autonomous' decisions that we treat as 'adequate decision making' we are not being practical.[128] According to Beauchamp and Childress, we should regard some decisions as autonomous even when they do not meet an exacting standard. They want a way for people to qualify as deserving respect for their decisions 'even when they have *not* reflected on their preferences at a higher level.'[129] They claim that a problem with such exacting requirements for autonomy, including second-order-desire theories, is that 'few choosers, and also few choices, would be autonomous.'[130] The term 'autonomous' is being used here in a way that means qualifying as deserving protection.

There may seem to be some common ground between a procedural and an evaluative concept of autonomy. In Beauchamp and Childress's account of autonomy some aspects which illustrate the way in which autonomy is a procedure also demonstrate the fact that autonomy is being used as an evaluative concept. This does not mean that the procedural and the evaluative concept cannot be separated. It may show that Beauchamp and Childress are not being consistent. They are swapping between concepts. An evaluative concept of autonomy is quite different from the procedural concept. The evaluative concept promotes autonomy as a value. As noted earlier, autonomy in the procedural sense is a constraint not grounded in a specific value given to autonomy. The crucial thing of an evaluative concept, that distinguishes it from the procedural and a descriptive concept of autonomy is that it implies an ethical conclusion. If something is labeled autonomous it follows by definition that it ought to be respected. And it is people's evaluations that determine what counts as 'autonomous.'

We saw earlier that Beauchamp and Childress do not want autonomy to be conceived as a psychological state. Some theories of autonomy have certain standards or requirements that agents and their actions need to meet before they will be deemed autonomous. For instance, some theories require agents to reflect on their preferences at a higher level in order for their decisions to qualify as deserving respect. Beauchamp and Childress, however, do not make these kinds of demands.[131] They argue that the acceptance or rejection of a desire may be 'motivated by an overriding desire that is simply *stronger*, not more *rational* or *autonomous*.'[132] Therefore, on the Beauchamp and Childress' view, a descriptive psychological account of what it means to be autonomous or to make an autonomous decision is not helpful. They claim that rigorous standards and exacting requirements for autonomy are a 'problem' and they want ways for more choosers and more choices to qualify as autonomous.[133] In effect, what they want is for more choosers and more choices to qualify as deserving respect.

There is some evidence that in the fourth edition of their book, Beauchamp and Childress begin by deciding which choices they think ought to be protected and not overridden paternalistically and those are the decisions they want to call autonomous. They claim that people who are not generally considered autonomous; even some patients in institutions who need to be taken care of by others and have been declared legally incompetent 'may still be able to make autonomous choices.'[134] They are referring to things like preferences about food,[135] refusing 'some' medications, and choosing to make telephone calls. Clearly these are choices we would think it wrong to override. Beauchamp and Childress, however, call these 'autonomous' choices. In the discussion of various kinds of choices which they want protection for, we can see why Beauchamp and Childress do not support a descriptive psychological account of autonomy. Choices such as those just mentioned, which have not been accepted or repudiated at a higher level, would not qualify for protection.

Because Beauchamp and Childress's approach to formulating the concept of autonomy is an evaluative one (they want more choices protected) they proceed by offering examples of actions which may be ruled unworthy for protection from the perspective of a descriptive psychological view of autonomy. These are actions legislated from without in the sense that they comply with the authority of institutions, tradition or community. Beauchamp and Childress are operating with an account of autonomy for which they claim these actions are compatible. For instance, they argue that a Jehovah's Witness who refuses a recommended blood transfusion may be submitting to the authority of a religion but that that person's refusal is autonomous. They list some other actions which we would be loathe to overrule: 'Virtuous conduct, role responsibilities, acceptable forms of loving, charitable behaviour' and even 'respect for autonomy.' These kinds of actions or 'moral notions' they claim, usually derive from cultural traditions but are nevertheless chosen autonomously.[136] They claim that there is no fundamental inconsistency between autonomy and acting on reasons that are not entirely a person's own reasons. It is sufficient that the person views something as a 'legitimate source of direction'; if it is something they choose to accept.[137] This is not the same thing as critical reflection or second-order preferences as specified in a descriptive or psychological account. Beauchamp and Childress seem to be endorsing people's preferences and whatever choices people make. When they say a choice or action is autonomous they mean that the person who chooses or acts should not be interfered with and if they are interfered with a violation of autonomy has occurred.

From the third edition of their book, Beauchamp and Childress introduce the principle of respect for autonomy. This seems to be a way to avoid having to specify content in their notion of autonomy. The emphasis seems to shift from the meaning of autonomy to the idea of respect. Beauchamp and Childress do not focus on autonomous persons or choices. In the fourth edition they claim that '[b]eing autonomous is not the same as being respected *as* an autonomous person'[138] (my emphasis). There is significance in the word 'as.' It suggests that autonomy, or a clear idea of what autonomy is, is not a prerequisite for the principle of respect for autonomy to apply. 'To respect an autonomous agent' Beauchamp and Childress claim, is 'at a minimum, to acknowledge that person's right to hold views, to make choices, and to take actions based on personal values and beliefs.'[139] They claim that as well as obligations of nonintervention, in some contexts respect includes 'obligations to build up or maintain others' capacities for autonomous choice while helping allay fears and other conditions that destroy or disrupt their autonomous actions.'[140] In answer to the question: 'Why is such respect owed to persons?' Beauchamp and Childress invoke Mill and Kant (see above for a detailed discussion of this), but, they are not embracing a Kantian metaphysical concept of autonomy and they do not want to endorse a content full descriptive psychological view of autonomy of the kind that derives from Mill. Beauchamp and Childress want ways for more rather than fewer choices to qualify as deserving of respect but there is a limit in that they do not want it to cover what they call 'nonautonomous persons':[141]

> The principle should not be used for persons who cannot act in a sufficiently autonomous manner (and cannot be rendered autonomous) because they are immature, incapacitated, ignorant, coerced, or exploited.[142]

There is a difficulty for Beauchamp and Childress because without embracing a detailed descriptive standard there is no way to know when a decision is to be regarded as within the reach of what they call 'ordinary; or 'normal choosers' and whether it is a meaningful decision in the sense that they would regard it as worthy of respect. The decision could be one that is made by someone who is ignorant or exploited and not worthy of respect on their view. To get around this Beauchamp and Childress offer 'typical examples' of nonautonomous persons who fit the criteria: 'Infants, irrationally suicidal individuals, and drug dependent patients.'[143] Decisions made by these people can be overridden paternalistically, they claim.

In their discussion about paternalism in the fourth edition of their book, Beauchamp and Childress argue that the question about whether a person is substantially autonomous or substantially nonautonomous is a 'conceptual or empirical problem about the nature and conditions of autonomy.' This suggests a descriptive rather than an evaluative view; they claim it is 'not a problem about the moral grounds of intervention.'[144] And yet, in their discussion of autonomy it seems to be precisely that. Their concern seems to be with the grounds of intervention rather than the characteristics of autonomy. This is particularly evident when they refer to choices made by people who could be considered incompetent and to choices which could be considered substantially nonautonomous on conceptual empirical grounds but which Beauchamp and Childress want to qualify as deserving protection nevertheless. According to Beauchamp and Childress, there is a close connection between the concept of competence in decision making and the concept of autonomy. They claim that there is a striking similarity in the criteria for each and they argue that competency judgments have a distinctive evaluative element. They claim that competency judgments are not only empirical findings:

> For example, a person who appears irrational or unreasonable to others might fail a psychiatric test, and so be declared incompetent. The test is an empirical measuring device, but normative judgements determine how the test will be used to sort persons into the two classes of competent and incompetent. They are normative judgements because they concern how persons ought to be or may permissibly be treated.[145]

Beauchamp and Childress are doing much the same thing in their discussion of respect for autonomy. They do not want to give specific content to the idea of autonomy because that can lead to a standard that is too demanding to be practical and some actions which they think deserve respect and protection would not qualify. Instead, they make an evaluative judgment about what qualifies as deserving respect.

Beauchamp and Childress are not consistent in their use of the principle of respect for autonomy. As well as appealing to a Kantian concept of autonomy, they seem to be mixing and confusing descriptive psychological, procedural, and evaluative elements. This is confusing and not conducive to a consistent or coherent view of autonomy.

CONCLUSION

I have separated the different concepts of autonomy that are being referred to in contemporary discussions because in order to have a proper discussion about autonomy it is better not to be confused by shifting concepts. We have seen some of the problems of mixing concepts in particular by looking at Beauchamp and Childress. Next we need to critically analyse the different concepts to decide which sense of autonomy is important and applicable to the clinical context.

NOTES

1. Kant, *Groundwork*, 120 (452).
2. Kant, *Groundwork*, 125–56 (457–58).
3. Kant, *Groundwork*, 121 (453), 123 (455).
4. Kant, *Groundwork*, 124 (456).
5. Kant, *Groundwork*, 75 (408).
6. Kant, *Groundwork*, 75 (408).
7. O'Neill, *Constructions of Reason*, 76. Quoting from Iris Murdoch, *The Sovereignty of Good*, 80.
8. O'Neill, *Constructions of Reason*, 67n1, 76.
9. Kant, *Groundwork*, 76–77 (408–409).
10. Kant, *Groundwork*, 77 (409).
11. O'Neill, *Constructions of Reason*, ix.
12. O'Neill, *Constructions of Reason*, ix.
13. O'Neill, *Constructions of Reason*, 66.
14. Rousseau, *The Social Contract*, 20–21.
15. Rousseau, *The Social Contract*, 11.
16. Kant, *Groundwork*, 106 (438).
17. O'Neill, *Constructions of Reason*, 44.
18. Immanuel Kant, *Idea for a Universal History with a Cosmopolitan Purpose*, in *Kant Political Writings*, ed. Hans Reiss, trans. H. B. Nisbet (Cambridge: Cambridge University Press, 1991, 2nd ed.), 44
19. Kant, *Idea for a Universal History*, 44.
20. Rousseau , *The Social Contract*, 20.
21. Kant, *Idea for a Universal History*, 46.

22. Kant, *Idea for a Universal History*, 46.

23. Hans Reiss ed., *Kant Political Writings*, trans. H. B. Nisbet (Cambridge: Cambridge University Press, 1991), 3.

24. Immanuel Kant, "On the Common Saying: 'This May Be True in Theory, but It Does Not Apply in Practice,'" in *Kant Political Writings*, ed. Hans Reiss, trans. H. B. Nisbet (Cambridge: Cambridge University Press, 1991, 2nd ed.), 81.

25. Lewis W. Beck, "Kant and the Right to Revolution," in *Immanuel Kant: Critical Assessments* vol.III, ed. Ruth F. Chadwick (London: Routledge, 1992), 401–402.

26. Beck, "Kant and the Right to Revolution," 405.

27. Kant, "On the Common Saying," 82–83.

28. Kant, "On the Common Saying," 83.

29. Beck, "Kant and the Right to Revolution," 401.

30. Kant, "On the Common Saying," 81.

31. Rousseau, *The Social Contract*, 20–25.

32. Andrew Levine, *The General Will: Rousseau, Marx, Communism* (Cambridge: Cambridge University Press, 1993), 160; Andrew Levine, *The Politics of Autonomy: A Kantian Reading of Rousseau's Social Contract* (Amherst: University of Massachusetts Press, 1976), chapters 1–2.

33. Levine, *The General Will*, 160–63.

34. Kant, *Groundwork*, 84 (416).

35. O'Neill, *Constructions of Reason*, 67n1.

36. Thomas E. Hill, Jr., "The Kantian Conception of Autonomy," in *The Inner Citadel: Essays on Individual Autonomy*, ed. J. Christman (New York: Oxford University Press, 1989), 91.

37. David A. J. Richards, "Rights and Autonomy" in *The Inner Citadel: Essays on Individual Autonomy*, ed. J. Christman (New York: Oxford University Press, 1989), 208.

38. See Schneewind, *The Invention of Autonomy*, 515. Kant's conception of autonomy is embedded in a 'metaphysical psychology.' This presupposes that we are 'rational agents' with a kind of freedom which is 'out of the domain of natural causation.'

39. Mill, *System of Logic*, 554.

40. L. C. Becker and Charlotte B. Becker, ed., *Encyclopedia of Ethics* (New York: Garland Publishing Inc., 1992), 1039.

41. *The Belmont Report*, 5.

42. Beauchamp and Childress, *Principles of Biomedical Ethics*, 1979, 1st ed., 56–57.

43. Beauchamp and Childress, *Principles of Biomedical Ethics*, 1994, 4th ed., 121; and Beauchamp and Childress, *Principles of Biomedical Ethics*, 2001, 5th ed., 58.

44. Beauchamp and Childress, *Principles of Biomedical Ethics*, 1994, 4th ed., 123.

45. Beauchamp and Childress, *Principles of Biomedical Ethics*, 2001, 5th ed. 59.

46. Beauchamp and Childress, *Principles of Biomedical Ethics*, 1994, 4th ed., 123; and Beauchamp and Childress, *Principles of Biomedical Ethics*, 2001, 5th ed., 59.

47. Beauchamp and Childress, *Principles of Biomedical Ethics*, 1889, 3rd ed., 69.

48. Beauchamp and Childress, *Principles of Biomedical Ethics*, 1994, 4th ed., 123; and Beauchamp and Childress, *Principles of Biomedical Ethics*, 2001, 5th ed., 59.

49. Beauchamp and Childress, *Principles of Biomedical Ethics*, 1994, 4th ed., 126; and Beauchamp and Childress, *Principles of Biomedical Ethics*, 2001, 5th ed., 64.

50. Beauchamp and Childress, *Principles of Biomedical Ethics*, 1994, 4th ed., 126; and Beauchamp and Childress, *Principles of Biomedical Ethics*, 2001, 5th ed., 64.

51. Beauchamp and Childress, *Principles of Biomedical Ethics*, 1994, 4th ed., 127; and Beauchamp and Childress, *Principles of Biomedical Ethics*, 2001, 5th ed., 64.

52. Beauchamp and Childress, *Principles of Biomedical Ethics*, 1994, 4th ed., 121; and Beauchamp and Childress, *Principles of Biomedical Ethics*, 2001, 5th ed., 58.

53. Beauchamp and Childress, *Principles of Biomedical Ethics*, 1994, 4th ed., 122–23; and Beauchamp and Childress, *Principles of Biomedical Ethics*, 2001, 5th ed., 59–60.

54. Robert Young, *Personal Autonomy: Beyond Negative and Positive Liberty* (London: Croom Helm, 1986), 8.

55. Young, *Personal Autonomy*, 9.

56. Young, *Personal Autonomy*, 8.

57. Young, *Personal Autonomy*, 109.

58. Young, *Personal Autonomy*, 8, 109.

59. Dworkin, *The Theory and Practice of Autonomy*, 9–20.

60. Dworkin, *The Theory and Practice of Autonomy*, 6.

61. Dworkin, *The Theory and Practice of Autonomy*, 19–20.

62. Dworkin, *The Theory and Practice of Autonomy*, 17.

63. Dworkin, *The Theory and Practice of Autonomy*, 18.

64. Dworkin, *The Theory and Practice of Autonomy*, 15–16.

65. Richard Lindley, *Autonomy*, (London: Macmillan, 1986), 6.

66. Lindley, *Autonomy*, 69–70.

67. Lindley, *Autonomy*, 67.

68. Harry G. Frankfurt, "Freedom of the Will and the Concept of a Person," *Journal of Philosophy* 68 (1971); reprinted in *The Inner Citadel: Essays on Individual Autonomy*, ed. John Christman (Oxford: Oxford University Press, 1989), 63–76. (Gerald Dworkin's 'hierarchical' view predates Frankfurt's). Dworkin notes in the introduction of *The Theory and Practice of Autonomy*, that Frankfurt's article was published shortly after his own "Acting Freely," but, acknowledges Frankfurt's paper has been 'extremely influential.' Lawrence Haworth, *Autonomy: An Essay in Philosophical Psychology and Ethics* (New Haven: Yale University Press, 1986), 3–4, also develops an account of autonomy as a psychological idea involving different levels of desires or what he calls 'critical competence.' Haworth acknowledges his debt to Dworkin and Frankfurt as being amongst several writers who greatly influenced his conception of autonomy.

69. Frankfurt, "Freedom of the Will," 64.

70. Frankfurt, "Freedom of the Will," 64.

71. Frankfurt, "Freedom of the Will," 68.
72. Frankfurt, "Freedom of the Will," 67.
73. Frankfurt, "Freedom of the Will," 69.
74. Frankfurt, "Freedom of the Will," 70.
75. Diana T. Meyers, *Self, Society, and Personal Choice* (New York: Columbia University Press, 1989), 43.
76. Diana T. Meyers, *Self, Society, and Personal Choice*, 26.
77. Diana T. Meyers, *Self, Society, and Personal Choice*, 26.
78. Meyers is referring to essays that predate the book length accounts of both Dworkin and Young. The essays are: Gerald Dworkin, "Autonomy and Behaviour Control," *Hastings Center Report* 6 (1976): 23–28.; Robert Young; "Compatibilism and Conditioning," *Nous* 13 (1979): 361–78; and "Autonomy and Socialization," *Mind* 89 (1980): 565–76. In the preface of his book, Dworkin claims that the view expressed there has 'undergone considerable revision.'
79. Meyers, *Self, Society, and Personal Choice*, 40, 42.
80. Robert Young, review of *Self, Society, and Personal Choice* by Diana T. Meyers, *Australasian Journal of Philosophy* 68 (1990): 354. Young thinks there is not really the gulf between Meyer's views and those of the writers from whom she is trying to distance herself. He argues that '[s]ometimes that gap is made to seem greater because of indifferent exposition of opponents' views.'
81. Meyers, *Self, Society, and Personal Choice*, 42–45.
82. Meyers, *Self, Society, and Personal Choice*, 47–48.
83. Meyers, *Self, Society, and Personal Choice*, 50–53.
84. Bernard Berofsky's account of autonomy—Bernard Berofsky, *Liberation from Self: A Theory of Personal Autonomy* (Cambridge: Cambridge University Press, 1995), 4, 10—is also a psychological account. It admits degrees of autonomy. There is some similarity with the accounts discussed here. One of the conditions Berofsky requires for autonomy is personal integrity. He claims that before the idea of an agent's autonomy can be broached, he or she 'must have some internal coherence.'
85. I also refer to this approach as a 'notion' of autonomy because it is perceived as a 'notion' of autonomy in some contemporary bioethical discussions. This is explained in the course of this chapter.
86. Mill, *On Liberty*, 8–9.
87. Engelhardt, "Basic Ethical Principles in the Conduct," 28.
88. Engelhardt, "Basic Ethical Principles in the Conduct," 22.
89. Engelhardt, "Basic Ethical Principles in the Conduct," 22.
90. H Tristram Engelhardt, Jr., *The Foundations of Bioethics* (New York: Oxford University Press, 1986), 68–72.
91. Engelhardt, *The Foundations of Bioethics*, 1986, 1st ed., 72–73.
92. Engelhardt, *The Foundations of Bioethics*, 1986, 1st ed., 69.
93. Engelhardt, *The Foundations of Bioethics*, 1986, 1st ed., 68.
94. Engelhardt, *The Foundations of Bioethics*, 1986, 1st ed., 69.

95. Engelhardt, *The Foundations of Bioethics*, 1986, 1st ed., 72.

96. H. Tristram Engelhardt, Jr., *Bioethics and Secular Humanism: The Search for a Common Morality* (Philadelphia: Trinity Press International, 1991), xiii—xv.

97. Engelhardt, *Bioethics and Secular Humanism*, 119.

98. Engelhardt, *The Foundations of Bioethics*, 1986, 1st ed., 72.

99. Engelhardt, *The Foundations of Bioethics*, 1986, 1st ed., 73.

100. Engelhardt, *The Foundations of Bioethics*, 1986, 1st ed., 81, 85.

101. Engelhardt, *The Foundations of Bioethics*, 1986, 1st ed., 85.

102. Engelhardt, *The Foundations of Bioethics*, 1986, 1st ed., 116.

103. Engelhardt, *The Foundations of Bioethics*, 1986, 1st ed., 78, 85.

104. Engelhardt, *The Foundations of Bioethics*, 1986, 1st ed., 86.

105. Engelhardt, *Bioethics and Secular Humanism*, 115, 118.

106. H. Tristram Engelhardt, Jr., *The Foundations of Bioethics*, (2nd ed.) (New York: Oxford University Press, 1996, 2nd ed.) xi.

107. Meilaender, *Body, Soul, and Bioethics*, 29.

108. Meilaender, *Body, Soul, and Bioethics*, 18–19, 53.

109. Meilaender, *Body, Soul, and Bioethics*, 3, 18.

110. Meilaender, *Body, Soul, and Bioethics*, 12, 13.

111. Meilaender, *Body, Soul, and Bioethics*, 52.

112. Beauchamp and Childress, *Principles of Biomedical Ethics*, 1994, 4th ed., 123; and Beauchamp and Childress, *Principles of Biomedical Ethics*, 2001, 5th ed., 59.

113. Beauchamp and Childress, *Principles of Biomedical Ethics*, 1994, 4th ed., 4.

114. Beauchamp and Childress, *Principles of Biomedical Ethics*, 1994, 4th ed., 181; and Beauchamp and Childress, *Principles of Biomedical Ethics*, 2001, 5th ed., 57, 104.

115. Beauchamp and Childress, *Principles of Biomedical Ethics*, 1994, 4th ed., 181.

116. Beauchamp and Childress, *Principles of Biomedical Ethics*, 1994, 4th ed., 128; and Beauchamp and Childress, *Principles of Biomedical Ethics*, 2001, 5th ed., 65–66.

117. Beauchamp and Childress, *Principles of Biomedical Ethics*, 1994, 4th ed., 128–29; and Beauchamp and Childress, *Principles of Biomedical Ethics*, 2001, 5th ed., 65–66.

118. Beauchamp and Childress, *Principles of Biomedical Ethics*, 1994, 4th ed., 142.

119. Beauchamp and Childress, *Principles of Biomedical Ethics*, 2001, 5th ed., 77, 107fn41. In the 5th edition of their text Beauchamp and Childress seem to be distancing themselves from or qualifying some of the claims they made in earlier editions. In the 5th edition Beauchamp and Childress say that 'since the 1970s, the primary justification advanced for requirements of informed consent has been to protect autonomous choice, a loosely defined goal that is often buried in broad discussions of protecting the rights of patients and research subjects.' They also refer to an article that casts doubts on a justification of informed consent based on con-

siderations of autonomy. And, they add that '[H]istorically, we can claim little beyond the fact that a general, inchoate societal demand has emerged for the protection of patients' and subjects' rights, particularly their autonomy rights.' I am arguing that Beauchamp and Childress have influenced the way others in the field have come to view the concept of autonomy and their influence on the way others have come to view the idea of autonomy referred to in contemporary bioethics is still considerable despite any changes or corrections made in the 5th edition of *Principles of Biomedical Ethics*.

120. R. M. Hare, *Sorting Out Ethics* (Oxford: Clarendon Press, 1997), 55, 59.

121. R. M. Hare, *The Language of Morals* (Oxford: Clarendon Press, 1992, [first published 1952]), 114.

122. Michael Tooley, *Abortion and Infanticide* (Oxford: Clarendon Press, 1983), 35–36.

123. Tooley, *Abortion and Infanticide*, 35.

124. Beauchamp and Childress, *Principles of Biomedical Ethics*, 1994, 4th ed., 181; and Beauchamp and Childress, *Principles of Biomedical Ethics*, 2001, 5th ed., 57, 104.

125. Beauchamp and Childress, *Principles of Biomedical Ethics*, 1889, 3rd ed., 69; Beauchamp and Childress, *Principles of Biomedical Ethics*, 1994, 4th ed., p.123; and Beauchamp and Childress, *Principles of Biomedical Ethics*, 2001, 5th ed., 59.

126. Beauchamp and Childress, *Principles of Biomedical Ethics*, 1994, 4th ed., 121.

127. Beauchamp and Childress, *Principles of Biomedical Ethics*, 1994, 4th ed., 123; and Beauchamp and Childress, *Principles of Biomedical Ethics*, 2001, 5th ed., 59.

128. Beauchamp and Childress, *Principles of Biomedical Ethics*, 1994, 4th ed., 123.

129. Beauchamp and Childress, *Principles of Biomedical Ethics*, 1994, 4th ed., 122; and Beauchamp and Childress, *Principles of Biomedical Ethics*, 2001, 5th ed., 59.

130. Beauchamp and Childress, *Principles of Biomedical Ethics*, 1994, 4th ed., 123; and Beauchamp and Childress, *Principles of Biomedical Ethics*, 2001, 5th ed., 59.

131. This is a change that comes about in the 4th edition. They claim that 'serious problems' confront this kind of theory (4th. ed. p.122). In the 3rd edition they held the view that autonomy is 'a concept that is properly linked to reflective individual choice' (3rd. ed., p.71).

132. Beauchamp and Childress, *Principles of Biomedical Ethics*, 1994, 4th ed., 122; and Beauchamp and Childress, *Principles of Biomedical Ethics*, 2001, 5th ed., 59.

133. Beauchamp and Childress, *Principles of Biomedical Ethics*, 1994, 4th ed., 122–23; and Beauchamp and Childress, *Principles of Biomedical Ethics*, 2001, 5th ed., 59.

134. Beauchamp and Childress, *Principles of Biomedical Ethics*, 1994, 4th ed., 121; and Beauchamp and Childress, *Principles of Biomedical Ethics*, 2001, 5th ed., 58.

135. Re. preferences about food. Contrast this with Kant's metaphysical concept of autonomy in the section 'autonomy and choice' in chapter 1 above. For Kant these kind of choices do not warrant respect.

136. Beauchamp and Childress, *Principles of Biomedical Ethics*, 1994, 4th ed., 124.

137. Beauchamp and Childress, *Principles of Biomedical Ethics*, 1994, 4th ed., 124; and Beauchamp and Childress, *Principles of Biomedical Ethics*, 2001, 5th ed., 60.

138. Beauchamp and Childress, *Principles of Biomedical Ethics*, 1994, 4th ed., 125. This sentence which begins the section on the principle of respect for autonomy is dropped in the 5th edition. The rest of the paragraph remains the same.

139. Beauchamp and Childress, *Principles of Biomedical Ethics*, 1994, 4th ed., 125; and Beauchamp and Childress, *Principles of Biomedical Ethics*, 2001, 5th ed., 63.

140. Beauchamp and Childress, *Principles of Biomedical Ethics*, 2001, 5th ed., 63.

141. Beauchamp and Childress, *Principles of Biomedical Ethics*, 1994, 4th ed., 127.

142. Beauchamp and Childress, *Principles of Biomedical Ethics*, 1994, 4th ed., 127.; and Beauchamp and Childress, *Principles of Biomedical Ethics*, 2001, 5th ed., similar wording p. 65.

143. Beauchamp and Childress, *Principles of Biomedical Ethics*, 1994, 4th ed., 127; and Beauchamp and Childress, *Principles of Biomedical Ethics*, 2001, 5th ed., 65.

144. Beauchamp and Childress, *Principles of Biomedical Ethics*, 1994, 4th ed., 279.

145. Beauchamp and Childress, *Principles of Biomedical Ethics*, 1994, 4th ed., 133; and Beauchamp and Childress, *Principles of Biomedical Ethics*, 2001, 5th ed., similar wording p.70.

5

CRITICAL ANALYSIS OF THE DIFFERENT CONCEPTIONS OF AUTONOMY

IS THE METAPHYSICAL OR KANTIAN ACCOUNT OF AUTONOMY ONE THAT IS APPLICABLE IN THE CLINICAL CONTEXT?

In Kant's metaphysics, duty, rationality, good will, and universal law constitute a cluster of ideas, each of which depends for its meaning on the other. This means that part of being an autonomous choice is that it be a rational choice, that it accord with duty, and that it display a good will. And the maxim of the choice must be capable of being willed by all rational beings so as not to contradict their status as ends in themselves. Although connected, these terms of course do not have the same meaning.

Kant's emphasis on duty is a central part of his metaphysical concept of autonomy, but the idea of agents acting from duty, with reason as the determining ground of the will is not transferable into the clinical context without difficulty. Rationality has relevance where questions of autonomy arise, but the idea that duty has a role in the clinical context is not obvious. In fact, the idea that a doctor might reject a patient's decision as not being autonomous because it does not accord with duty seems extraordinary. In the medical setting, autonomous actions and choices are more likely to be viewed and assessed in terms of psychological notions such as deliberation, desires, and competency. However, Kant's concept of 'duty' and that relied on in contemporary discussions are not the same.

We have seen that for Kant, the ideas of duty, autonomy, reason, and morality are all linked. Duty is something we cannot escape if reason is in control and when we act for the sake of duty or from reason, our actions have moral worth. Our actions are autonomous and we are free from the influence of anything but our own reason—we are not caused. When we act from self-interest on the other hand, we are acting contrary to duty irrespective of how 'useful' these actions may be.[1] When we are acting from inclination and desire, we are at the mercy of outside forces and we are heteronomous. This suggests that a majority of choices in the clinical setting would fail to qualify as autonomous on the grounds that they are contrary to duty. Before we decide that Kant's view is unsuitable for the clinical context we should consider the way in which his notion of duty is linked to the notion of rationality.

For Kant, when we are faced with various options there is one option that, for rational beings, has a particular irresistibility or compulsion. We feel an obligation because there is something in the moral law and something in us that responds to it—reason compels our respect. In Kant's metaphysics, therefore, 'duty' has a specific metaphysical meaning. Acting from duty means acting from reason alone and Kant has a specific idea of what rationality means. Like his notion of duty, Kant's notion of rationality is also different to the conventional view.

In the clinical setting rationality is mostly used in a descriptive and an evaluative way. It is a description of what it means to be functioning successfully in everyday life and it refers to characteristics of a psychological nature which tend to be viewed positively.[2] When we say someone is rational we generally mean something like—this person deliberates, weighs options, and chooses a particular course of action. Simultaneously, we are often making a judgment that the person has chosen well. For Kant, rationality is not used in either of these ways because rationality is not viewed in terms of calculating particular ends. This also typifies Kant's account of autonomy which does not consist in acting for the sake of ends. Kant's metaphysical concept of autonomy and his sense of rationality are not empirically discernible. Reason or rationality is about producing a will that is good.[3] Consistency and rationality come about when we act as the categorical imperative commands and it is the 'form' of an action that matters for Kant.

Kant's view implies that a patient who acts contrary to duty has a will that is not good and that person is not autonomous. However, in the clinical setting there seems to be something inappropriate and distasteful about a concern with whether the patient is acting from duty and with the goodness of the patient's will. In order to assess Kant's notion of autonomy in the clinical context I will consider the kind of things which would not count as autonomy because they are contrary to duty and all that that entails on the Kantian account. On Kant's view, the decision made by the woman in the following example is contrary to duty and does not qualify as deserving respect:

> Ms. B is a thirty-four-year-old unmarried television news commentator who has never had any children. She takes pride in her appearance, which she also considers to be important for her job success and in her relationships with men. She is established in her career and she enjoys sexual relationships with a variety of male friends. When taking a shower, she notices an approximately two centimeter lump in her right breast. It appears to be freely floating and not fixed to the muscle behind the breast. On consulting her physician, she is referred to a surgeon who examines her and finds no clinical evidence of metastases to the lymph nodes but concludes from a mammography of the lump that it is very likely a malignant tumor. The surgeon recommends that a surgical biopsy be performed and that the patient receive a modified radical mastectomy if the frozen section indicates malignancy.
>
> The biopsy is performed and malignancy is indicated but Ms. B rejects the surgeon's recommendation. She has read that a simple excision of the area of the breast where cancer is found, followed by radiotherapy, often produces results as good as those available through a modified radical mastectomy. What she has read about the psychological impact of mastectomies on the patient, which includes depression and distaste for intercourse, concerns her very much. Furthermore, she thinks that a mastectomy will prevent her from continuing to live a sexually satisfying life because she won't be able to attract men with whom she can have those sorts of relationships.[4]

Ms. B is acting contrary to duty in Kant's sense because in choosing the less radical treatment she is acting on a maxim that, according to Kant, cannot become a universal law. For Kant, sex outside of marriage breaks the moral laws. The maxim of Ms. B's decision would take the form of something like: 'From fear I make it my principle that I will do anything I can to maintain my ability to attract sexual partners,' or 'If I want to attract men with whom to have sexual relationships, I should not have a mastectomy.' On Kant's view, this kind of response is a conditioned one which is made from desire or fear, not from duty. Kant would say: 'This maxim cannot possibly hold as a universal law of nature and is therefore entirely opposed to the supreme principle of all duty.'[5] When Ms. B acts on this kind of maxim she is, according to Kant, making herself into 'object of enjoyment' and hence into a 'thing.' And then 'anyone may treat [her] as they please, because [she] has thrown [her] person away.'[6]

For Kant we have duties toward our bodies in respect to sexual impulse. He claims that sexual love by itself is 'nothing more than appetite' and it is a 'degradation of human nature.' Sexual desire by a man for a woman is not directed toward the fact that the woman is human; that is of no concern. The object of his desire is her sex and that means that humanity is degraded: 'sexual love makes of the loved person an Object of appetite; as soon as that appetite has been stilled, the person is cast aside as one casts away a lemon which has been sucked dry.'[7] According to Kant, sexual intercourse within marriage is the only form of sexual indulgence that 'is possible without degrading humanity and breaking the moral laws.' It is only in marriage that 'one devotes not only sex but the whole person.'[8]

Translating Kant's ideas to Ms. B and to the clinical context, Ms. B is not autonomous and her wishes can be overridden. Surely though, this is not the way we want health care professionals to assess patients' decisions. In Ms. B's situation the treatment choice is more likely to be something we think she should decide in terms of the interventions available, the likelihood of a cure and the possibility of prolonging life. We probably think that she also needs to look at what is known of the possible side effects and the known consequences of treatment and to rate all of these things in terms of the way she wants to live her life.

Kant's emphasis on duty and the good will suggests that doctors should not respect the choices of patients who make these kinds of choices; choices which are contrary to duty and which are not the manifestation of a good will. But, do we really want doctors to morally assess patients' choices in this way? It seems inappropriate for health professionals to concern themselves with *morally* assessing the reasons which form the basis of the patient's choices. The moral assessment contemplated by the nurse in the following case certainly seems inappropriate:

> A twenty-five-year-old theology student who is completing her doctoral dissertation on the influence of John of Leiden upon sixteenth-century Protestantism, finds that she is pregnant by a close friend, also a graduate student, who is completing his dissertation on seventh-century Sanskrit love poetry. Ms. D consults her physician, seeking an abortion. She explains that a pregnancy at this time would interrupt her graduate work and complicate that of her boyfriend, whom she expects eventually to marry. The nurse who is present while Ms. D is being examined by the physician believes she should interrupt Ms. D's conversation with the physician and ask Ms. D whether in all of her theological studies she has reflected on the notion of responsible sexual activity.[9]

Someone who objects to abortion might think that nurse's response is not inappropriate. However, abortion is not the issue here. Ostensibly the nurse's moral assessment is to do with an inconsistency between the patient's beliefs and actions. On Kant's view, it follows that the nurse should respond in the same way if Ms. D was seeking treatment for a sexually transmitted disease rather than an abortion. But surely we would think it outrageous if health care professionals assessed patient's reasons for action by checking whether patients are acting only on the maxim through which they can at the same time will that it should become a universal law.

The question of who should make these kinds of assessments and whose conception of goodness will be used is also pertinent. If Kant's notion of autonomy is used in the clinical context there are cases where we might not agree with the views of others or with Kant's view of what constitutes duty or what constitutes a good will. Consider the patient with a life-threatening illness who bases treatment decisions on a desire to recover sufficiently to maintain the impression, within her workplace, of someone who enjoys good health. In other words, she wants to carry out a deception in terms of her professional life. On Kant's view, this is a lie. Since Kant condemns all lying, he would think that it is 'reprehensible' and a 'violation of man's duty to himself merely as a moral being (to humanity in his own person).'[10] But perhaps the person with the life-threatening illness suspects that knowledge of her condition will endanger her chance for continued employment. Her illness will cause her to be seen as unreliable and poor value in terms of further training and promotion. Although there are laws to protect people against discrimination of this kind, given that she is ill, the patient may not have the time or the energy to push for the enforcement of these laws.

Again, it is outrageous to think that the physician of a patient with a life-threatening illness should concern him or herself with the details mentioned in order to assess whether the patient's wishes can be respected. On Kant's view, the doctor would have to conclude that the patient acts contrary to duty; her will is not good, she is not autonomous, and her wishes do not deserve respect. There seems to be something wrong here. We generally think that it is more appropriate for doctors to view their patients in terms of medical need, rather than in terms of moral goodness?

Suicide as a Violation of Duty

Although there may be a certain noble or heroic appeal to Kant's ideas about autonomy, those ideas seem excessive and unnecessary for the clinical setting, especially when illness intrudes. In contemporary bioethics discussions, appeal to the principle of autonomy is often used to justify euthanasia or physician-assisted suicide, but Kant's metaphysical concept of autonomy cannot be used to justify ending lives in this way. We see this by way of one of Kant's own examples which is directly relevant to the clinical context. Kant describes a man who contemplates suicide because he feels sick of life as the result of a series of misfortunes. The man has suffered 'disappointments and hopeless misery' which have quite taken away his taste for life. He is wretched and longs for death.[11] The following case about a man whose life is full of misery fits Kant's description:

> Mr. A is a fifty-two-year-old diabetic who has been blind for five years and impotent for seven years because of his disease. He now appears to be developing renal failure, and he has difficulty in walking because of poor circulation to his legs. He has been living alone since his divorce three years ago. He concludes that it is not worth continuing life as it is and decides one day not to take his insulin. He is fairly sure that he will be dead before anyone discovers him. He has few friends or others who are likely to visit his apartment.[12]

The preservation of our lives is surely something that everyone wants but, for Kant, to preserve one's life is a duty and it is only when we protect our lives *'from the motive of duty'* rather than from inclination or fear (in conformity with duty) that the maxim of our action has moral content.[13] In Kant's example, the man at the point of despair still possesses enough reason to ask whether taking his life would be contrary to duty. He applies the test of the categorical imperative to his maxim and asks: 'Can the maxim of my action really become a universal law of nature?' His maxim or principle of self-love cannot become a universal law because it contradicts itself.[14] According to Kant, the 'use of the power of a free will for its own destruction is self-contradictory . . . to use life for its own destruction, to use life for producing lifelessness, is self-contradictory.'[15]

The maxim used by Mr. A when he contemplates suicide is the maxim Kant attributes to his own example of someone contemplating suicide: 'From self-love I make it my principle to shorten my life if its continuance threatens more evil than it promises pleasure.'[16] It is also the maxim used by a person with a terminal illness who rejects the opportunity to prolong his life:

> Mr. Jones is a sixty-seven-year-old retired farmer who lives alone and has no close relatives. Two years ago he had a skin lesion, which proved to be a malignant melanoma, and was treated with surgery and chemotherapy. However,

his cancer has recently recurred and is now more widespread than before. At the time of his current admission he is judged to be terminally ill. His physicians are recommending further debulking surgery and another course of chemotherapy, feeling these procedures may afford him appreciable relief from pain and possibly extend his life by a few months. Mr. Jones has declined these treatments, however, and says that he simply wants to go home and await his death.

Mr. Jones has no cognitive impairment and he has been seen by a psychiatric consultant who judges he is not clinically depressed.[17]

On Kant's view, the maxims of Mr. A and Mr. Jones cannot become universal law. Neither Mr. A nor Mr. Jones is autonomous and their wishes do not deserve respect. Kant concedes that there is something attractive in the thought that we can take our own life 'if we are so minded,' but he argues that misery does not give us the right to take our own lives: 'suicide is in no circumstances permissible.' For Kant suicide is not compatible with the idea of humanity as an end in itself and he is harshly critical of anyone contemplating suicide:

> We are, therefore, horrified at the very thought of suicide; by it man sinks lower than the beasts; we look upon suicide as carrion, whilst our sympathy goes forth to the victim of fate. . . . Humanity in one's own person is something inviolable. . . . If he disposes over himself, he treats his value as that of a beast. He who so behaves, who has no respect for human nature and makes a thing of himself, becomes for everyone an Object of freewill. We are free to treat him as a beast, as a thing, and to use him for our sport as we do a horse or a dog, for he is no longer a human being; he has made a thing of himself, and, having himself discarded his humanity, he cannot expect that others should respect humanity in him.[18]

The autonomous person, according to Kant, in this kind of situation where life is wretched and full of misery, is the man who 'still preserves his life without loving it—not from inclination or fear but from duty; then indeed his maxim has a moral content.'[19] Those who fail to act in this way cannot be regarded as autonomous. Clearly this is not the way we think patients should be assessed and treated in the clinical context, and this is not the sense of autonomy appealed to as a justification for euthanasia.

In the medical setting, in situations where the question of a patient's autonomy arises, particular ends are central. Discussion focuses on rationality or competence in terms of the specific ends of particular patients or broad goals such as well-being. And it is generally only when a patient refuses or chooses contrary to recommended treatment that the patient's rationality or competence is questioned and autonomy becomes an issue.

In contemporary discussions, Kantian autonomy is often viewed as a competing value with paternalism, but as we have seen, Kant's metaphysical view actually requires people to act in ways we would ordinarily call paternalistic. What has gone wrong here? Isaiah Berlin offers an explanation in Kantian terms through the tradition of Rousseau and Kant that leads to the idea of 'two selves.' Kant's metaphysical view involves the idea of rational beings having two viewpoints in so far as they belong to both the physical world and the intellectual world and that leads to the idea of a higher or moral self within each of us. We have both a physical desiring self and a rational self. This is described by Berlin as a self which dominates and something which is 'brought to heel.' The dominant self is identified with reason, my 'higher nature,' my 'real' or 'ideal' or 'autonomous' self and is contrasted with the 'irrational impulses' and 'uncontrolled desires' of my 'lower' or 'empirical' or 'heteronomous' self.[20] According to Berlin, the idea of two selves makes it easy for me to coerce others seemingly for their own sake, not mine:

> I may declare that they are actually aiming at what in their benighted state they consciously resist, because there exists within them an occult entity—their latent rational will, or their "true" purpose—and that this entity, although it is belied by all that they overtly feel and do and say, is their "real" self, of which the poor empirical self in space and time may know nothing or little. . . . Once I take this view, I am in a position to ignore the actual wishes of men or societies, to bully, oppress, torture them in the name, and on behalf, of their "real" selves.[21]

Berlin's objection is a political one but it has relevance for the clinical context. Berlin seems to be suggesting that this is a distortion or an abuse of the idea of two selves whereas we have seen that Kant's ideas actually require physicians to act paternalistically. Although Berlin's objection seems to be about disguising bad motives as good ones it shows that when decisions seem not to be based on reason, the idea of the two selves can be invoked to justify interventions by health professionals. An example of this exists when health professionals have a conception of rational action that is at odds with that of the patient. Young unmarried women who have been persuaded to relinquish their babies for adoption may have faced this kind of pressure. Having the baby adopted may be presented as the choice of the rational self; the choice which the young woman, as a rational being, will see is a good decision in the long run. The young woman may be counseled into believing that the decision to give the baby up is the best solution for the baby and for herself. It may also be presented as a decision which will free her from the encumbrances of the emotional self:

> I felt it was wrong to be pregnant and even worse to be sad about it. . . . I was muddled, exhausted, convinced that I was no good, because I hadn't wanted to give up my baby. The baby's father had dumped me, so my self-esteem was not great. But the counseling I received about relinquishing finished me off. . . . If someone had told me to kill myself, I"d have said, "OK. That sounds right." But I wouldn't have taken the initiative to do it myself. I wouldn't have thought *any* idea I had was any good.[22]

Young pregnant women are no longer pressured or encouraged to give their babies up for adoption, but the kind of situation that existed when that was the case illustrates Berlin's point. When a doctor and a patient have different values, the idea of two selves can be used to 'bully' and 'oppress' patients 'in the name, and on behalf, of their "real" selves,' or simply to override their wishes.

It seems that using the Kantian metaphysical concept of autonomy in the clinical context allows physicians to act in ways that seem quite antithetical to the idea of respect for autonomy. Overwhelmingly, the conclusion about the fitness of Kant's metaphysical conception of autonomy for the clinical setting is that it fails. Ironically, ideas such as rationality, consistency, and respect which are central to Kant's view, are also ideas that help show why we should respect or value autonomy. But, as we shall see, these ideas can only do that when used in ways that are contrary to Kant's metaphysics. It follows that, isolated from Kant's metaphysical view and Kant's specific metaphysical meanings, these ideas must be justified on different grounds. There is then no basis at all for reference to Kant.

IS THE PSYCHOLOGICAL CONCEPT OF AUTONOMY APPLICABLE TO THE CLINICAL CONTEXT?

There are many things about a psychological account of autonomy that make it suitable for the clinical context. Autonomy construed in this way is a feature of moral agents and this has relevance in the clinical context. Rational deliberation is called for when patients are required to make decisions relating to treatments and other aspects of their care and some of these decisions may have major life-altering significance. Rational deliberation and competency to decide are psychological notions and are closely connected to autonomous decision making.

We have seen that existing well-developed theories of autonomy rely on psychological descriptions of agents and their character.[23] On a psychological conception of autonomy people may be autonomous in varying degrees but it is something that is, to some extent, empirically discernible. Autonomy is a capacity that people possess and it is observable in what they say and do. As a theory of autonomy the psychological conception is easily understood. It produces a detailed picture of the autonomous person or the autonomous decision that in turn serves as a measure to assess the autonomy of particular patients in particular circumstances. It is a separate question as to whether we should respect autonomy but if we do value it highly the psychological account helps us to judge when we can or cannot intervene in the choices patients make.

A psychological account of autonomy has distinct features and it has practical applications in the clinical context. I will discuss some of those applications but we should keep in mind, as we saw earlier, that when we talk about the psychological concept of autonomy we are talking about a group of approaches. There are a number of psychological accounts of autonomy so the question of whether a person is or is not autonomous depends on the particular psychological conception being used. There are, however, some characteristics of persons or requirements that these accounts have in common. As we have seen, some notion of rationality, self-control, and consistency are common to most psychological accounts.

The psychological notion of autonomy is a positive concept. It is more than negative liberty or freedom. According to Robert Young, autonomous persons, as well as being free, make choices and act in ways that are expressive of their own preferences and aspirations. Autonomy is something that 'has to be worked for.'[24] Gerald Dworkin also argues that autonomy is more than negative freedom or liberty. He claims it is a 'richer notion' in the sense that it is about activity: 'It is tied up with the idea of being a subject, of being more than a passive spectator of one's desires and feelings.'[25] The point I am making is that the psychological notion of autonomy (in the sense of it being a positive concept) is useful for the clinical context. A psychological concept of autonomy is not restricted to a narrow account of human freedom. It concerns more than voluntariness and it takes account of individual preferences and the fact that persons are complex beings. A psychological concept gives us criteria for judging what counts as autonomous action. Autonomy judgments are not arbitrary—that is they do not depend on different speakers. They are made in accordance with the preferences and values of particular patients and this is helpful and relevant in the context of patient care.

A psychological account of autonomy is descriptive, not evaluative, but the characteristics of psychological autonomy are such that it seems to be something that many people regard as an ideal. Autonomy is an active thing in the sense that it requires deliberation and intentional action. This is something that can be discerned and measured, and to the extent that in the clinical context it has instrumental and intrinsic value, it can be promoted. To some extent a psychological notion of autonomy gives guidance to what the patient regards as well-being or at least as a desirable outcome of treatment. Therefore, if autonomy is valued and promoted it coincides with the aims of patient care.

When autonomy is seen as a psychological concept, autonomy can be compromised by psychological factors. We can fail to be autonomous because of irrational fears, because we lack knowledge or self-control or because we want something that undermines our deeper purposes and concerns.[26] Just as there are psychological limitations such as irrationality that interfere with our autonomy there are positive requirements that we need in order to be autonomous. According to Young, rationality, strength of will and self-awareness or self-knowledge are often put forward as positive requirements of the autonomous person.[27] Young claims that in order to be autonomous, as well as the absence of constraints, we need the positive element of self-determination. On Young's view this involves the 'capacity to do those things that figure prominently in one's life plan' and an awareness of and acceptance of the desires and principles on which we act. He also claims that there is a 'strong connection between autonomy and self-realisation (or self-fulfillment).'[28] All of this is relevant in the clinical context when patient's decisions come under scrutiny. There is something substantive to assess.

In the clinical context there are times when questions of autonomy become particularly important. Situations where patients refuse treatment or go against their physician's recommendation are especially contentious. As well as giving us a guide as to what an autonomous person looks like, psychological accounts of autonomy have something to say about the manner in which a person will go about making an autonomous decision. Before considering any decisions where there is disagreement about whether or not to respect a patient's wishes, it is instructive to look at decisions which are comparatively straight forward. According to most psychological accounts, autonomous people deliberate in a rational way which is in accordance with a set of stable values. What follows is one description of how, according to descriptive psychological accounts of autonomy, an autonomous person or someone who chooses autonomously, acts. In this case the patient is a woman who has been hospitalized for a biopsy to determine the nature of a lump in her breast:

> She knows that vigorous controversy exists within the medical profession about the various ways of dealing with malignancy—ranging from radiation and chemotherapy without surgery to radical mastectomy—and she knows that some physicians, but not all, favor performing a mastectomy immediately upon a diagnosis of malignancy, while the patient is still under the anesthesia that was employed in order to do the biopsy. She hopes for a negative finding, fears a positive finding, and resolves that if malignancy is found, she will look carefully into the therapeutic options, in consultation with several physicians, before deciding which treatment to elect. Since she knows that treatment standards in such cases vary to some extent from city to city, she sees the matter as involving a certain amount of fashion, and she determines that in a matter of such importance to her, the decision will be made on the most rational grounds she can establish, rather than on the basis of the city she happens to be in.[29]

An extra feature is that a psychiatrist has described the patient as having a sound and balanced sense of herself and her circumstances. Although the patient may, in the end, go against the treatment her doctor recommends for her, she is acting in a way that is consistent for an autonomous person within the framework of a psychological notion of autonomy. Despite the fact that her doctor argues that this matter is so complex that even the medical community cannot agree on the best treatment and that her understanding is deficient if she thinks she can make a better decision, the patient can still be autonomous according to a psychological notion of autonomy. The objection that fully informed consent cannot be achieved or that knowledge or understanding is 'imperfect' does not mean that it is 'inadequate' for the patient's purpose.[30] Patients' desires and preferences which are inevitably a part of the psychological notion of autonomy have an important role in the sense that they help to justify patient care decisions. In an instrumental conception of rationality it is rational for patients to pursue their desired ends and the utility of the outcome is related to their preferences and desires.

The psychological account also provides us with a picture of what an autonomous person is *not* like. It is probably easier to define a nonautonomous person than it is an autonomous one. When autonomy is a kind of 'psychological maturity' those who lack this can be deemed not autonomous and it is easier to identify the lack of this characteristic than to identify the exact type or amount of psychological maturity that constitutes autonomy. Young children, those who conform unthinkingly or rebel impulsively, do not have psychological maturity and it is relatively easy to make the pronouncement that they are not autonomous. Common paradigms of nonautonomous persons are drug addicts and compulsive gamblers.[31] To this list Beauchamp and Childress add 'irrationally suicidal individuals.'[32]

Frankfurt's idea of the 'wanton' also fits into the category of the nonautonomous. He claims that even though a wanton may have and use rational faculties of a high order, 'the essential characteristic of a wanton is that he does not care about his will.' A person is moved to act according to a desire which is either the will that person wants or a will that person wants to be without. For a wanton the desires and motives that move him to action are a matter of indifference.[33] It is by default that the wanton lacks autonomy. A more radical idea about a lack of autonomy is described by Diana Meyers. She claims that someone who is concerned only with other people's expectations, who adopts a life plan in deference to others, and does not attend to signs of internal discord, exhibits a lack of autonomy.[34] Although she claims that this does not entail that the person is nonautonomous in all circumstances, choices made in this way that do not reflect the true or authentic self are deemed not autonomous.[35] Meyer's view is an example of how the psychological theory of autonomy can be filled out to give a picture of what an autonomous person is like and what nonautonomous persons or choices are like. This exacting standard of autonomy is helpful in the sense that it is discernible and assessable but it may also have unwelcome implications in the clinical context. In a later section I will examine these difficulties and the ways Meyers may be able to get around them. At this point I am trying to bring to light those concepts of autonomy which seem most promising and which are worth further discussion and exploration. More specifically, in this section I am considering the ways in which the psychological concept *is* applicable and *can* be useful in the clinical context.

We cannot always take patients' decisions at face value and assume that they are autonomous. Especially when decisions lead to grave or irreversible consequences we should look beyond patients' first-order desires. According to Dworkin, autonomy is an activity which involves our ability to have preferences about preferences insofar as we can reflect upon and adopt attitudes toward our first-order desires. This activity is an important feature of human action and an ability which seems to be distinctively human. He claims that we ignore a crucial feature of persons if we think that autonomy consists only in the promotion of first-order desires. We are complex beings to the extent that: 'one may not just desire to smoke, but also desire that one not have that desire.'[36] We have the ability to scrutinize our first-order motivations and to change them.[37] This has relevance in the clinical context.

The patient who refuses treatment may do so because his or her expected quality of life does not warrant prolonging it and the treatment itself may be burdensome. We could, and often do conclude that the decision of a patient in this situation is expressive of his own preferences and call it autonomous. However, a patient who refuses an effective life-saving treatment may do so because of an irrational fear about the recommended treatment. A descriptive psychological account of autonomy is applicable in this kind of situation when we are trying to decide whether to respect the patient's views. It helps us to distinguish autonomous decisions from those that are not autonomous and it provides justification for exerting pressure or even overruling decisions. Intervention of this kind does not have to be seen as a violation of autonomy. It can be justified in terms of autonomy itself.

In the example that follows, Gert, Culver, and Clouser claim that 'almost everyone' would agree that the patient's refusal of treatment should be overruled even though the patient is competent in the sense that she understands and appreciates the information given:

> A depressed woman, phobic about receiving electroconvulsive therapy (ECT), cannot bring herself to consent to the procedure, despite her agreement with her doctors' opinion that she may die without ECT, her avowal that she does not want to die, and her acknowledgment that ECT would likely prevent her death. She understands and appreciates everything her doctors tell her, but she has a fear, which she herself calls "foolish," that prevents her from consenting.[38]

If we understand autonomy as a psychological concept and if we value autonomy, we can justify intervening in the patient's first order desire.[39]

A psychological concept of autonomy has a special role in the clinical context in the sense that it is a central value in the doctor patient relationship. Autonomy, psychologically construed, as well as the care and fate of our bodies, is basic to medical care. The significance of this conception of autonomy in the clinical context is explained by Charles Fried:

> The doctor's prime and basic function is not so much the prevention of death (which is not in his power) but the preservation of life capacities for the realization of a reasonable, realistic life plan. As in particular cases conflicts arise and decisions must be made between various capacities and between the risk

of death and the impairment of various capacities, the doctor must see himself as the servant, not of life in the abstract, but of life plans of his patients.[40]

Dworkin also argues that our goals and values are tied up with our bodies and with our identity as persons. Decisions about treatments, the probabilities of cure or extension of life, considerations about side effects, judgments about how our body will look to others after surgery, and whether to die at home or in a hospital are 'not technical, medical judgements.' He claims that failure to respect our wishes in these matters is a 'particularly insulting denial of autonomy' [41] In other words, the idea of autonomy is at the heart of a patient-centered view of medicine.

A psychological account of autonomy is consistent with a subjective patient-centered view of medicine as opposed to medical paternalism. It fits with the idea that the moral significance of informed consent involves more than disclosure and the idea that health professionals should be guided in their disclosures by the unique or specific informational needs of the particular patient.

IN SUMMARY

A descriptive psychological account of autonomy seems especially well suited to the clinical context. The characteristics of psychological accounts of autonomy are consistent with contemporary ideas about the doctor/patient relationship and a patient centred view of medicine. The significance of the psychological notion of autonomy for the medical setting is that, to the extent that it is empirically discernible, it provides a basis on which health care professionals can judge whether patients' decisions are autonomous. This guides us in knowing which decisions should be respected and which can be overridden—or something in between. The fact that psychological accounts of autonomy are useful and practicable in the clinical context does not, of course, mean that they are free of problems. I will discuss the problems in a later section.

IS A PROCEDURAL APPROACH TO AUTONOMY APPLICABLE IN THE CLINICAL CONTEXT?

Before focusing on the principle of autonomy as a procedural notion, it is worth looking at the way in which the principles referred to in contemporary bioethics discussions,[42] were developed as a model for ethics. This will help us understand autonomy as a procedural concept, the reason why some people think it has come to dominate bioethics, and it will help us understand the role and usefulness of the procedural concept of autonomy in the clinical context.

The development of some of the contemporary principles of biomedical ethics can be viewed as a procedural thing. According to Jonathan Moreno, the commission that produced *The Belmont Report* was 'consensus oriented'[43] and it was charged with conducting 'a comprehensive investigation and study to identify the basic ethical principles which should underlie the conduct of biomedical and behavioural research involving human subjects' and with developing 'guidelines which should be followed in such research to assure that it is conducted in accordance with such principles. . . .'[44] Prior to this there had been an assortment of codes and rules governing research. There was the Nuremberg Code of 1947, the Helsinki Declaration of 1964 (revised in 1975), and the 1971 United States Department of Health, Education and Welfare guidelines (codified into Federal Regulations in 1974).[45] Because this assortment of rules was difficult to interpret the commission was charged with formulating 'broader ethical principles [to] provide a basis on which specific rules may be formulated, criticized and interpreted.'[46] This was then meant to frame 'in a more general and useful way the moral concerns that underlay the diverse, ambiguous, and (sometimes) conflicting rules' of the many ethical codes covering research using human subjects. According to Gert, Culver, and Clouser it is 'very likely' that, for the commission, the principles that were identified accomplished another crucial purpose as well as generalizing and encapsulating moral considerations applicable to research using human subjects: 'They made possible a consensus in a setting where a more detailed account of morality would probably never have been agreed upon.'[47] In other words, concern with public policy and consensus helps brings into play a procedural concept of autonomy.

As we saw earlier, the lack of protection for subjects of research was part of what led to the setting up of the National Commission for the Protection of Human Subjects. It was a situation that called for rules and regulations with principles to justify the rules rather than a contentful ethics or reliance on moral education to tell us what kind of persons we ought to be. An immediate response was required.[48] Revelations of abuses in research, scientific advances, and new medical research were pressing issues and the National Commission was directed by Congress to develop principles that would function at a procedural level.

This model of ethics, in which principles provide action guidance, was attractive to many people hoping to develop an ethics for medical practice. One of the members of the National Commission suggests that some of the appeal of the principles came from their propensity for resolving problems. Albert Jonsen claims that Congress, which set up the commission, and the public, had a desire to see 'the chaotic world of biomedical research reduced to order by clear and unambiguous principles.'[49]

Bioethics and Problem Solving

A procedural approach to autonomy is common in bioethics but whether this is a useful notion of autonomy for the clinical context is another matter. To the extent that medicine and bioethics are concerned with problem solving, there is an emphasis on process and procedures and the procedural approach to autonomy has a role in this.

As we saw earlier, Gilbert Meilaender claims that the increasing focus of bioethics on public policy has led to a move from a substantive to a procedural approach to ethics. The result, according to Meilaender is a bioethics without content; a bioethics which has become a defense of autonomy. To be a person, he claims, is about being an 'autonomous chooser,' so with nothing substantive to agree on we can only agree to respect everyone's autonomy.[50]

Like Meilaender, Pellegrino and Thomasma hold the view that there has been a move in contemporary bioethics to a procedural approach. They also argue that bioethics has become a problem-solving exercise. For most of its history, they claim, medical ethics has been concerned with 'a series of deeply held beliefs about the right and the good and the norms of medical behaviour.'[51] Procedures did not eclipse content: 'Moral principles and moral reasoning were not neglected, but they were always grounded in some notion of the good as an end for human life.'[52] According to Pellegrino and Thomasma, contemporary medical ethics has become focussed on the process of decision making and normative claims are shunned. The result of this, they claim, is that ethics assumes a 'neutralist stance' and loses its 'practical value as a guide for living.'[53]

Pellegrino and Thomasma claim that it was the reshaping of medical ethics by philosophy and contemporary philosophers that led to the focus on problem solving with the subsequent loss of content. When our attention is on the decisions we make and on the process, the emphasis is no longer on the kind of person we are. With the input from philosophy and philosophers, questions of medical morality became the subject of analysis, justification, and argumentation and this transformed medical ethics into a problem-solving exercise or what Pellegrino and Thomasma call 'quandary ethics.' Quandaries, they claim, create a demand for practical resolutions and philosophy provides a useful analytical framework for that. Pellegrino and Thomasma acknowledge a certain inevitability about a procedural approach to ethics in a pluralistic society: 'there is more likelihood of agreement with secularists on procedure than on substantive normative ethics'[54] but they argue that the ethics of character and virtue is 'the central issue in medical as well as in any other form of ethics.' They maintain that unless we have a theory of the good life and the good society, there is 'no check on political expediency.'[55]

In other words, Pellegrino and Thomasma want a bioethics and a notion of autonomy with content. A descriptive psychological account of autonomy would not satisfy them, however. They have a particular substantive view (a theological or religious view) in mind: 'To be silent about one's beliefs . . . [t]o suppress the religious perspective, means tacitly to accept secular and civic religion as the final determinants of morality,'[56] and although they believe that 'procedure and substance are not neatly separable' they claim it is 'useful and important to disengage them' for practical or 'heuristic purposes.' Although they claim 'it is distressing even to think that a physician would exploit a patient's illness to proselytize'[57] they see the procedural approach in terms of an opportunity to proselytize:

> Christian physicians must comprehend more clearly how important procedural ethics has become as a meeting ground in which believers and nonbelievers have a reasonable possibility of agreeing . . . it offers concrete opportunity for frequent and practical dialogue with colleagues, families, and patients who may hold other beliefs or none at all. Engaging in this dialogue as a Christian is part of the vocation of transforming the contemporary culture, of which John Paul II has spoken so often as incumbent on each of us in accord with the station in life we occupy.[58]

Pellegrino and Thomasma are not advocates for, or defenders of, a procedural approach to autonomy but they seem prepared to exploit the prevalence of the procedural approach in bioethics. The role Pellegrino and Thomasma envisage for a procedural concept of autonomy is a way for Christian physicians to 'reconcile profession and faith in a secular, pluralistic society.'[59] This role offers nothing of use for the clinical context. It is not motivated by benefit to patients and it does not resolve conflicts or disputes. Pellegrino and Thomasma's view of ethics is one with content. They are concerned with what they claim might be 'in fuller development, a theology of medical ethics.'[60] The point I am making is that a procedural approach can be exploited for a purpose but it need not be a purpose that is useful for or even relevant to the clinical context.

Gert, Culver, and Clouser, also view bioethics as being concerned with problem solving. They argue that the four principles which make up the dominant view of biomedical ethics are often treated as a problem-solving tool: 'it has become fashionable and customary to cite one or another of these principles as the key for resolving a particular biomedical ethical problem.' According to Gert, Culver, and Clouser, the dominant view or 'theory' (although not a theory) in bioethics is Beauchamp and Childress's four principles or what has come to be labeled 'principlism.'[61] Gert, Culver, and Clouser note that it is not so much the approach of Beauchamp and Childress that their criticism is focused on, but the 'widespread popularization of principlism' or a 'paradigmatic form of principlism.' They say that by the fourth edition of *Principles of Biomedical Ethics,* Beauchamp and Childress have accommodated criticisms of past editions and have changed their theoretical account considerably. Gert, Culver, and Clouser's criticism is leveled at people who have gone to conferences and workshops and become 'imbued with principle talk.' They claim that the early editions of Beauchamp and Childress's text, nevertheless, have been influential in shaping the 'paradigmatic form of bioethics' which persists. According to Gert, Culver, and Clouser, the 'centrepiece' of principlism is the principle of autonomy which is cited more frequently than the other principles and has come to dominate bioethics discussions. The principle of autonomy has 'taken on a life of its own' they claim.[62]

Autonomy and Public Policy

A procedural approach to autonomy acts as a check on the authority of others to encroach on or interfere with individuals. In a secular pluralistic society a procedural notion of autonomy is practical and useful insofar as it resolves conflicts and generates tolerance.

When different people have different convictions, social collaboration in the form of public policy requires distinguishing between a public and a private sphere of morality. The public sphere coincides with a procedural approach to morality and a procedural concept of autonomy whereas private sphere morality involves questions about the 'good life' and ideals of character. The answers to these questions have content and because of that content, substantive conflict can occur. Public morality on the other hand emphasizes procedures for us to follow which enable us to reach consensus or agreement concerning moral conflicts.[63] A procedural notion of autonomy prevents the imposition of private convictions as public requirements. Quite apart from the difficulty in deciding whose views would apply, intrusions of this kind are surely something we would abhor. For instance, in the case of the pregnant theology student mentioned earlier, a procedural approach to autonomy means that the doctor, the nurse, or anyone else who takes exception to the idea of an abortion cannot stop her from having an abortion if that is what she competently chooses.[64] This is the case even if those who oppose abortion are in the majority. A procedural approach to autonomy also means that others cannot force her to have an abortion if she does not choose to have an abortion. It protects persons from unwanted medical interventions and it constrains others from encroaching on patients' freedom to choose for themselves.

What the procedural notion of autonomy does not do is provide us with answers of a substantive kind. It does not tell us whether it is right or wrong to seek an abortion in a given situation.[65] Although a procedural notion of autonomy generates moral authority to prevent others from interfering with a person's choice it does not provide moral authority to support or promote a particular choice. It does not have a standard by which the choice measures up to or fails to measure up to.

A procedural notion of autonomy commits us to not interfering with others without their consent and this has an important function in the clinical context. Regulatory standards in human subject research also employ a procedural notion of autonomy as a limit or a check on interventions. Gaining informed consent amounts to a procedural approach to autonomy. The notion of informed consent also functions as a moral framework on which people can agree.

Informed Consent

Informed consent is a process in which patients decide whether or not to undergo a particular medical procedure and it is a process by which physicians and investigators can ensure freedom from some forms of legal liability. Autonomy is usually cited as the underlying value or basis of informed consent but that is not necessarily the real basis of the legal doctrine. The focus of a procedural notion of autonomy is more to do with regulation of the consent seeker's behavior.

Jay Katz and George Annas both express dissatisfaction with the fact that the doctrine of informed consent is a procedure in which we do not have to understand autonomy as a value.[66] They argue that fear of legal liability rather than autonomy may be the guiding value and their arguments suggest that there is something amiss in the fact that autonomy is not recognised as a value in the procedure. Both argue that concessions to patient autonomy are often a procedure for physicians to escape legal liability rather than a response to medical considerations or the patient's interests. Katz claims that the impetus for the requirement of informed consent came from law rather than medicine and likewise, Annas claims that the most important ethical requirement in medicine came through the courts rather than being recognized as an ethical value.[67] These arguments suggest that, in the medical context, there is something important about giving consideration to a patient's interests. This in turn suggests that although a procedural approach to autonomy such as observance of the doctrine of informed consent is being followed, something important may be missed. There is something incongruous about the idea that fear of legal liability generates the 'morality of mutual respect' referred to by Engelhardt.[68] Jay Katz argues that the impact of law means that although the medical profession may bow to the doctrine of informed consent and its underlying value they do not necessarily accept it.[69] The question is does it matter if physicians don't accept the underlying value of informed consent?

A defender of a purely procedural approach may argue that as long as physicians follow the procedure of informed consent, the private views physicians hold about giving consideration to patients' interests and the underlying value of informed consent are of no account. As long as they follow the procedure we have the basis for avoiding social strife and conflict.

It is important to note that in talking about a procedural approach or notion of autonomy I am not referring to any one writer. There are a variety of procedural approaches and some are purer than others. My attack is on a purely procedural approach but it is not clear that any writers hold strictly to that. It is clear however, that at times a purely procedural approach is what some seek or aspire to.

In the clinical context do we want a notion of autonomy that does more than resolve conflicts? The procedural approach misses altogether ideas about individuality and character. These are the aspects which suggest that autonomy is part of what it means to be a person. As we saw earlier, Mill claims that individuality is the 'privilege and proper condition of a human being'[70] and '[e]ach is the proper guardian of his own health, whether bodily, *or* mental and spiritual.'[71] On Mill's view, ideas about autonomy and what it means to be a person are connected. Concern with personhood is also important and relevant in the clinical context, but a procedural approach to autonomy does not address this. The procedural concept does not allow psychological considerations, so it has nothing to say about the psychological characteristics of a person or the standard of deliberation that is required in order to give informed consent.

Does it matter if the notion of autonomy is an empty process, or do we need a substantive account of autonomy and a notion of informed consent with content? Patients' choices have content and sometimes it is very difficult to ignore the content. When the procedural approach is aspired to, the content of a person's choice does not matter. *Consent* is the focus. Consent is the 'right-making condition—i.e., to act rightly, one must act with the permission of those on whom one acts' and to act on persons without their consent makes an action wrong.[72] These right/wrong-making conditions do not have content but that does not mean that a person's choice has no content. In the clinical context this can cause confusion. The public policy/public sphere of morality cannot always be kept separate from the private sphere of morality. It is in terms of the content or concrete understandings of the good life that people know what things are worth living or dying for.[73] When individuals deliberate and make decisions which may have life-altering consequences, those decisions have content. What is more, proponents of the procedural approach to autonomy need a descriptive psychological account behind it or they are really only talking about mere *agreement* and they ought not to be talking about informed consent.

The following cases show that the content cannot be dismissed and that procedures or agreement are not all that matter. By 'content' in this context I do not mean the specific content of the patient's decision—say, whether or not to accept the form of treatment that offers the best chance of prolonging life—but the content of the account of autonomy in so far as it refers to psychological considerations such as competency, understanding and rationality which seem to have a role in determining whether consent is valid. In this first case, the patient satisfies the standard procedure for entering a clinical trial, and on the surface there seems no reason to question the validity of the consent:

Following a suicide attempt, a young man with a long history of tumultuous relationships and difficulty controlling his impulses is admitted to a psychiatric hospital. After a number of days, a psychiatrist approaches the patient, explaining that he is conducting a research project to determine if medications may help in the treatment of the patient's condition. Is the patient interested, the psychiatrist asks? The answer: 'Yes, I'm willing to do anything that might help me.'

The psychiatrist returns over the next several days to explain the project further. He tells the patient that two medications are being used along with a placebo: medications and placebo are assigned randomly. The trial is double blinded: that is, neither physician nor patient will know what the patient is receiving until after the trial has been completed. The patient listens to the explanation and reads and signs the consent form.[74]

On the basis of what the patient then says, his understanding is apparently flawed. When asked why he agreed to be in the study the patient's response is 'disquieting.' He believes the medication he will receive will be the one most likely to help him and he has ruled out the possibility that he might receive a placebo. We may think that he has just failed to understand the methodology. A female subject in another study demonstrates better this kind of flawed understanding. Despite her ability to understand the overall methodology and to spontaneously describe a randomized, double-blind study with a placebo group this woman also distorts an important part of the experiment:

> When asked directly . . . how *her* medication would be selected, she said she had no idea. She then added, "I hope it isn't by chance," and suggested that each subject would probably receive the medication she needed. Given the discrepancy between her earlier use of the word "random" and her current explanation, she was then asked what her understanding was of "random." Her definition was entirely appropriate: "by lottery, by chance, one patient who comes in gets one thing and the next patient gets the next thing." She then began to wonder out loud if this procedure was being used in the current study. Ultimately, she concluded that it was not.[75]

Questions about people's decisions are hard to avoid when there seems to be a lack of competency or understanding. The next example is a very extreme case which shows that a purely procedural approach is absurd. Prior to signing a consent form, a twenty-eight-year-old woman had been given an explanation of ECT and why it was being recommended. She signed the form without hesitation and then took part in a test of patient capacity for understanding. When asked to explain the purpose of the treatment and why it was recommended for her, she responded: 'Paul McCartney, nothing to zero.'[76]

This example shows that by simply putting her signature or her mark on the consent form, a patient may be capable of completing the formal procedure in some sense but not in a way that anyone would want to regard as satisfying a requirement for informed consent or autonomous decision making. The last example poses a difficulty for the procedural account because a purely procedural approach to autonomy does not demand rationality or understanding and it does not depend on any notion of ideal moral agents. It simply requires agreement or consent from subjects. Informed consent however, is more than agreement or consent; it involves psychological considerations.

To conclude, relying on a purely procedural concept of autonomy does have advantages for the clinical context. When consent or agreement becomes the focus we do not have the problem of deciding what constitutes autonomy. We do not have to decide whether autonomy requires rationality and we are spared the added problem of defining the kind or level of rationality that constitutes autonomous choice. Nevertheless, while consent is a vital part of the doctor patient relationship, irrational consent by patients or consent made without understanding is meaningless. Defenders of a procedural approach to autonomy have no way of excluding the woman who merely puts her mark on the consent form.

Engelhardt is probably the major proponent of the procedural approach to autonomy. He seems to vacillate between notions of consent or simple agreement and informed consent. Engelhardt raises the issue of whether we should respect all decisions or only those that appear sound and well reasoned. As part of his discussion of free and informed consent, he presents a case for the right to be left alone and concludes: 'the fact that individuals' choices are troublesome, bizarre, and tragic does not of itself mean that one may use force to stop them.'[77] He focuses on the idea of the right 'most valued by civilized men' (protection for an individual's beliefs, thoughts, emotions, and sensations) by referring to American law, legal decisions, and the American Constitution and he draws attention to the idea that nothing suggests that an individual possesses this right 'only as to *sensible* beliefs, *valid* thoughts, *reasonable* emotions, or *well-founded* sensations.' Engelhardt emphasizes the idea that 'foolish, unreasonable and even absurd ideas' should be respected and he argues that the content of a choice need not be 'rationally grounded or argued for.'[78] At the same time he also argues that an individual needs to affirm and endorse his or her choice in the sense of understanding and appreciating the circumstances of the choice. He argues for this in procedural terms of a 'right to be left alone': According to Engelhardt 'To justify successfully the right to be left alone in one's choices, one need only show that the choice is one of a moral agent: a rational, self-conscious individual, who freely chooses a particular action or omission.'[79] The difficulty with this is that it gives content to the notion of an autonomous person.

Although for Engelhardt the notion of autonomous choice may have no content[80] he relies on a contentful notion of moral agents in order for a consent to be valid. It is difficult to understand this contentful notion of moral agents as anything other than a contentful notion of an autonomous person and we are confronted with the question about rationality. The answers to these questions have content and substantive conflict can occur—for example, we could construct an argument for the view that the Jehovah's Witness who refuses treatment is rational, or we could just as plausibly argue that the Jehovah's Witness is not rational.

In his most recent writing Engelhardt stops using the term autonomy. This shift reflects an attempt to deal with the problems that beset a purely procedural approach to autonomy. We saw earlier that he drops the 'principle of autonomy' in favor of the 'the principle of permission' so that his argument will not be misunderstood as a 'libertarian manifesto celebrating the value of freedom.' He prefers the 'principle of permission' because it is meant to indicate that 'secular moral authority' is derived from the permission of individuals and his concern is with the process not a substantive view of autonomy: 'what is at stake is not some value possessed by autonomy or liberty.'[81] The change in terminology removes some ambiguity but does not resolve the difficulties of pursuing a procedural notion of autonomy.

Also in the second edition of *The Foundations of Bioethics*, Engelhardt refers constantly to 'profound' or 'fundamental' tensions at the roots of bioethics. According to Engelhardt, 'for those who recognize the concrete values that should guide the good life, secular morality is a wasteland without moral content, without the possibility of moral guidance, and with the possibility of such serious moral failures as suicide and euthanasia.'[82] Therefore, in the health care setting which has no single authoritative view of the good life and of the concrete goals of medicine, Engelhardt envisages a central role for free and informed consent in creating common understandings or resolving conflict. However, in trying to maintain a purely procedural approach to autonomy, even though we saw earlier that having a notion of consent without giving any content to the nature of the consent is simply *agreement,* Engelhardt needs some way to eradicate the content. He does this by trying to break the connection between the notion of informed consent and liberal ideas: 'Free and informed consent thus plays its central role not so much out of a commitment to a liberal ideal, but out of a despair regarding the possibility of discovering a concrete view of the goals of health care in a secular, pluralist context.'[83] Engelhardt may be able to distance the idea of informed consent from the liberal ideal but informed consent and notions of autonomy can have another kind of substantive content. Unacknowledged psychological content still remains.

James Childress also grapples with the problem of trying to avoid a substantive account of autonomy. He tries to explain how the notion of 'respect' and the 'principle of respect for autonomy' get around this problem. He claims that the principle of respect for autonomy does not presuppose an ideal of personal autonomy and also that the attitude of respect that is fitting for an autonomous choice does not depend on the content of the choice. He also claims that even though content is not what counts, there is no inconsistency involved in criticizing those choices.[84] These claims show the strains involved in trying to keep to a purely procedural notion of autonomy. Psychological assumptions cannot be avoided and rationality becomes an issue when we want to criticize a choice.

The procedural approach to autonomy is applicable to the clinical context in the sense that it is a constraint on action. It ensures a kind of negative liberty, but as we have seen, it is less substantive than Mill's arguments about liberty which include ideas about individuality. To be more than a constraint requires a concept that is more than a procedural one. Beauchamp and Childress do not want to embrace a descriptive psychological account of autonomy and they oppose the idea of autonomy as a character ideal. In the fourth edition they want an account of autonomy that is 'adequate to identify what is protected by rules of informed consent, informed refusal, truth telling, and confidentiality.' For their 'objectives,' they want an account to 'fill out and qualify the nature and importance of respect for autonomy.'[85] In the fifth edition of their text they renounce further a descriptive psychological account of autonomy. They say: 'We use the concept of autonomy in this chapter to examine individuals' decision making in health care and research, especially informed consent and refusal.' Gone is the reference to 'what is protected by the rules of informed consent, informed refusal, truth telling.' They simply say: 'This account is essential to our objectives in subsequent chapters, which fill out and qualify the principle of respect for autonomy.'[86] Nevertheless, a purely procedural approach is difficult to sustain and their notion of respect includes ideas that are psychological in nature.

A purely procedural approach to autonomy breaks down because of the need to say what informed consent or an autonomous decision really is. There seems to be two aspects to the procedural approach—the 'liberal neutrality' sense where no particular vision of the good life is endorsed, and the procedure to gain informed consent. Both are necessary to a procedural approach—a neutralist stance is necessary to avoid conflict about visions of the good life and the notion of informed consent is the framework on which people can agree and provide moral authority for medical interventions. However, a procedural approach needs a descriptive psychological view to back it up or it ceases to be a notion of informed consent, and becomes just 'Did this patient make this mark on the consent form?'

IS AN EVALUATIVE APPROACH TO AUTONOMY APPLICABLE IN THE CLINICAL CONTEXT?

Although it is a separate question whether we should respect autonomy after we decide what autonomy is, the fact that the characteristics of psychological autonomy such as rationality and consistency are traits that we view in a positive way, the word 'autonomy' is sometimes used with evaluative content. We may start with a psychological account and then start to use 'autonomy' in a way that builds in positive evaluation.

Even though we may try, like Beauchamp and Childress, to concern ourselves with the question of why we should respect autonomy rather than the question of what constitutes autonomy, it is not easy to divorce ourselves from the idea that autonomy is a kind of desirable psychological state. Gerald Dworkin argues that the idea of autonomy is used in an 'exceedingly broad fashion' and it is related to and equated with many different things but the idea that 'autonomy is a feature of persons and that it is a desirable quality to have' is something that seems to be 'held constant' from author to author.[87] This implicit assumption that autonomy is good means that although there may be a reluctance to give the term descriptive content, moral content persists. The evaluative notion of autonomy depends on the speaker's evaluations and it follows by definition that something ought to be respected once it is labeled autonomous.

In bioethics and in the clinical context autonomy is sometimes used in a way that gives the actions or choices of particular persons a stamp of approval. Simply naming a person, action or choice as 'autonomous' implies that it qualifies as deserving respect. It suggests also that these persons and choices should not be interfered with and interference if it does occur is a violation of autonomy. Those who value autonomy or self-determination and are committed to the idea of patient rights or rights to autonomy often use the term in an evaluative way. Conversely, those who use an evaluative notion of autonomy may indicate that a choice can be paternalistically overridden by denying the choice is autonomous.

We have seen that the development of contemporary bioethics has had an influence on the different notions of autonomy that have developed. This gives us insight into the reasons why bioethics is sometimes treated as a political movement rather than a neutral field of inquiry. Gert, Culver, and Clouser argue that the search for 'genuinely' autonomous actions and choices 'invites a kind of activism' which promotes the choices and actions which are regarded as 'autonomous.' An increasing awareness of a markedly paternalistic medical profession, an increase in alternative treatments, and situations where it is rational to refuse life-prolonging treatments are some of the reasons for the interest in patient autonomy or self-determination. Gert, Culver, and Clouser claim there is an 'overwhelming political appeal' in invoking the principle of autonomy and allowing patients to make their own treatment decisions and the idea of autonomy has become 'the banner' under which forces rally to 'gain for patients more control over their own health care.'[88]

Jonathan Moreno has analyzed the differences between bioethics as a strictly academic pursuit and bioethics as a movement for social reform. In my view and in terms of Moreno's distinction, the way in which we understand the concept of autonomy makes a difference to whether we see bioethics as an area of study or as a social reform movement, and that perhaps accepting an evaluative concept pushes bioethics toward being an advocacy movement.[89]

Moreno claims that autonomy or self-determination is a prominent and abiding theme in bioethics and, '[i]nsofar as self-determination is a theme that is, in fact, part of the way bioethics is understood, and insofar as bioethics strives to advance this theme in its critical and prescriptive activities, bioethics is a movement.' In this sense bioethics is an 'agent of social change, of social reform' and according to Moreno, social reform movements can develop into 'advocacy movements.' There is a point at which commitment is 'qualitatively transformed into commitment to an agenda' and the person with the commitment becomes an 'advocate.' Moreno argues that an example of this is the patients' rights movement that is characterized by a commitment to autonomy or self-determination.[90]

Moreno illustrates the distinction between a social reform movement and an advocacy movement by referring to the Hastings Center which is a bioethics research institute and the Hemlock Society which is an advocacy organization for the rights of the terminally ill. According to Moreno, the Hastings Center engages in critical analysis and while there is usually an underlying concern with self-determination, it is satisfied with raising questions. The Hemlock Society on the other hand has an agenda of self-determination. Its role is in supporting specific legislation to implement self-determination and its role does not involve criticism of the agenda.[91] Moreno argues that 'in presenting a reasoned defence of their views, [bioethicists] are implicitly prepared to entertain other views, and this is mandatory in their role as bioethicists.'[92] The advocate, he claims, simply promotes the idea of autonomy without questioning or analyzing it. I want to suggest that one thing that may make bioethics seem to be an advocacy movement rather than critical analysis, is the way in which we understand autonomy. First of all, the distinction between social reform and advocacy movements is not as clear cut as Moreno suggests. To the extent that ethics committees exist and function to protect the interests of patients[93] they could be viewed as advocates with an agenda of patient autonomy—but they are not confined to using an evaluative concept of autonomy.[94] Bioethics may seem to be an advocacy movement when we understand autonomy simply as a label for something good or something we don't want to interfere with because we make it impossible to have a critical discussion of whether we should advance patient autonomy. Instead, we make it almost inevitable that we will seek to advance that which is labeled autonomous.

An evaluative concept of autonomy has no content and, as we saw earlier with the procedural concept of autonomy, there are problems with a concept of autonomy that has no substantive content. It is important to note, however, that the evaluative concept is contentless in a different way from the procedural concept. Although the procedural concept has no substantive content about the good life, it involves an interest in resolving conflicts and there is the idea of a procedure to grab onto, e.g., patient of adult years with an IQ above a certain minimal level and signs the consent form. As we shall see, the evaluative concept of autonomy is more radically contentless than that.

How can a contentless principle guide action? And, on what basis can we resolve conflicts when a contentless idea of autonomy comes into conflict with other ethical principles? These questions have significance in the clinical setting when issues of patient autonomy arise.

A contentless principle cannot guide action. If we are using an evaluative notion of autonomy and we are trying to decide what decisions ought to be respected we have to decide on grounds other than the specific content of an individual's decision. What are these other grounds? It is a speaker's evaluations that determine what counts as 'autonomous.' In other words, determinations of autonomy depend on the speaker's judgments, even arbitrary judgments. This seems to be at odds with the reasons for the beginning of the contemporary bioethics movement, the reaction against violations of what would commonly be understood as autonomy and the concern for vulnerable subjects. Although the use of an evaluative concept of autonomy promotes autonomy as a value it does not mean that using the concept in this way actually protects the interests of patients or subjects—or tells us how to protect their interests. In fact, arbitrary evaluations in the clinical setting can lead to violations of autonomy and once again vulnerable people can be endangered.

Problems arise when autonomy is treated evaluatively and comes into conflict with other principles such as beneficence. The refusal of a blood transfusion by a Jehovah's Witness illustrates the conflict between autonomy and beneficence as well as the fact that arbitrary evaluations are doing the work because contradictory conclusions can be reached simultaneously by different people. Conflict and contradictory conclusions occur when one person argues that: 'the transfusion must not be given because this is an autonomous decision and as such it should be respected' and another claims: 'the transfusion must be given to save the patient's life.' It is also consistent with an evaluative approach to recommend treatment on the basis of judging the decision *not* autonomous. The Jehovah's Witness example illustrates the limitations of an evaluative notion of autonomy.

The refusal of a blood transfusion by a Jehovah's Witness is often cited as a classic example of an autonomous choice. This happens when people start with the idea of a choice that they would be loath to override. A case in point is Beauchamp and Childress who hold the view that even though some choices may be deemed unworthy according to a descriptive psychological account of autonomy they nevertheless deserve respect: 'individuals can exercise their autonomy in choosing to accept an institution, tradition, or community that they view as a legitimate source of direction.'[95] They cite the refusal of blood as an exercise of autonomy.[96]

In deciding whether or not to respect the Jehovah's Witness's choice, the evaluative concept of autonomy actually does no work. In trying to resolve such cases we tend to rely on a substantive—that is descriptive—account of autonomy. I will look at the question of autonomous action and Jehovah's Witness's refusal of treatment in more detail in a later section. In terms of an evaluative approach however, in order to assess the function and usefulness of an evaluative concept of autonomy I will consider some more examples where there is disagreement about whether to respect patient's choices. As well, I will examine an argument that rejects a psychological concept of autonomy in favor of what amounts to an evaluative approach. We can then ask if taking an evaluative approach helps in the clinical context.

Priscilla Alderson argues that interpretations of autonomy in which autonomous persons are usually regarded as rational, independent, mature, and competent can work against the interests of vulnerable patients because they offer no defence against harm for people with limited autonomy. Alderson argues for this in the context of sick children and consent.[97] Her arguments coincide with the evaluative concept of autonomy used by Beauchamp and Childress. Beauchamp and Childress do not argue specifically for treating children as autonomous agents, but the arguments of Alderson and others have impacted on their analysis of autonomous action which they discuss in terms of normal rather than ideal choosers. In some ways children and the elderly fit their idea of normal choosers. Beauchamp and Childress argue that understanding and independence (two of the conditions of autonomous action), are exhibited by many children and many elderly patients to a greater or lesser extent, and in the context of normal choosers they cite Alderson's article about children's consent.[98]

Alderson argues that sick children are 'often distressed, dependent, and immature' but this apparent lack of autonomy should not exclude them from the consent process. She argues for 'broader interpretations' of autonomy which will 'allow serious acceptance of children's views' and uses the example of Sarah who asks for her treatment to be stopped:

> After long, intensive, but unsuccessful treatment for leukaemia, Sarah aged six said to her mother one morning, "I don't need to get well any more, I want to go home." Her decision was immediately respected.[99]

In this example the decision to respect the child's wishes seems an entirely reasonable decision and we could easily, with little hesitation, decide to call it an autonomous choice.[100] If the child's treatment offered some chance of recovery, however, other considerations are not so easily dismissed.

In this case the decision about what action should be taken is influenced by the consequences of regarding the decision as autonomous or regarding the decision as not autonomous. We can easily accept the child's wishes because her situation seems futile. However, if the situation was not futile and treatment offered a good chance or even some chance of recovery, respect for the child's decision (stopping treatment) may be viewed differently. It may be seen as pandering to the child's fear and immaturity with the result that she will surely die. Here it is the bad consequences of treatment and the idea of burdensome treatment that seem to be influencing judgments. Sarah's desire to stop treatment would be viewed differently if treatment could benefit her. This shows us that an evaluative notion of autonomy does no work in guiding us.

In situations where a descriptive psychological notion of autonomy is thought to be of limited use, an evaluative notion of autonomy is not the answer. An evaluative approach will not protect patients' interests. On a psychological account of autonomy, a child's wishes need not be paternalistically overridden. Where children are concerned, the decision about what action to take can be decided differently. Parental consent on behalf of the child may be the thing that guides action so even though the child may be considered nonautonomous, her wishes can still be respected.

Alderson's view correlates with Beauchamp and Childress's view that reliance on a rigorous psychological standard will mean that a lot of decisions may not qualify as deserving respect. We saw earlier that Beauchamp and Childress want a way for people to qualify as deserving respect for their decisions even when those decisions have not been evaluated at a higher level. They think there are some decisions that should be regarded as 'autonomous' although they may not be especially consistent or authentic. Alderson provides us with another example of treating autonomy as an evaluative concept. As before, it is a case in which a judgment about whether a choice ought or ought not to be respected is made and then the choice is called 'autonomous' or 'not autonomous' accordingly.

Again, in the context of children's consent, Alderson discusses the idea that some actions deserve respect and are autonomous. Ironically she introduces the following case with a statement suggesting instrumental rationality and a kind of authenticity (aspects of some descriptive psychological concepts of autonomy) are worthy of esteem:

> In my present research on children's consent, parents tell me that their children "will go through tremendous levels of pain to get where they want to." Ten-year-old Amy had months of painful treatment, with complications, to increase her very small stature. Just before yet another operation, she spoke for many [children] when she said, "I know I want this operation. I know it hurts a lot. But it's so important to me that I don't really want to think about the problems. I just think about what it will be like to be taller." Her mother said, "This had to be Amy's decision. No one else can make this kind of choice for her."[101]

Using psychological criteria, it would be quite easy to argue that this choice is not autonomous. Limb lengthening is a 'long and arduous undertaking' which can involve up to three years of pain with complications occurring 'to some degree in almost 100% of cases.' One of the complications that can occur carries with it the possibility of death or amputation. At the present time, it is not known whether the potential benefits of the procedure outweigh the risks.[102] It is not clear that Amy has information about these risks and implications. Her obvious immaturity also has relevance. She shows no recognition of the risks of treatment and there is no evidence that she has evaluated risks and benefits so there is nothing to support the view that her choice is autonomous. The question of whether she can comprehend and assess the impact of ideas (hers and others) about what is 'normal' in terms of stature is also an issue. On a psychological account of autonomy her choice does not demonstrate sufficicient understanding.

A psychological concept helps us resolve the question about whether or not to respect this patient's wish to have her short stature treated medically—that is, if we also value autonomy. An evaluative concept does not help. 'solutions' arrived at by relying on an evaluative concept often tell us more about the person trying to resolve the issue than they do about autonomous action. On an evaluative concept we take into account the consequences of regarding the decision as autonomous and various other factors of which questions of whether the patient's wishes are autonomous and the nature of decision making might be part, but only part. Then, according to our evaluations and judgements, well considered or arbitrary, we decide whether we think the patient's decision is to be respected and therefore autonomous.

An evaluative concept of autonomy mixes and distorts ideas and values. It does not fit with the critical philosophical nature of bioethics and it is not helpful in the clinical context. The evaluative concept has no content and yet it implies ethical conclusions. It can confuse arguments and mislead because it inevitably suggests that a decision or person has satisfied some psychological criteria. To recap—when the term is used evaluatively it is the value judgments of the person using the term that determines its application.

NOTES

1. And even though our action may accord with duty. Kant, *Groundwork*, 65 (397).

2. Ruth Macklin, *Man, Mind, and Morality: The Ethics of Behaviour Control* (Englewood Cliffs, Prentice Hall, Inc., 1982), 39.

3. Kant, *Groundwork*,.64 (396).

4. This is based on a case presented in Baruch A. Brody and H. Tristram Engelhardt, Jr., *Bioethics Readings & Cases* (New Jersey: Prentice-Hall, 1987), 324–25.

5. Kant, *Groundwork*, 80 (422).

6. Kant, *Lectures on Ethics*, 127.

7. Kant, *Lectures on Ethics*, 163–64.

8. Kant, *Lectures on Ethics*, 167.

9. Brody and Engelhardt, *Bioethics Readings & Cases*, 240.

10. Kant, *The Doctrine of Virtue*, 92.

11. Kant, *Groundwork*, 65–66 (398).

12. Brody and Engelhardt, *Bioethics Readings & Cases*, 375.

13. Kant, *Groundwork*, 65 (397–98).

14. Kant, *Groundwork*, 80 (422).

15. Kant, *Lectures on Ethics*, 148.

16. Kant, *Groundwork*, 80 (422).

17. This case had been altered slightly from a case discussed in *A Casebook in Psychiatric Ethics*, Group for the Advancement of Psychiatry (New York: Brunner/Maxel Publishers, 1990), 17.

18. Kant, *Lectures on Ethics*, 151.

19. Kant, *Groundwork*, 66 (398).

20. Berlin, "Two Concepts of Liberty," 132.

21. Berlin, "Two Concepts of Liberty," 133.

22. Merry Bloch Jones, *Birthmothers: Women Who Have Relinquished Babies for Adoption Tell Their Stories* (Chicago: Chicago Review Press, 1993), 18, 38.

23. These accounts of autonomy were listed and detailed in an earlier section. They are the theories of Gerald Dworkin, Robert Young, Richard Lindley, Harry G. Frankfurt, Diana T. Meyers, and Bernard Berofsky.

24. Dworkin, *The Theory and Practice of Autonomy*, 19–20; Young, *Personal Autonomy*, 9.

25. Dworkin, *The Theory and Practice of Autonomy*, 107, 112.

26. Robert Young, *Personal Autonomy*, 49–50.

27. Robert Young, *Personal Autonomy*, 34.

28. Robert Young, *Personal Autonomy*, 49.

29. Samuel Gorovitz, *Doctors' Dilemmas* (New York: Oxford University Press, 1982), 34.

30. Gorovitz, *Doctors' Dilemmas*, 40–42.

31. Hill, "The Kantian Conception of Autonomy," 92.

32. Beauchamp and Childress, *Principles of Biomedical Ethics*, 1994, 4th ed., 127; and Beauchamp and Childress, *Principles of Biomedical Ethics*, 2001, 5th ed., 65.

33. Frankfurt, "Freedom of the Will," 67–69.

34. Meyers, *Self, Society, and Personal Choice*, 50.

35. Meyers, *Self, Society, and Personal Choice*, 44–53.

36. Dworkin, *The Theory and Practice of Autonomy*, 15.

37. Dworkin, *The Theory and Practice of Autonomy*, 16. There are different versions of descriptive psychological theories of autonomy and there are important differences between them—for example, Alfred Mele in *Autonomous Agents: From Self-Control to Autonomy* (1995) discusses this aspect of Dworkin's view in a different light, pp. 146–53 and 170. These different accounts of autonomy will be discussed in more detail in a later chapter.

38. Bernard Gert, Charles Culver and K. Danner Clouser, *Bioethics: A Return to Fundamentals* (New York: Oxford University Press, 1997), 134.

39. Intervention covers a range of pressures from more talk or rational persuasion to declaring the patient incompetent. The manner of intervention is also important—for example, rational persuasion versus coercion

40. C. Fried, *Medical Experimentation: Personal Integrity and Social Policy* (New York: Elsevier, 1974), 98 in *The Theory and Practice of Autonomy*, Dworkin (Cambridge: Cambridge University Press, 1988), 113.

41. Dworkin, *The Theory and Practice of Autonomy*, 113.

42. I am referring to the principles identified in *The Belmont Report* and those identified in *Principles of Biomedical Ethics* by Beauchamp and Childress—that is, the principle of respect for persons, the principle of justice, the principle of beneficence, the principle of respect for autonomy, and the principle of nonmaleficence

43. Jonathan D. Moreno, *Deciding Together: Bioethics and Moral Consensus* (New York: Oxford University Press, 1995), 73.

44. National Research Act Sec. 202 (a)(1)(A) July 1974. In *Practical Decision Making in Health Care Ethics: Cases and Concepts*, Raymond J. Devettere (Washington: Georgetown University Press, 1995), 406.

45. *The Belmont Report*, 1, footnote.

46. Gert, Culver, and Clouser, *Bioethics: A Return to Fundamentals*, 73–74, quoting from *The Federal Register* 44. no.76 (Wednesday, April 18, 1979): 23,193.

47. Gert, Culver, and Clouser, *Bioethics: A Return to Fundamentals*, 73–74.

48. Gert, Culver, and Clouser, *Bioethics: A Return to Fundamentals*, 406–407

49. Albert Jonsen, "American Moralism and the Origin of Bioethics in the United States," *Journal of Medicine and Philosophy* 16 (1991): 115–29, quoted in Devettere, *Practical Decision Making*, 408.

50. Meilaender, *Body, Soul, and Bioethics*, 29, 52.

51. Edmund D. Pellegrino and David C. Thomasma, *The Christian Virtues in Medical Practice* (Washington D.C.: Gerorgetown University Press, 1996), 12.

52. Pellegrino and Thomasma, *The Christian Virtues*, 7.

53. Pellegrino and Thomasma, *The Christian Virtues*, 9.

54. Pellegrino and Thomasma, *The Christian Virtues*, 100.

55. Pellegrino and Thomasma, *The Christian Virtues*, 15.

56. Pellegrino and Thomasma, *The Christian Virtues*, 2.

57. Pellegrino and Thomasma, *The Christian Virtues*, 1.

58. Pellegrino and Thomasma, *The Christian Virtues*, 100.

59. Pellegrino and Thomasma, *The Christian Virtues*, 1.

60. Pellegrino and Thomasma, *The Christian Virtues*, 3.

61. Gert, Culver, and Clouser, *Bioethics: A Return to Fundamentals*, 71–72; K. Danner Clouser, "Common Morality as an Alternative to Principlism," *Kennedy Institute of Ethics Journal* 5 no.3 (1995): 221.

62. Gert, Culver, and Clouser, *Bioethics: A Return to Fundamentals*, 77.

63. Brendan Minogue, *Bioethics: A Committee Approach* (Boston: Jones and Bartlett Publishers, 1996), 169–70.

64. On a purely procedural approach they would not even try to persuade her because the content of a person's choice does not matter. A purely procedural approach has nothing to say about the standard of the patient's deliberation or understanding.

65. Engelhardt, *Bioethics and Secular Humanism*, 116. Perhaps no concept of autonomy does this. I am referring to the procedural approach to autonomy which, on Engelhardt's view in *The Foundations of Bioethics*, 1986, 1st ed., 71, 'justifies the process for generating content' as opposed to the 'principle of beneficence' which 'identifies the content of the practice of morality' and 'supports the concrete moral goals to which medicine ought to be directed.'

66. Annas, "The Dominance of American Law," 86–87; Katz, "Informed Consent: Must It Remain a Fairy Tale?" 69–91.

67. The Nuremberg Code with its emphasis on informed voluntary consent nevertheless came to us through the courts. Also, see Baruch A. Brody, *The Ethics of Biomedical Research: An International Perspective* (New York: Oxford University Press, 1998), 34. Even the World Medical Association's Declaration of Helsinki which emphasises the interests of patients/subjects, was, according to Brody, 'designed to meet the threat that inappropriate research posed both to the integrity and the reputation of the research enterprise.'

68. Engelhardt, *The Foundations of Bioethics*, 1986, 1st ed., 72–73.

69. Katz, "Informed Consent: Must It Remain a Fairy Tale?" 71.

70. Mill, *On Liberty*, 51.

71. Mill, *On Liberty*, 11.

72. H. Tristram Engelhardt, "Bioethics Reconsidered: Theory and Method in a Post-Christian, Post-Modern Age," *Kennedy Institute of Ethics Journal* 6, no. 4 (December, 1996): 340.

73. Engelhardt, *The Foundations of Bioethics*, 1986, 1st ed., 54.

74. Paul S. Appelbaum, Loren H. Roth, Charles W. Lidz, Paul Benson, and William Winslade, "False Hopes and Best Data: Consent to Research and the Therapeutic Misconception," *Hastings Center Report* 17, no.2 (April 1987): 20.

75. Appelbaum et al., "False Hopes and best Data," 22.

76. This case has been adapted from a case in Loren H. Roth, Alan Meisel, and Charles W. Lidz, "Tests of Competency to Consent to Treatment" in *Psychiatry and Ethics: Insanity, Rational Autonomy, and Mental Health Care*, ed. Rem B. Edwards (New York: Prometheus Books, 1982), 201–11, 205–206.

77. Engelhard, *The Foundations of Bioethics*, 1986, 1st ed., 266.

78. Engelhard, *The Foundations of Bioethics*, 1986, 1st ed., 264–65. Referring to the dissent written by Justice Brandeis in *Olmstead vs. United States* and the dissenting opinion of Justice Burger while a member of the Circuit Court of the District of Columbia which was developed as a gloss on Brandeis's dissent in *Olmstead*.

79. Engelhard, *The Foundations of Bioethics*, 1986, 1st ed., 266.

80. Again, "content" as used here refers to the content of the notion or account of autonomy, and not to the content of the patient's choice

81. Engelhard, *The Foundations of Bioethics*, 1996, 2nd ed., xi.

82. Engelhard, *The Foundations of Bioethics*, 1996, 2nd ed., 288.

83. Engelhard, *The Foundations of Bioethics*, 1996, 2nd ed., 290.

84. James Childress, *Practical Reasoning in Bioethics* (Bloomington: Indiana University Press, 1997), 60–61. There is a distinction to be made between the idea of a substantive account of autonomy that demands a particular ideal of a way of life—that is, a particular content for the choices that the person makes, and an account that gives content to the notion of what it is to make an autonomous choice—that is, 'content' can refer to the criteria for an autonomous decision and it can also refer to the actual content of the decision. Childress seems to be rejecting both substantive ideas but in wanting to be able to criticize some choices he embraces the substantive idea of what it is to make an autonomous choice (a descriptive psychological account of autonomy)

85. Beauchamp and Childress, *Principles of Biomedical Ethics*, 1994, 4th ed., 120.

86. Beauchamp and Childress, *Principles of Biomedical Ethics*, 2001, 5th ed., 57.

87. Dworkin, *The Theory and Practice of Autonomy*, 6.

88. Gert, Culver and Clouser, *Bioethics: A Return to Fundamentals*, 82.

89. An advocate falls into a special categrory of social reformer. An advocate is committed to an agenda. See Jonathan D. Moreno, *Deciding Together: Bioethics and Moral Consensus* (New York: Oxford University Press, 1995), 145–46.

90. Moreno, *Deciding Together*, 145–46.

91. Moreno, *Deciding Together*, 146.

92. Moreno, *Deciding Together*, 146–47.

93. Susan M. Wolf, "Ethics Committees and Due Process: Nesting Rights in a Community of Caring," *Maryland Law Review* 50, no.3 (1991): 820–21. Ethics committees may claim to serve patient interests or to protect the institution. Some committees favor the needs of one or the other and some alternate between the two.

94. Members of ethics committees may determine that someone is nonautonomous and they might also analyse and discuss what constitutes autonomy

95. Beauchamp and Childress, *Principles of Biomedical Ethics*, 2001, 5th ed., 60.

96. Beauchamp and Childress, *Principles of Biomedical Ethics*, 1994, 4th ed., 24 and; Beauchamp and Childress, *Principles of Biomedical Ethics*, 2001, 5th ed., 60.

97. My discussion of autonomy has centered on adults. I do not include infants or young children in the class of what could be described as psychologically

autonomous persons—at least not without considering that issue in detail and I am not doing that here.

98. Beauchamp and Childress, *Principles of Biomedical Ethics*, 1994, 4th ed., 123n5; and Beauchamp and Childress, *Principles of Biomedical Ethics*, 2001, 5th ed., 59n3.

99. Priscilla Alderson, "Consent to Children's Surgery and Intensive Medical Treatment," *Journal of Law and Society* 17, no. 1 (Spring, 1990): 57–58.

100. More information about why Sarah said what she did would help a clinician here but Alderson does not provide us with this additional kind of information.

101. Alderson, "Consent to Children's Surgery," 55.

102. Ravi Savarirayan, "The Long and the Short of It: Ethics of Surgical Limb Lengthening in Dwarfs," February 2004. Unpublished. Personal communication.

III

THE SEARCH FOR A BETTER, MORE DEFENSIBLE THEORY

6

CAN A GOOD DESCRIPTIVE PSYCHOLOGICAL ACCOUNT OF AUTONOMY BE ACHIEVED?

After critically analyzing the four concepts of autonomy which I have identified, it seems that the descriptive psychological account is the one that stands up best. In the clinical context, there seems to be a need for a descriptive psychological account. However, it is not without problems. In order to see whether a good psychological concept can be achieved I will begin with an assessment of the psychological notion of autonomy in its various forms. I will categorize the various theories in terms of what they base autonomy on and I will identify the prerequisites according to particular categories of psychological autonomy for judging persons or particular choices to be autonomous or nonautonomous. I will also look at the questions or concerns influencing particular theorists.

In some way, these theories all address the question of the autonomy or the lack of autonomy possessed by members of certain kinds of religious sects. Some descriptive psychological theories view these people as a paradigm case of the nonautonomous person. At least one descriptive psychological account, however, says that these people are really autonomous. In terms of the way the various psychological theories work, it will be useful to examine the various treatments of members of religious sects. This will be one of the tasks I undertake in assessing the various psychological theories of autonomy.

PSYCHOLOGICAL THEORIES OF AUTONOMY IN CATEGORIES

Psychological theories of autonomy are spelled out in terms of the psychology of an agent. Preferences and desires, capacities and competencies, notions of the self, life plans, and rationality have a central role in this. A descriptive psychological theory of autonomy helps us to identify an autonomous person or an autonomous choice but it does not tell us how to act. As I have noted previously, the question of whether we should value or respect autonomy is a separate question and it is not addressed in this section. Here I am categorizing and assessing the various theories.

In an earlier section I critically assessed the descriptive psychological notion of autonomy and identified some examples of what an autonomous or nonautonomous person is like according to the descriptive psychological account of autonomy in general. My concern back then was in deciding whether a descriptive psychological conception of autonomy, in comparison with a metaphysical, a procedural and an evaluative notion, was applicable and useful to the clinical context. In this section, having decided that the descriptive psychological account seems the most promising, I will try to work out which is the best version. In order to do that, I will begin by analyzing and categorizing the various psychological accounts. Then, in the next section, I will use some test cases to evaluate the different versions in terms of how they fit the clinical context.

Most descriptive psychological accounts of autonomy can be described as well developed in the sense that they give us a clear picture of what it is to be an autonomous person, what it takes to make an autonomous decision, or what counts as an autonomous decision. I will be categorzing the accounts under the headings of hierarchical, historical, life plan, and authentic self views of autonomy. In addition, there are syncretist accounts of autonomy which amalgamate elements of these versions—they are composite accounts which are coherent and do not contain conflicting elements. Some other accounts are more aptly described as critique accounts. The conception of autonomy that is advanced in a critique account may not make a coherent whole or count as a well-developed theory of autonomy itself, but it provides a useful commentary on other psychological accounts.

Hierarchical Approval Accounts of Autonomy

This view of autonomy is sometimes referred to as the higher and lower order desire view or the split-level view of the self. Dworkin and Frankfurt's theories are the two best-known accounts which can be described as hierarchical although there is more than one component to Dworkin's theory. Richard Lindley and Lawrence Haworth have descriptive psychological accounts of autonomy which can also be classed as hierarchical.[1] I have outlined the main theories earlier and I will now discuss and assess the descriptive hierarchical psychological view of autonomy.

The hierarchical psychological account of autonomy is an advance on the idea of autonomy as absence of interference or not being constrained in what we want to do. In an earlier section I have said why that will not do. The hierarchical account introduces the idea of reflection, specifically critical reflection. Both Dworkin and Frankfurt are concerned with more than voluntariness.

I noted earlier that Frankfurt does not use the word 'autonomy' but what he describes fits with a descriptive psychological account of autonomy. Frankfurt's concern with 'freedom of the will' and 'the concept of a person' is a concern with the set of characteristics that are essential to persons and according to Frankfurt they are characteristics which distinguish persons from other creatures:

> Human beings are not alone in having desires and motives, or in making choices. They share these things with members of certain other species, some of whom even appear to engage in deliberation and to make decisions based upon prior thought. It seems to be peculiarly characteristic of humans, however, that they are able to form what I shall call "second-order desires" or "desires of the second order."
>
> Besides wanting and choosing and being moved *to do* this or that, men may also want to have (or not to have) certain desires and motives ... Many animals appear to have the capacity for what I shall call "first-order desires" or "desires of the first order," which are simply desires to do or not to do one thing or another. No animal other than man, however, appears to have the capacity for reflective self-evaluation that is manifested in the formation of second-order desires.[2]

For Dworkin, too, the capacity for second-order reflection captures something important and distinctive about human agents.[3] I will focus on Dworkin's account as the representative hierarchical conception of autonomy. Dworkin's account seems to be the most detailed and well developed of the hierarchical accounts. To recapitulate, Dworkin says:

> Putting the various pieces together, autonomy is conceived of as a second-order capacity of persons to reflect critically upon their first-order preferences,

> desires, wishes and so forth and the capacity to accept or attempt to change these in light of higher-order preferences and values. By exercising such a capacity, persons define their nature, give meaning and coherence to their lives, and take responsibility for the kind of person they are.[4]

Procedural independence is an aspect of Dworkin's account. Dworkin argues that second-order reflection is not the 'whole story' of autonomy. There are influences such as 'hypnotic suggestion, manipulation, coercive persuasion, subliminal influence and so forth' which can affect a person's reflective and critical faculties. Procedural independence ensures that our first-order desires are consistent with autonomy: 'Spelling out the conditions of procedural independence involves distinguishing those ways of influencing people's reflective and critical faculties which subvert them from those which promote and improve them.'[5] Dworkin also speculates that 'as people critically reflect on the procedural independence or lack of it in the ways in which they acquire their tastes and preferences, they will change those preferences that they discover are the result of manipulation or deception.'[6] Therefore, for Dworkin, in addition to second-order reflection, autonomy includes:

> some ability to alter one's preferences and to make them effective in action. Indeed to make them effective partly because one has reflected upon them and adopted them as one's own.[7]

Dworkin is not suggesting that the condition of procedural independence by itself is enough and that we can do away with the need for second-order reflection. It seems that it is necessary to subject one's preferences and desires to critical reflection in order to maintain procedural independence. We want to be able to identify persons who are coerced, but also, we want to be able to distinguish between two people who are coerced. Some people may choose to be coerced as a means of motivation. In that kind of situation the significance of the distinction in first- and second-order motivations is evident. Dworkin claims that a theory of autonomy would be deficient if it did not recognize these different levels and, to illustrate this, he offers us the contrast between a patient who is deceived by his doctor against his will and another who wants his doctor to lie to him if cancer is diagnosed.[8]

Dworkin says that the 'process of reflection ought to be subject to the requirements of procedural independence'[9]but the requirements of procedural independence are not easy to determine. Dworkin does not give us a lot of detail about procedural independence and he adds to the confusion by introducing further terms such as 'substantive independence' and 'substantive dependence.'

He says that in using the term 'procedural independence,' what he means is 'roughly' the 'absense of causal influences that interfere with our thinking correctly; for example, hypnosis, brain washing, and the like' and he uses the term 'substantive independence' to mean 'exercising a capacity for critical reflection.'[10]

For Dworkin it is not the content of a choice that counts. His procedural independence requirement means that the person must be capable of the right sort of self reflection. In other words, an autonomous person's reflection must not be manipulated or coerced. A person counts as autonomous on Dworkin's view even if that person does whatever their mother, their friends, their leader, or their priest tells them to do—as long as that is how that person decides they want to conduct their life.[11] Dworkin claims '[i]n my conception, the autonomous person can be a tyrant or a slave, a saint or sinner, a rugged individualist or champion of fraternity, a leader or follower.'[12] This suggests that Dworkin would count as autonomous a Jehovah's Witness who embraces the Jehovah's Witness way of life. Dworkin asks how a person could be considered not autonomous when 'he is leading just the kind of life he thinks is worth leading.'[13] For Dworkin, autonomy is contentless in the sense that he does not want to endorse a substantive view of the good life:

> There is nothing in the idea of autonomy that precludes a person from saying, "I want to be the kind of person who acts at the command of others. I define myself as a slave and endorse those attitudes and preferences. My autonomy consists in being a slave."[14]

Presumably a Jehovah's Witness would want to be the kind of person who acts at the command of God as interpreted from biblical texts by the Jehovah's Witness religion. Dworkin thinks that it is coherent to act at the command of others and to be autonomous. He adds that we cannot argue against this on the grounds of autonomy:

> The argument will have to appeal to some idea of what is a fitting life for a person and, thus, be a direct attempt to impose a conception of what is "good" on another person.[15]

Nevertheless, a person who is indoctrinated and has their reflections manipulated and coerced would not count as autonomous for Dworkin.

Substantive independence is not a requirement of Dworkin's account. Substantive independence means that a person must not 'defer independent judgment.'[16] The opposite of substantive independence is substantive dependence—e.g., a selfish person (substantively independent) as opposed to a caring person (substantively dependent). Dworkin claims that if autonomy is thought of as substantive independence, a selfish person who does not allow the needs of others to interfere with his plans or projects is more autonomous than the benevolent person.[17] Dworkin complains that notions of autonomy which insist on substantive independence do not just rule out promising, worship, obedience to command, and conformity to the law, but commitment and loyalty as well.[18] Persons who are either substantively independent or substantively dependent can count as autonomous on his view.

Although Dworkin's notion of autonomy is without content, this does not mean that it is not a descriptive psychological account of autonomy. Descriptive psychological conceptions of autonomy do have content of the type which is given in terms of the psychological features of autonomous persons, e.g., second-order capacity to reflect etc. The kind of content Dworkin rejects is moral or value-laden content. An instance of the kind of substantive content he rejects is, the idea that to be autonomous one must be a 'self-sufficient, independent, person relying on his own resources.' This is the kind of content that 'one can attempt to justify as worthy of admiration.'[19] It is also the idea of giving content to life plans that Dworkin rejects.[20] Morally or evaluatively neutral may be a better way to describe Dworkin's account of autonomy because it does have content in a descriptive psychological sense. On Dworkin's view, people's choices have content but we cannot focus on that in our determination of autonomy. The content, however, is reflected on by agents themselves.

Despite the fact that Dworkin argues for a conception of autonomy that requires procedural independence, and he does not insist on substantive independence, he does believe there is some connection between autonomy and substantive independence[21]:

> Although there are no a priori truths about the content of an autonomous person's values, one can speculate about psychological and sociological connections. It seems plausible that those who practice in their daily life a critical reflection on their own value structure will tend to be suspicious of modes of thought that rely on the uncritical acceptance of authority, tradition, and custom. They will be disposed to value the kind of substantive independence ranked so highly by philosophers like Mill and Humboldt.[22]

According to Dworkin's conception of autonomy therefore, it is possible to be a Jehovah's Witness while being autonomous, but there is something in the idea of autonomy involving critical reflection and procedural independence which may lead people considering such a choice to decide against it. Despite this, there is nothing in his conception to rule out autonomously choosing to be a Jehovah's Witness.

How does this conception of autonomy fare in the clinical context? An implication of Dworkin's view is that the decisions made by an autonomous person have no specific content[23] but an autonomous person has a particular sort of reflection. On this basis, it seems reasonable to assume that we can discern whether a person is autonomous or not. The example of a Jehovah's Witness who refuses a blood transfusion is one way to illustrate how Dworkin's hierarchical conception of autonomy works in the clinical context.

Dworkin concedes that there is a sense in which the wishes of the Jehovah's Witness are not really hers. Nevertheless, he thinks we should respect her wishes: 'I certainly may think that her life is not a very good one, but it does have a claim on me.'[24] In terms of his descriptive psychological theory of autonomy Dworkin explains why he would not reject the Jehovah's Witness's claim to be respected.[25] He distinguishes between two senses in which the Jehovah's Witness's wishes are not her own. First, he concedes that her wishes are not her own in some things: 'she has not independently reflected upon the command that she solicit from door to door.' But, he also argues that 'she has decided that she wants to define her life as a follower of the way. For her, the Lord's wishes *are* her commands.' According to Dworkin, the Jehovah's Witness 'attributes value to obedience.' Her decision, therefore, 'reflects a fundamental commitment' as to 'how she wants to live her life, what kind of person she wants to be.' Some things she has 'autonomously abandoned,' but, she is still an 'autonomous person.'[26]

The hierarchical account certainly helps us to identify autonomous choices and nonautonomous choices. It is also compatible with other values such as obligation, commitment, and promising. There are, however, some objections to aspects of Dworkin's account[27]—in particular, his appeal to higher order levels of reflection. The most serious objection to Dworkin's view is that either acts of critical reflection are autonomous or an infinite regress to higher levels of critical reflection threatens and nothing explains where the autonomy comes from. Dworkin addresses these objections but not entirely satisfactorily as we will see in the chapters that follow.

Historical Psychological Theories of Autonomy

Historical theories of autonomy focus on the 'manner' in which an agent comes to have a set of desires. John Christman develops a 'historical' account of autonomy as a 'replacement theory' for the 'received model.' He argues that the generally accepted model (some kind of hierarchical theory which utilizes notions of higher and lower order desires) is defective. The 'key element' in his replacement theory is: 'the agent's acceptance or rejection of the process of desire formation or the factors that give rise to that formation, rather than the agent's identification with the desire itself.'[28] The emphasis seems to be on the idea that 'the agent would not have rejected the desires in light of the processes' rather than that the person approved of the processes.[29]

Christman devotes considerable attention to conditions that hinder or obstruct autonomy. To 'motivate the contours of the new model' he says 'we should imagine a person who seems (intuitively and pretheoretically) an obvious case of someone lacking autonomy' and he invites us to imagine a friend or family member spending two intensive weeks with a religious cult. Few signs of her former self remain and she mindlessly mouths the credo of the sect. He then asks what sort of claims we would have to make if we were required to justify our judgment about the lack of autonomy. Christman claims that we would consider the conditions under which the person's 'character change' has taken place and we would speculate about the way in which these conditions are incompatible with autonomy. If the new cult member 'did not submit to the regimen of "programming" with the full knowledge of its nature and effects; i.e., it was not part of a strategy of self-change that might have included a decision to pursue a new lifestyle,' she lacks autonomy.[30] According to Christman, what matters is not the agent's evaluation of a desire at a particular time, but what the agent 'thinks about the *process* of coming to have the desire, and whether she resists that process when (or if) given the chance.' The agent's 'participation' in the process of preference formation is important for the determination of autonomy and the conditions which define autonomy must capture the idea that 'the agent was in a position to resist the development of a desire and she did not.'[31] Christman argues that we are justified in judging the new cult member nonautonomous if she was prevented from reflecting on the process of preference formation. If the cult was controlling her sleeping and her eating, denying her contact with friends and relatives, exploiting her emotional vulnerabilities, and playing on her fears, or if she submitted to these processes because of 'inconsistent beliefs, faulty reasoning or self-deception' we can say that she lacks autonomy.[32]

Christman has two cognitive requirements for autonomy. These relate to the reasons that a person does not resist the formation of a desire or value. The first is 'minimal rationality.' He argues that 'only minimal "internal" conditions for rationality (like consistency of beliefs and desires) would be plausible as conditions for autonomy.'[33] He claims that this requirement is 'in some ways too stringent itself' but it is needed to capture 'the necessity that the autonomous person is not being guided by *manifestly inconsistent* desires or beliefs.'[34] Christman claims that his approach differs from some accounts of autonomy which depend on questions of rationality and which are complicated by the variety of requirements for rationality. He claims that his distinction between 'internalist' and the more stringent 'externalist' conditions which need to be confirmed by objective evidence parallels a distinction between 'subjective' and 'objective' rationality made by Richard Brandt.[35] Brandt calls an act 'subjectively rational' if it is 'based on the full use of beliefs rationally supported by the evidence the agent actually had at the time.' An act that falls short of objective rationality is not necessarily irrational.[36] Christman's use of Brandt's distinction suggests a way in which desires which are not rational in themselves can be considered rational. Brandt advances a process of 'cognitive psychotherapy' which is a way of detecting and eliminating desires acquired through defective processes. Irrational desires extinguish under cognitive psychotherapy and any desire which will not extinguish is considered to be a rational desire. Christman's reference to Brandt suggests that something like this is going on.

Christman wants to 'develop and defend' a 'threshold of normal autonomy.'[37] He argues that to demand more or to argue for an 'externalist' rationality condition which requires objective evidence is too exacting. Even the requirement for internal consistency is in some ways too demanding he claims: 'few of us have examined all our beliefs and preferences and tested them' to such a standard.[38] His notion of autonomy seems to be one of autonomy relative to evidence. Christman's argument for minimal internal rationality is meant to rule out, amongst the preferences and beliefs that are easily brought to consciousness, those which are in obvious conflict.[39]

Self-awareness is Christman's other cognitive requirement for autonomy. It rules out self-deception in the process of preference formation. It is also rules out people with defective cognitive mechanisms such as those with severe neuroses and 'most cases' of weakness of will. Underlying the self-awareness requirement is the 'rough idea' that in order to act autonomously a person needs to be 'in tune with the settled aspects of herself that apply to the judgment at hand.' According to Christman, the 'process' of self-determination is 'absent or incomplete' if the '"self" doing the "governing" is dissociated, fragmented, or insufficiently transparent to itself.'[40] In order for the agent's motivating desires and beliefs to be subject to reflection, they must be transparent and easily brought to consciousness.[41] For Christman, the self-awareness requirement means that an agent is not autonomous if she has manifestly inconsistent beliefs and the inconsistency is 'buried' by the agent's 'tactics of not focusing her awareness on the suppressed belief.'[42] Christman claims that 'the test for autonomy is met when the agent would not resist the processes' of desire formation and a 'lack of resistance' is not the product of 'irrationality or self-deception.'[43]

Christman makes a distinction between 'not resisting' and the converse of identifying: '"[I]dentification" is a relation between the judging person and her *desire*, while "not resisting" is a relation between the person and the *process* of coming to have the desire.'[44] He also reminds us of 'the new cult member' and claims that one of the reasons we think she lacks autonomy is that 'although she may well (retrospectively) *not* disapprove of the development of her desires, we are inclined to presume that this second-order acceptance is also the result of her conditioning.' For a person to be autonomous on Christman's historical view, 'it must be true that during the processes where she might have resisted these developing desires, she wasn't also under the influence of manipulating factors' that affect her reflective capabilities. If the cult member suffered fear and anxiety because she was harangued relentlessly by the cult leader to the point that her level of anxiety prevented her from stepping back to reflect on the process of change she was undergoing, she lacks autonomy. According to Christman, 'hypnosis, some drugs, and certain educational techniques' are examples of influences which disturb the conditions necessary for autonomy because they can undermine a person's ability to evaluate the processes by which they come to develop a desire or value.[45] Christman claims that certain indicators of the presence of 'reflection-constraining factors' and the failure of capacities necessary for autonomy can be listed. These indicators include failure to bring salient aspects of a desire to consciousness, failure of concentration, and failures in judgment and they are all 'symptoms of the general failure of self-awareness and rationality that autonomy demands.'[46]

Christman claims that his historical account of autonomy is not simply a matter of identifying the factors that inhibit critical reflection on the process of desire formation. The reason he resists this simplification is that people often subject themselves autonomously to influences that severely undercut their reflective capacities. They sometimes submit to hypnosis in order to quit smoking and this is autonomous on his view unless an agent's 'judgment and evaluations of her states are *all* the product of these influences.' According to Christman, the thing which distinguishes 'autonomy-supporting processes from heteronomous ones is whether the agent was inhibited in her ability to reflect on her own mental states and the forces that affect them.'[47]

Christman concedes that a purely historical model of autonomy has some problems and is in need of further development. In response to one criticism that a purely historical theory is not sufficient for autonomy he adds an extra, nonhistorical condition that applies to the occurrent rationality of the agent. Christman admits that it is possible for an agent to be autonomous with respect to the development of a desire but that she can still be nonautonomous relative to a desire.[48] A case in point is that of a willing addict. Christman therefore adds a nonhistorical condition to the conditions that define autonomy:

An agent P is autonomous relative to some desire (value, etc.) D at time t if and only if:

1. P did not resist the development of D (prior to t) when attending to this process of development, or P would not have resisted that development had P attended to the process.
2. The lack of resistance to the development of D (prior to t) did not take place (or would not have) under the influence of factors that inhibit self-reflection.
3. The self-reflection involved in condition (i) is (minimally) rational and involves no self-deception. And,
4. The agent is minimally rational with respect to D at t (where minimal rationality demands that an agent experience no manifest conflicts of desire or beliefs which significantly affect the agent's behavior and which are not subsumed under some otherwise rational plan of action).[49]

Christman concludes that this model can still be understood as a 'historical' model of autonomy because it is still centrally concerned with the development of desires and values rather than identification with a desire. And the idea that an agent would not reject a desire or value 'in light of the processes' that gave rise to them is, according to Christman, 'an important hypothetical test for autonomy.'[50] He adds that one of the implications of his conception of autonomy is that people can be autonomous despite having desires for 'subservient, demeaning, or even evil things and lifestyles.' For Christman, it is the *origin* of the desire that matters in judgments of autonomy so if an agent has *good reasons* for a particular desire it can be autonomously formed.[51]

Christman's addition of the nonhistorical condition was partly in response to criticisms and examples presented by Alfred Mele.[52] Mele asks us to consider the case of Alex. This case suggests that there is more to being autonomous relative to a desire than being autonomous in terms of its development. Alex has developed a strong desire for hard work. He believes there is a correlation between hard work and success and he has 'carefully monitored and nurtured the development of this propensity in (at least) a minimally rational way and without self-deception.' At no time was he subject to reflection-constraining factors. Years later when Alex marries and has a young child he finds his desire for hard work is causing trouble. His wife complains that he does not spend enough time with his family and Alex himself, after rational non-self-deceived reflection, now judges that he would be better off shedding his desire for hard work for a less rigorous work schedule. Nevertheless, 'against his better judgement' he 'persists in his rigorous routine.' According to Mele, even though Alex satisfies Christman's historical conditions he has 'become a slave' to the original desire and he is 'victimized' by its continued presence.[53]

Christman responds by conceding that a purely historical account of autonomy is insufficient and adds the nonhistorical condition to address cases of 'occurrent conflict' so that agents who have conflicting desires and are 'clearly not fully autonomous' are not mislabeled as autonomous. Christman argues that the internal conflict suffered by Alex makes him a 'fractured and divided' self who is not autonomous.[54] According to Christman, where a conflict of desires 'exhibits a noticeable effect on behavior,' there is a loss of autonomy.[55] He argues that the addition of the nonhistorical condition allows 'mildly conflicted individuals' to remain autonomous but rules out those like Alex who have what he calls 'manifestly conflicting desires (and beliefs in support of those desires) both to work relentlessly and also not to do so in order to spend more time in other pursuits.'[56] Unless an agent really cannot help taking on more tasks and working longer hours, in which case he/she seems more like an 'addict,' the description of Alex fits that of a lot of people. There are many people who want both to have time for their family and for getting a lot of work done. How do we decide whether an individual with conflicting desires is acting autonomously or not? Despite the fact that Alex may want to work less, there may be occasions when he makes an autonomous decision to work longer. And how do we differentiate between 'mildly conflicted individuals' and those who are 'fractured and divided'?

Even though Christman's idea of autonomy is meant to be at the level of preferences and to be assessed in terms of the formation of a single desire rather than a whole way of living, his minimal rationality requirement is not very effective when localized to a particular desire—given that there seems to be other areas of irrationality that may obstruct autonomy. The added nonhistorical condition addresses the problem in part but creates other problems. There are common situations where a minimal rationality requirement does not seem to be met. For instance, many Christians believe that God is omnibenevolent and omnipotent, yet know that there is evil in the world and cannot think of any of the sophisticated philosophical arguments that attempt to reconcile these apparently inconsistent beliefs.[57] Christman may say that the internal conflict does not preclude autonomy because it does not exhibit a noticeable effect on behavior or he may class it with other forms of 'self-manipulation' which agents sometimes use to 'achieve their goals.'[58] He argues that there are some human goods such as commitments to religious practices and values which are 'incompatible with constant reconsideration' and that these 'connections can be maintained only if one refuses, to some extent at least, to repeatedly subject one's commitments' to 'scrutiny from a point of view outside of the commitment.'[59] The point is that while Christman wants to restrict the assessment of autonomy to single desires it is not necessarily the case that the notion of minimal rationality can be similarly compartmentalized or restricted to preferences in a meaningful way. Would we really want to say that the reflection of someone whose life is guided by an inconsistent belief set meets a minimal rationality requirement? Christman's minimal rationality requirement seems to be more demanding than he wants.

His self-awareness requirement and the ban on self-deception may also be stronger than he wants. The ban on self-deception seems to rule out illusions that facilitate effective functioning and which are useful in terms of autonomy. One example is that of a person who tells himself there is no danger in learning to drive—'knowing that without this bit of self-deception, he would never take the first lesson.'[60] Research has shown that illusions such as exaggerated perceptions of control and unrealistic optimism are normal human characteristics and that these positive illusions are especially useful and adaptive in conditions where a person is threatened.[61] The requirement for self-awareness and the ban on self-deception means that a lot of people may come out nonautonomous in relation to the decisions they make, particularly when illness threatens.

Christman claims that the addition of the nonhistorical condition prevents determinations of autonomy being prejudiced in favor of 'attitudes of constant self-scrutiny and self-control which may conflict with the rational goals of many individuals.'[62] Conflicts do not negate autonomy if they belong to some 'otherwise rational and autonomous plan of action' and rationality is understood as 'the lack of manifest behavior-affecting conflicts which are not subsumed under an otherwise rational (and autonomous) plan of self-development.'[63] He claims that the addition of the nonhistorical condition does not negate the historical nature of his account because its principal conditions still concern the development of desires and values.[64] The 'kind of authenticity' he claims autonomy demands, 'are factors over and above the occurrent attitude that an agent has toward her desires and values.' And the extra condition is to do with the 'agent's occurrent ability to rationally act on her desires.'[65]

Finally, for Christman, autonomy is a richer notion that needs to be distinguished from freedom. He claims freedom is generally taken to be the absence of restraints of various kinds (internal or external, positive or negative), that stand between an agent's desires and actions. Christman is concerned with autonomy 'at the level of preferences' which means that he views autonomy as 'an additional component of an account of free action' and he argues that something crucial is left out of account if we do not consider influences other than restraints. For instance, influences that 'induce a person to *prefer* something they otherwise would not.'[66] Subliminal advertising has this kind of influence. It taints the preference that guides action although a person is not restrained from acting or even from performing some alternative action. What renders the agent unfree is that 'she would not *prefer* any other action.'[67]

Even though there are problems, the historical approach to autonomy explains some typical ways in which a person can lack autonomy and it shows the relevance of personal history to a conception of personal autonomy. It may capture something important that is overlooked in other accounts.

Berofsky's Critique of Hierarchical and Historical Accounts

Gerald Dworkin has reviewed Berofsky's book, which critiques hierarchical and historical accounts of autonomy and is somewhat critical of it. He credits the book with making a definite contribution to the literature on autonomy and then quotes Christine Korsgaard with respect to opposing philosophical views:

> The correct view is not going to be the one left standing when the contradictions and absurdities of all the others have finally been exposed. It is going to be the one that answers best to the human concerns which motivate the study of philosophy in the first place.[68]

Although Berofsky's account seems not be a coherent whole and cannot be classed as a well-developed descriptive psychological theory of autonomy I want to use his discussion of autonomy for its value as a critique of hierarchical and historical accounts, specifically his treatment of Jehovah's Witnesses.

Berofsky describes his theory of autonomy as 'liberation from self' and he claims it is nonhierarchical and nonhistorical. He also claims that his conception of autonomy 'is the one idea of personal autonomy that survives conceptual and empirical scrutiny.'[69] According to Berofsky, it is not necessary that 'autonomous agents' engage in the evaluation of the motives that incline them to action. He argues that even the demand that 'identification' be rational is of little use and he rejects the idea that the self is located on the reflective level. Instead he locates autonomy at the level of action or engagement in the world.[70]

Like other theorists, Berofsky is concerned with 'impediments to autonomy.' He claims that in order to characterize these we have to understand 'the way these barriers can form' and to do that we must turn to psychology.[71] Looking at the way barriers form seems like a historical consideration but Berofsky explicitly rejects a historical notion of autonomy.[72] He claims that, in part, his case rests on a repudiation of other accounts.[73]

Positive freedom is a necessary but not sufficient requirement for autonomy according to Berofsky, and positive freedom is a descriptive psychological requirement because it is comprised of a set of personal traits or intellectual and physical competences. The psychological aspect of positive freedom encompasses intellectual competences such as 'capacities for memory, perception, calculation, reasoning, information processing, and the elimination of irrational and inconsistent belief sets.'[74] He also claims that a 'free agent is free of debilitating physical infirmities, addictions, and severe stress.' For Berofsky, it seems, a patient with these afflictions cannot be a free agent or autonomous. While he is not claiming that freedom and autonomy are the same thing, he does claim that autonomy is dependent upon freedom.[75]

According to Berofsky, the need to identify the 'internal differences' between 'genuine autonomy' and the heteronomy of the addict is misguided. He argues that the addict's heteronomy can be explained in terms of features of his life which are 'grounded in his current condition' and which have nothing to do with the origin of his addiction.[76] Berofsky is concerned with 'current' interactions and capacities.[77] He claims that historical conditions or the process which leads to a person's current will is not relevant to determinations of autonomy. He claims it is reasonable to object to the process without having qualms about the results. Berofsky is not convinced that the 'actual or hypothetical endorsement of the *process* by which one arrived at one's current state' is important. He asks us to imagine we are deprogramming a Jehovah's Witness or a cult member to an autonomous life style. Resistance to the deprogramming would not surprise us. He also questions the idea that our success should depend on the 'cooperation of our charges.'[78]

If there are any qualms, the 'relevant matter' according to Berofsky, is 'the current capacity to change.' The 'current autonomy of an agent' according to Berofsky, is 'essentially to do with the current relation of that agent to the world.'[79]

For Berofsky, the 'core' of his new conception of autonomy is 'objectivity.'[80] It is about our response to the world and it involves the 'capacity for flexible response.'[81] It means being 'open to the world' and 'responding to it in an appropriate manner.'[82] Berofsky explains the idea of objectivity in terms of something that 'rigid persons' lack. He does not appeal to paradigm cases but his many references to the 'rigid ' person suggest that for Berofsky, the 'rigid' person is a kind of paradigm case of the nonautonomous person. He views Jehovah's Witnesses as the embodiment of the rigid person. Rigid persons and Jehovah's Witnesses lack objectivity. According to Berofsky, Jehovah's Witnesses and rigid persons do not respond to the world by an objective and relevant examination of its relevant features. They invoke principles instead: 'the world for them is a place to apply, not test their convictions.'[83]

Berofsky refers to Bruno Bettelheim's observation that in concentration camps Jehovah's Witnesses displayed extraordinary integrity and inner strength through their internalized ideals. Berofsky, however, argues that Jehovah's Witnesses lack autonomy because they lack the willingness to defend their principles or revise them in accordance with relevant evidence and objective data. Although they are able to retain their faith and in some circumstances they may be better able to preserve their identity than autonomous persons, that is not sufficient grounds to count them as autonomous. Berofsky argues that the 'comforts of group solidarity and subjective certainty' may be useful in times of crisis, but that does not constitute autonomy.[84]

In contrast to Dworkin and some others, Berofsky seems to be defending a substantive ideal. Berofsky's account has a sense of what we should believe if we looked at the 'relevant evidence.' His idea of engagement with the world and objectivity involves the notion of an agent 'whose beliefs "track" the true' and who 'adjusts his beliefs in light of the actual state of the world.'[85] If Berofsky is saying that Jehovah's Witnesses are not really autonomous, this implies that there is no violation of autonomy in giving blood to a Jehovah's Witness who clearly refuses a blood transfusion. Although that is what his view suggests, Berofsky does not want to be committed to the idea that we can simply override the wishes of the Jehovah's Witness. He reminds us that on his account autonomy is a matter of degree and even a Jehovah's Witness therefore, has 'some autonomy.' He holds the view that a Jehovah's Witness 'ought not to surrender even this small amount if he needs to do so in order to retain those other values resident in his group.' Berofsky adds: 'There are values provided by a cohesive community that are unavailable outside that community. . . . It is a wonderful thing to live one's own life, but there is surely *something* to be said for living *our* life.'[86] This is an example of the kind of content Dworkin rejects; that which we try to 'justify as worthy of admiration.'[87]

In a review of Berofsky's book, Gerald Dworkin comments on Berofsky's commentary of Dworkin's own account of autonomy and Berofsky's use of the terms 'procedural independence' and 'substantive independence.' Because they are using the terms differently, Dworkin compares the difference between his view and Berofsky's view in terms of the autonomy of Jehovah's Witnesses. Berofsky seems to be slipping toward what I call an evaluative concept of autonomy:

> We both agree that the person who becomes a Jehovah's Witness (Berofsky's example) is no longer thinking for herself (exercising her capacity for critical reflection). We both also agree that such a person still has the capacity; she has not had a lobotomy. We also presumably, both agree that the decision reflects a fundamental commitment by the person as to how she wants to live her life, what kind of person she wants to be. But I claim what she has autonomously abandoned still leaves her an autonomous person, while Berofsky believes that she has autonomously abandoned her autonomy.[88]

Dworkin suggests that Berofsky is going beyond what is required of a psychological account of autonomy because he is smuggling in the answers to other questions such as: 'Is it a good thing to be autonomous? Why? How does autonomy ground (if it does) the claims of others to our moral attention?'[89]

So what exactly are the descriptive psychological requirements of Berofsky's account? Berofsky's account does not give us a clear criterion. His concern is with the way that 'autonomy is achieved'; with the way an agent engages in his or her world—in his or her 'current environment.'[90] The following points will help provide a fuller picture of what Berofsky's account is about.

Berofsky acknowledges that we could have 'greater autonomy' if we could increase our intelligence, remove innate infirmities, and eliminate 'emotional barriers to a full participation in a wide range of satisfying relationships and activities.'[91] However, we cannot do this and that indicates that we have 'maximal or ideal autonomy in mind.' He argues that the idea of ideal autonomy is incoherent or irrelevant[92] but it does not invalidate the fact that there are different people who have different degrees of autonomy. He claims that we identify differences in autonomy 'in terms of differences in rationality, independence, objectivity, or personal integrity.'[93]

Berofsky seems to be suggesting that the idea of 'ideal autonomy' is a 'value-laden' notion that involves a conception of 'flourishing.' He argues that the failure of a rational, independent person to flourish 'does not clearly tell against her autonomy.' We cannot say that people who are content and lead very simple but narrow lives are obviously nonautonomous.[94]

According to Berofsky, there are three minimal conditions' or 'core components' for autonomy. These are independence, rationality, and personal integrity. He claims that the only problematic condition is the third, but argues that 'a disintegrated self cannot be autonomous.'[95] An individual 'must have some internal coherence or unity before we can even broach the subject of his autonomy,' he claims.[96] Then, the independent rational and integrated agent needs tools of freedom and knowledge. The agent then does not, according to Berofsky, have to embody ideals such as 'flourishing, morality or self-expression.' The 'rejection of liberation' Berofsky argues is 'essentially a reversion to dependence, the very antithesis of autonomy.'[97]

Berofsky has one exception to what he calls 'the principle of the irrelevance of history.'[98] He decides that an appeal to history must be introduced in order to distinguish 'what might have been' from 'what never could be.'[99] Rather than something like Christman's historical condition, this seems to be a distinction between physical possibility and physical impossibility.

Berofsky's view has some inconsistencies and his claim to have 'the' theory that 'survives conceptual and empirical scrutiny' does not come to fruition. Some of the inconsistencies are that Berofsky argues that his account is nonhistorical and yet, he 'seems to reinstate an origins requirement.'[100] He argues that autonomous persons 'must be independent, not just from the pernicious influence of others, but from the pernicious influence of their own earlier lives'[101] and this seems to be a historical consideration. Also, as we saw in Berofsky's discussion of Jehovah's Witnesses, despite the fact that he rejects a 'value-laden account of autonomy,'[102] he introduces an evaluative element.[103]

Despite these problems and the fact that Berofsky's account seems not to be a coherent whole and cannot be classed as a well-developed descriptive psychological theory of autonomy, his ideas are interesting, useful, and relevant in terms of assessing autonomy and other views.

Life-Plan Accounts of Autonomy

In an earlier section, I outlined Robert Young's and Diana Meyers' views of autonomy involving life plans. In this section I will show what an autonomous person and a nonautonomous person is like according to the life-plan view. I will focus on Young's account which is predominantly about life plans. While Meyers' account involves life plans it is somewhat different and I will categorize it differently—as the authentic self account of autonomy.

I noted in the earlier section that Young claims '*lives* are the primary referents in talk of autonomy'[104] His account is therefore a global one like Dworkin's account. Life plans are central to his conception of autonomy and he introduces two types of autonomy—'occurrent' autonomy, ('autonomy of the moment') and 'dispositional' autonomy which he describes as 'the more important' sense of autonomy where the focus is on the person's 'life as a whole.'[105] Young's aim is to flesh out a 'positive' conception of autonomy which is not simply to be equated with independence and which will involve more than 'freedom from' others.[106] To be autonomous is to 'author one's world.'[107]

According to Young, autonomy is an ideal that has to be worked at and that requires certain positive qualities. Rationality, at least in the sense of not being seriously irrational is a requirement. Strength of will is also needed. For Young, this amounts to a 'preparedness to carry through with one's plans and desires.'[108] Self-knowledge is also needed. However, Young notes that though self-knowledge helps us to resist manipulation by others and helps in overcoming some inner obstacles like self-deception, simply getting to know a flaw is not to eliminate it.[109]

An autonomous person enjoys a life that is 'unified, orderly, and free from self-defeating conflict over fundamentals' and the more one is able to 'direct one's own life' in this way, the 'greater the degree of one's autonomy.'[110] To this end, choices about career, life style, and what he calls 'dominant pursuits' are the areas of 'prime importance.'[111]

Young discusses a lack of autonomy in terms of dispositional concerns. Without rationality, dispositional autonomy is out of reach. Rationality is therefore a 'positive requirement for autonomy.' [112] Skid-row alcoholics, anyone who is insanely deluded, very young children, and those who are irrationally obsessed with someone or something are considered heteronomous because they lack rational qualities like judgment, reflection, calculation, and planning which is necessary to order their lives in 'a manner which is not fundamentally self-defeating.'[113] According to Young, a distressed, painracked, terminally ill patient who is unable to deliberate or order their thoughts, also fits this picture.[114]

Young claims that rationality has an 'important, but not exclusive place in the achievement of autonomy.'[115] He thinks there are some ways in which we can see the significance of being rational without having to talk in terms of a 'highly developed capacity for calculation' or 'penetrating logical analysis' as requirements for autonomy. Although being seriously irrational seems to interfere with autonomy he claims that when one 'tries to put the point more positively, matters are not as straightforward.'[116] Rather than opt for the 'trappings of a forensic approach to reasoning' Young thinks we can see the relevance of rationality to autonomy in the sense that being rational can mean coherence between a person's 'general purposes' and actions. Also, autonomous persons do not accept uncritically the advice given by others. Rationality is therefore an important safeguard given the extent that we rely on the advice and information of others.[117] This is particularly relevant in the medical setting.

Young's conception of autonomy can accommodate the idea that although a person's preference may seem irrational it may demonstrate personal integrity or authenticity constitutive of that person.[118] He argues that we should not judge Jehovah's Witnesses as heteronomous because they violate the notion of rationality 'endorsed by philosophers.'[119] It seems that the preferences of a Jehovah's Witness who refuses a blood transfusion may be irrational in the sense that the decision is based on irrational beliefs[120] but it is not necessarily a heteronomous decision on Young's account. It can be autonomous in that it defines the person someone chooses to be. How is this so?

Like Berofsky, Young cites Bruno Bettelheim's account of the way in which individuals managed under the constraints of imprisonment by the Nazis. Jehovah's Witnesses were one group who managed to hang on to their integrity and who continued to exercise a degree of autonomy: 'They had, it seems, an inner strength that derived from their having resolutely determined to abide by standards they had previously followed.'[121] According to Young:

> However dimly we regard the inculcatory processes which led them to internalise the set of values they followed, and however unreasonable their continued adherence to those values may appear to us, in their conduct they clearly made them their own.[122]

The commands of their religion were 'so internalised as to become the Witness's own directive.'[123] Even though rigidity is generally considered a trait that disqualifies a person from being considered autonomous, on Young's view, to the extent that the Jehovah's Witnesses 'abided by principles that they had made their own,' they qualify as 'autonomous to a significant degree.'[124]

Young takes the paradigm case of the nonautonomous person according to the historical conception of autonomy and says these people are really autonomous. It is worth looking at Young's attitude to the importance of historical conditions and the role of history in his conception of autonomy. He places little importance on historical considerations and yet it seems that history must figure somewhere in a notion of life plans.

For Young it does not seem to matter how we come by our desires. By referring again to the Jehovah's witnesses who lived by principles which they 'made their own,' he claims that the idea of an 'emerging self' which shapes attitudes and commitments is a legitimate idea,' and this partially formed self 'contributes to the making of the developed self.'[125] This is 'despite doubts about such attitudes and commitments being arrived at autonomously.' According to Young, socialization may involve the imposition of attitudes and commitments but the 'impact of socialization' is not entirely predictable: 'It may encourage fundamental resistance to change. But then again it may not.'[126] He argues that although socialization may preclude our developing our motivations from the beginning the important thing is identification:

> It is open to us either to make them our own by identifying with them in our reflective judgings or by rejecting them. Once privy to such awareness it does not matter so much how one came to have one's particular desires, but whether one matches up effective and reflective preferred motivations.[127]

As noted earlier, some degree of self-knowledge and self-awareness is also necessary. The crucial thing for Young, however, is the 'following through on a plan.'[128] And, in determinations of autonomy, the emphasis on the 'following through' overshadows the manner in which a desire is formed:

> It is of some significance that we commonly resort to testing the genuineness of professed motivations by ascertaining the person's preparedness to follow through with his (or her) declared preference. It is just such tests, of what the legal tradition terms 'informed voluntary consent,' which provide the theoretical underpinning for the 'cooling off' periods now customary in consumer protection legislation, in the making and ratification of wills and in proposals

for advance declarations ('living wills') registering a preference for voluntary euthanasia. While such tests serve to protect individuals against giving in to aberrant (occurrent) desires, their premise is the responsible agency of persons. The autonomous are foremost among those to whom such agency may rightfully be attributed.[129]

Young's life-plan conception of autonomy seems more consistent with a hierarchical view[130] than a historical account such as Christman's.

Young has another example that shows that, for him and his life-plan view, history is not particularly important:

> Suppose S knows that heroin addiction causes severe physical harm and likely death before thirty years of age, but still chooses to take the drug because he wants the pleasure of the moment more than anything else. Assume, furthermore, that we independently have good grounds for believing S is emotionally stable and of sound reason.[131]

In this situation, because he values autonomy, Young supports intervention. For Young, 'strong paternalism is sometimes needed to preserve autonomy'[132] and intervention is justified because, even though there may be no defects in his decision making, the consequences of S's action would undermine his 'more dispositional commitments.' What this example shows is that if we are concerned with historical conditions, there seems to be nothing wrong with the development of S's desire—yet it clearly threatens his long-term autonomy.

In light of Young's opposition to things which threaten dispositional autonomy it is worth looking at his view of voluntary euthanasia. We may speculate whether he would oppose voluntary euthanasia on the grounds that the desire to end one's life is nonautonomous. On Young's account, the desire could be interpreted as a failure to 'follow through' on the life plan or as something that (if carried out) thwarts dispositional autonomy. Young stresses first of all that paternalistic interventions are 'instruments of last resort,' and then he argues that voluntary euthanasia is usually sought by those with 'incurable conditions':

> Generally speaking, their state of suffering requires them to make their request in advance by way of a "living will." . . . Such persons clearly have concluded quite reasonably that the fulfilment of further aspects of their life plan is now out of the question. Death for them would be a benefit. In acceding to their request for voluntary euthanasia, we preclude no significant future choices.[133]

Young holds that the 'informed voluntary consent' of advance directives or living wills which register a preference for voluntary euthanasia help ascertain a person's preparedness to *follow through* with his (or her) declared preference (my emphasis).[134] On Young's view, a decision made in conditions where death is not so clearly a benefit may be more problematic.

On Young's account there are inner as well as external obstacles to autonomy:

> One can fail to be autonomous because of one's inner fears, because one cannot violate norms one has internalised, because one allows elements in one's nature which will not admit of denial to be thwarted, because of lack of knowledge or awareness of one's motivations, or because of lack of self-control, just as one can fail because of systematic bullying or physical enslavement.[135]

Again, the focus for Young, is not on the development of desires but on the 'following through' of a plan: 'autonomy may on occasion be forsaken, not because of the dynamics of the unconscious, but for the want of the courage, honesty or effort of will by a person to forge his (or her) life into a life of his own.'[136] And, it is 'the will which holds the key' to 'opening the way for the exercise of autonomy' in the weak-willed person. Young distinguishes compulsiveness from weakness of will by claiming that the weak willed person 'could have done otherwise.' The weak-willed person is free but weak, whereas the compulsive is unfree in the sense that he does not have the capacity to 'have done otherwise.'[137] For Young, the idea of 'following through' puts the emphasis on prospective action rather than retrospective hypothetical assessment.

The emphasis on prospective action suggests that Young's account will be useful in the clinical context. As well as being a descriptive psychological account of autonomy, it may give action guidance in the sense that it can tell us what choices or actions are consistent with autonomy and should be respected (that is if we value autonomy). Young is concerned with the effect that a lack of 'inner coherence' or 'inner unity' has on autonomy. He thinks these effects are not always recognized. According to Young, a person has no 'unified life' in the 'fairly weak sense that is bound up with autonomy,' when the self is divided over which projects to engage in, or over the order in which to engage in them. Disarray results when someone fails to pursue 'what he would acknowledge to be more significant and more authentically "him" (or "her"). The person in truth identifies with the desire he (or she) sees as more important but lets other, lesser desires get in the way.'[138] In some cases new goals interfere with the completion of earlier goals but for

Young this is not incompatible with autonomy. This merely signifies an 'altered conception' of the life plan.[139] Choices or actions which seem out of kilter with what has gone before do not necessarily lack autonomy on Young's view, but, it is not clear how we can judge this and Young does not provide us with criteria for doing so.

To summarize, Young's account is useful in the clinical context in relatively straightforward situations. When things are more complicated it may not be so useful.

The Authentic-Self Account of Autonomy

Diana Meyers account of autonomy is most definitely a descriptive psychological account although she calls it a 'procedural account of personal autonomy.' She uses the term 'procedural' to indicate the 'way in which people arrive at [decisions].'[140] This involves the idea of 'autonomy competency':

> Autonomous people 'must be disposed to consult their selves, and they must be equipped to do so. . . . They must be able to 'pose and answer the question "What do I really want, need, care about, value etcetera?"; they must be able to act on the answer; and they must be able to correct themselves when they get the answer wrong.'[141]

On the idea of 'autonomy competency,' Meyers' account of autonomy is said to be the 'definitive' work.[142]

Meyers claims that her account has an additional component which hierarchical accounts of autonomy lack. This is a form of 'self-mastery' or 'self-regulation' which she calls 'self-definition.' Hierarchical accounts of autonomy require doing what we 'really' want or living in harmony with our 'true' or 'authentic' selves and that involves 'self-discovery' and 'self-direction.' She claims that the skills needed by higher-order theories: 'autobiographical retrospection, detection and reconciliation of conflicts within the self, and identification with preferred components of the self' are amongst the skills needed for 'autonomy competency' but that is not enough. It does not include the ability to 'institute changes' in accordance with our true selves.[143] According to Meyers: 'Whether or not a person is autonomous depends on whether or not the person possesses and successfully uses the skills comprised by the competency of autonomy.'[144]

Meyers' notion of self-definition is about more than just exercising a capacity.[145] She emphasizes the idea that self-definition is a 'reciprocal and dynamic process' which involves life plans and an evolving self-concept or 'true self.'[146] And she claims that the 'core of the concept of personal autonomy is the concept of an individual living in harmony with his or her authentic self.'[147]

Meyers' account of autonomy is a very demanding one. In terms of the examples she uses, her account certainly has something to say about autonomous living as an ideal but in a practical context such as the medical setting it may not be so useful. Meyers lists some of the things which lead us to distinguish an autonomous person from a person who lacks autonomy. She claims that we attribute autonomy in relation to 'the spirit in which' a person lives and the 'the way in which' that person makes decisions. The autonomous person 'demands much of life' and 'expects fulfillment, not merely success as it is conventionally understood.'[148] Here Meyers seems to be imposing her ideas of a good life on the notion of autonomy. Surely I could autonomously choose to pursue success rather than fulfillment.

For Meyers, a 'central feature of autonomous living' is 'episodic' and 'programmatic' self-direction:

> Autonomous episodic self-direction occurs when a person confronts a situation, asks what he or she can do with respect to it—the options may include withdrawing from it as well as participating in it in various ways—and what he or she really wants to do with respect to it, and then executes the decision this deliberation yields. Autonomous programmatic self-direction has a broad sweep. Instead of posing the question "What do I really want to do now?" this form of autonomy addresses a question like "How do I really want to live my life?" To answer this latter question, people must consider what qualities they want to have, what sorts of interpersonal relations they want to be involved in, what talents they want to develop, what interests they want to pursue, what goals they want to achieve, and so forth.[149]

According to Meyers, the decisions and ideas involved in the programmatic self-direction process add up to a life plan. A life plan is a 'largely schematic, partially articulated vision of a worthwhile life that is suitable for a particular individual.'[150] When formulated in accordance with a person's capabilities, inclinations, and feelings and there has been no coercive external pressures, life plans are autonomous.[151] According to Meyers, 'programatically autonomous people have autonomous life plans.'[152]

Meyers argues that a person's life plan can be violated without it being the case that the person has acted heteronomously. The reason for this is that the true self is in transition and some actions can be autonomous expressions of the 'evolving self.'[153] The exercise of 'autonomy competency' according to Meyers is: 'an ongoing sensitivity to one's self and a willingness coupled with an ability to deal with symptoms of discord within one's self.' It can also be exercized retrospectively in the sense that a person can certify conduct as autonomous by interpreting an unexpected outcome in terms of a revised life plan or a revised understanding of the self.[154]

According to Meyers' account it seems that just about anything could be interpreted as an autonomous action. The dynamic nature together with the possibility of frequent revisions of the self and of life plans means that it is not clear how autonomous action can be distinguished from heteronomous action. But Meyers does give some guidance about what a nonautonomous person and a nonautonomous choice is like.

Unwillingness or inability to 'reshape one's plans' indicates a lack of autonomy according to Meyers.[155] She claims that 'whether or not a person is autonomous or not depends on whether or not the person possesses and successfully uses the skills comprised by the competency of autonomy' and '[w]hether episodic or programmatic, what makes the difference between autonomous and heteronomous decisions is the way in which people arrive at them—the procedures they follow or fail to follow.'[156] Presumably, therefore, a lack of sensitivity to self and an inability to deal with discord in one's self indicates a lack of autonomy.

Meyers questions whether anyone can be autonomous without a life plan. However, she also claims that life plans can be alien if they are not 'selected autonomously' and not reconsidered. Life plans can be alien in the sense that they are imposed by others or adopted in deference to others. They are also alien if they are simply a demonstration of 'automatic conformity to popular conventions.' Although Meyers claims that life plans 'seem to be indispensable to autonomy,' she also argues that acting in accordance with a life plan that is alien implies nothing about autonomy.[157] Meyers also suggests that acting with an alien life plan is an indication of heteronomy.[158]

The apparent stringency of Meyers' account creates difficulties for the clinical context. In a different context—that of career choices—she tells us about Martin who chooses his life plan in deference to his parents. By the age of forty, Martin is a respected and wealthy surgeon but he has chosen medicine as a career simply because his parents expected it and he was taught to feel guilty if he did not meet his parent's expectations. On Meyers' view there is nothing to indicate that Martin is autonomous despite his outward success.[159] In fact, she claims that Martin's 'unwillingness' and 'inability' to reconsider his plans demonstrates his lack of autonomy. While Meyers claims that Martin is not autonomous, it is only in relation to his decision to become a doctor that she judges him not autonomous. She argues that his lack of autonomy in this area does not mean that he is in 'no way autonomous.' According to Meyers, Martin could make 'episodically' autonomous' medical decisions and he could even make 'episodic' autonomous decisions within his profession.[160] Meyers' account has greater difficulties, however, when a medical decision originates in what Meyers suggests is an alien life plan. Suppose a woman rejects mastectomy because she is worried about her partner's reactions. Would Meyers say she is nonautonomous because she is living her life in deference to others or that her decision can be overridden because it is not a reflection of her authentic self and therefore not an autonomous decision? Meyers may be able to get around this by claiming that the plan is not alien and the decision is a result of the reciprocal dynamic relationship between an evolving self and a revised plan. The problem is that it all becomes quite arbitrary and we lose any basis for judging what is autonomous and what is not autonomous.

Psychological Accounts That Are Functional

Jay Katz, Benjamin Levi, and Richard Lindley have descriptive psychological accounts of autonomy which are worth considering separately although they are not a separate category of descriptive psychological account.[161] My interest here is in the functional or practical nature of the views they put forward rather than which category of psychological autonomy their views fit. Although the views of these writers can be categorized as hierarchical in nature they each express doubt or uneasiness about the practicality of a hierarchical account[162] and Katz and Levi are more concerned with *respecting* patient autonomy than with the question 'What is autonomy?'

Katz's book *The Silent World of Doctor and Patient* was written before Dworkin's book on autonomy but Katz refers to one of Dworkin's early essays that later becomes a chapter in Dworkin's book.[163] Katz rejects an aspect of Dworkin's account that he interprets as 'artificial restrictions to conduct regulated primarily by reason.' He claims that traditional accounts of autonomy involve a number of psychological assumptions which require consideration, but go largely unacknowledged: 'In contrast to other definitions of psychological autonomy, mine is not solely "linked . . . to those higher forms of consciousness that are distinctive of human potential."'[164] Despite this comment, there seems to be no major inconsistency between the views of Katz and Dworkin.

Levi seems for the most part to endorse what Dworkin says,[165] but he has reservations about the decision-making process in hierarchical accounts. He asks: 'how can we tell whether the [higher-order desire] that endorses the [lower-order desire] is itself authentic, such that the identification is constitutive of autonomous decision-making. . . . How do we really decide what counts as a good or better reason?' According to Levi, decision making is 'mysterious' and 'we should be cautious of arrogant presumptions that we can qualitatively distinguish the various influences that generate a decision, much less an autonomous decision.'[166]

In *The Silent World of Doctor and Patient* Katz argues for a 'functional' or 'comprehensive' account of autonomy. This illustrates the way in which a psychological hierarchical account of autonomy can function in the clinical context—but Katz's purpose is not to defend or address problems with a hierarchical account of autonomy.[167] According to Katz, a 'functional' definition of autonomy should include recognition of unconscious motivational forces on behavior and an awareness of rational and irrational influences that play a part in decision making.[168] He argues that we need to recognize that some forces which influence decisions are not introspectively accessible and that in order to become 'freer' we need to acknowledge or at least appreciate the influence of these forces.[169]

What is the nature of the forces referred to by Katz? Irrational determinants, which Katz regards as a complication for traditional accounts of autonomy include the impact of unconscious impulses, fantasies, timelessness, and confusion of past and present realities, unmodulated emotions, unattainable and infantile conceptions, and disregard of facts. Another set of 'irrationalities' manifests itself in patients' 'overevaluation of the physician as an omnipotent healer' and physicians' 'underevaluation of the patient as a competent adult.'[170] These things, as well as ignorance, misconceptions, exaggerated fears, and magical hopes about diagnostic tests and therapeutic interventions are forces that can influence decisions.[171]

Katz is not suggesting that autonomous decision making needs to be free of unconscious influences or completely rational. He claims that this is neither possible nor desirable[172] and argues that although patients' decisions seem to be based on nonrational grounds we can lessen the impact of irrational and unconscious forces.

Katz claims that psychological autonomy is an ideal and argues that while human psychological capacities for autonomy are limited, awareness of influences that impinge on it can be significantly improved. In other words, autonomy can be promoted and enhanced through self-reflection and conversation with others.[173] He says that John Stuart Mill anticipates his views on the need for conversation and he uses Mill in support of the case for the imposition of dialogue:

> [Mill] eloquently argued that his "principle"—that "the sole end for which mankind are warranted, individually or collectively, in interfering with the liberty of action of any of their number, is self-protection"—is misunderstood if it is interpreted to require "selfish indifference, which pretends that human beings have no business with each other's conduct in life." He most insistently asserted instead that "[c]onsiderations to aid his judgment, exhortations to strengthen his will, may be offered to him, even obtruded on him, by others." Only after such an enforced conversation must individual men and women be allowed to be "the final judge," since "they have means of knowledge [about their feelings and circumstances] immeasurably surpassing those that can be possessed by anyone else."[174]

For Katz, the role of conversation (self-reflection and reflection with others) is not meant to go so deep as to unravel the roots of psychological motivations or analyze irrationalities. Instead, the role of conversation or what he sometimes calls the 'imposition of dialogue'[175] is to clarify misconceptions and misunderstandings.[176] This obligation to converse involves both physicians and patients and includes an awareness of the irrationality that physicians bring to decision making as well.[177]

Katz view fits the clinical context in the sense that it incorporates the obligation of health care providers to provide information. Assuming that conversation involves patients asking or being prompted to ask questions and physicians answering truthfully, conversation delivers the awareness of relevant information required by patients for making decisions:

> In conversation with one another, patients may uncover mistaken notions about their diseases and their treatment that they have held for a long time or have recently acquired through misunderstanding the import of their doctors' recommendations. Physicians may uncover the fact that their unconscious preferences and biases compelled patients to yield to their recommendations even though consciously they had intended otherwise. Without conversation, individual self-determination can become compromised by condemning physicians and patients to the isolation of solitary decision-making.[178]

Katz argues that 'the practice of medicine is beset by great uncertainty'[179] and 'the denial of uncertainty, the proclivity to substitute certainty for uncertainty, is one of the most remarkable human psychological traits. It is both adaptive and maladaptive, and therefore both guides and misguides.' There is a pervasive human need to give coherence to the world and we will even falsify data to fill in the gaps.[180] According to Katz, the uncertainty about available knowledge can be specified and:

> it may turn out that an acknowledgment of uncertainty will enhance physicians' therapeutic effectiveness, because it demonstrates honesty in the face of uncertainty and a willingness to be more engaged with their patients than is possible when communications are beset by evasions, half truths, and even lies.[181]

How does this tie in with the way in which a hierarchical account of autonomy can function in the clinical context? The extra reflection brought on by conversation gets patients to go 'second order' in their decisions. Katz 'functional' account is a descriptive psychological hierarchical account of autonomy which gives a role to conversation or dialogue as a practical aid for promoting or enhancing autonomy.

Katz thinks that the obligation to converse 'introduces an element of paternalism' but by making a distinction between *reflection* and *choice* he claims that 'it must also be recognised that [his] views about psychological autonomy and its accompanying obligations to reflect and converse seek to avoid paternalism and to strengthen patient self-determinism.'[182] According to Katz, '*choices* deserve to be honoured' unless there is 'substantial evidence of incompetence,' but *reflection* 'deserves to be treated differently.'[183] Katz uses conversation to promote what seems to amount to critical reflection and procedural independence, as referred to by Dworkin but gives ultimate weight to a patient's choice. In other words, unless a choice clearly lacks autonomy we should respect it and not override it—but considerations to aid judgment, exhortations to strengthen [the] will, may be offered, even obtruded.

Katz provides an example of how his functional account works. In a discussion of what he considers a '*rare* situation' when a patient's choice should not be respected, he describes exchanges between Mr. D (a patient who refuses routine diagnostic procedures), a psychiatric consultant, and a bioethicist. Katz tells us that unlike the bioethicist who supported Mr. D's choice, he 'might not have deferred to [the patient's] wishes'[184] He adds that he may have gone forward with the tests if the patient was unwilling to give reasons for the refusal.

Mr. D was a 'previously healthy sixty-six-year-old black man who had come to the emergency room suffering from an acute febrile illness of three day's duration.' He seemed critically ill and a chest X-ray showed that he had pneumonia. He was treated aggressively with antibiotics but his condition worsened. Mr. D's physicians wanted to do two 'uncomfortable but relatively routine diagnostic procedures' which they thought might establish the cause of his illness but Mr. D refused permission and when the physicians tried to explain the necessity of the procedures Mr. D became increasingly angry and agitated and began refusing even blood tests and X-rays. He deteriorated to the point where he seemed to be near death. During this time, the bioethicist conducted two forty-five-minute interviews with Mr. D. He asked Mr. D if he came to the hospital to be helped and Mr. D replied: 'I want to be helped. I want you to treat me with whatever medicine you think I need. I don't want any more tests and I don't want the breathing machine.'[185]

According to Katz, there was 'something incomprehensible' about Mr. D's wishes that 'begged for clarification' and Katz questions whether, without that clarification, we can really judge the state of Mr. D's autonomy. The psychiatric consultant considered Mr. D competent and aware of the 'gravity of his situation' but Katz thinks that there was a conflict between Mr. D's '"autonomous" wish to be cured and his "autonomous" refusal to undergo diagnostic tests'—and which deserves respect is not clear. Katz tells us what he would do instead of deferring to Mr. D's refusal:

> I would have impressed on him the necessity of our talking together. Indeed, I would have insisted . . . in order to clarify our respective positions. I would have promised him that I had every intention of ultimately respecting his wishes, but that I could not make an absolute promise to do so, for it could turn out that the acuteness and seriousness of his condition might require an intervention prior to our having made ourselves understood to one another. I would have added that I expected it to be an unlikely outcome, but that it could happen. . . . If in the midst of our talking together, Mr. D had "turned away." And bid me to "leave [him] alone," I would not have left his bedside. . . . I would have stayed with him and renewed my invitation to talk with one another. Had he continued to decline the invitation, I would eventually have been forced to tell him that I might very well order the tests, place him on a respirator, and resuscitate him if he refused to talk with me. "There is too much that we both do not understand," I would have added, "and you must not hide behind silence."[186]

The crucial thing for Katz is that the account of the interviews between Mr. D and the bioethicist and the psychiatrist 'are devoid of any data as to why Mr. D was so adamant in his refusal.' Katz says he would consider overruling a patient's choice when two conditions hold: 'One, the consequences of nonintervention pose grave risks to a patient's immediate physical condition *and* two, the process of thinking about choices is so seriously impaired that neither physician nor patient seem to know what one or both wish to convey to the other.'[187] Both of these conditions apply in the case of Mr. D.

The first condition Katz notes is necessary but not decisive. If he had intervened it would have been because he had no idea why Mr. D had decided what he did, not because he thought his decision was unwise or foolish. He adds that if Mr. D had refused tests on religious grounds because he was a Jehovah's Witness, he would 'still have talked with him but readily accepted his decision.'[188] Katz concludes that it is inevitable that there will be flaws in disclosure and consent but that 'should not lead to the imposition or acceptance of silence.'[189]

Benjamin Levi also has a functional psychological account of autonomy. Levi's concept of autonomy is presented in the context of a discussion about respecting patient autonomy and involves the idea of 'dialogue.' According to Levi, dialogue is a practical means for respecting patient autonomy.[190] He notes that there is a tendency for the term *'dialogue'* to be used interchangeably with *'conversation* or even *talk'* but suggests that dialogue is 'something special' in the sense that it is a kind of 'relation that we enter into' and it requires 'commitment and attention.'[191] Nevertheless, Levi's notion of dialogue seems to have much in common with the role Katz gives to conversation. Levi reminds us that it is unrealistic to think all situations in the medical setting lend themselves to full-fledged dialogue: 'philosophical discussions usually do not break out during the transition stage of labor or on the way to a cardiac arrest . . .'[192] but he points out that dialogue can promote autonomy and 'sometimes dialogue will prove useful in discerning whether a patient is in fact autonomous.'[193] According to Levi:

> dialogue encourages us to rethink our understandings of ourselves and our practices and has the potential to create greater meanings in our activities, relationships, and lives in general. Moreover, it has the potential to challenge and transcend the barriers that impede inquiry and communication and, ultimately, the resolution of conflict. . . . Dialogue keeps us on our toes, so to speak, by encouraging us to question ourselves and our understanding of the world.'[194]

In terms of a psychological account of autonomy, both Katz and Levi seem to be adopting Mill's view:

> If the cultivation of the understanding consists in one thing more than in another, it is surely in learning the grounds of one's own opinions. . . . He who knows only his own side of the case, knows little of [truth]. His reasons may be good and no one may have been able to refute them. But if he is equally

> unable to refute the reasons of the opposite side; if he does not so much as know what they are, he has no ground for preferring either opinion. The rational position for him would be suspicion of judgment, and unless he contents himself with that, he is either led by authority, or adopts, like the generality of the world, the side to which he feels most inclination.[195]

Richard Lindley also has a functional aspect in his account[196] and also quotes Mill to support his view—the Millian view which regards 'passion for truth as a good in itself, as a constituent element of autonomy' apart form any instrumental value it may have.[197] Lindley talks about 'theoretical rationality' and claims that 'full theoretical rationality requires a disposition to seek the truth, to ensure that one's beliefs are not false.' He calls this 'active theoretical rationality'—meaning an interest in or a commitment to truth. He says it is not meant to be a Cartesian quest for the foundation of beliefs but 'a disposition to question received wisdom' or 'any proposition one is inclined to accept; not just because this is a sound policy for realising one's goals, but out of concern for truth itself.'[198] According to Lindley autonomy requires more than rationally pursuing goals; it also requires that people not be 'deluded about the nature of their goals and the consequences of their actions.'[199] Lindley argues, following Mill, that the 'best defence against error' requires that one 'not only have good reasons for one's own opinion, but also give proper consideration to rival opinions':[200]

> He must know them [the opposing views] in their most plausible and persuasive form; he must feel the whole force of the difficulty which the true view of the subject has to encounter and dispose of; else he will never really possess himself of the portion of truth which meets and removes that difficulty.[201]

In this chapter I have categorized psychological accounts of autonomy as mainly hierarchical, historical, life plan, or authentic self accounts. In the chapter that follows I will use some challenging cases to test these accounts. The functional and practical nature of the accounts will figure in my discussion as well as in the improved version I propose for the clinical context.

NOTES

1. Richard Lindley, *Autonomy*, 66–67. Lindley's account involves a conception of rationality that is expressed loosely as 'do as well as you can' and the notion of higher-order preferences. Therefore, to be autonomous, a person's will 'must be as he wants it to be' and that 'must be in accordance with what he judges to be best.'

Lawrence Haworth, *Autonomy: An Essay in Philosophical Psychology and Ethics* (New Haven: Yale University Press, 1986), 3. Haworth acknowledges the influence of Dworkin and Frankfurt on his account of autonomy.

2. Frankfurt, "Freedom of the Will," 64.
3. Dworkin, *The Theory and Practice of Autonomy*, 19.
4. Dworkin, *The Theory and Practice of Autonomy*, 20.
5. Dworkin, *The Theory and Practice of Autonomy*, 18.
6. Dworkin, *The Theory and Practice of Autonomy*, 29.
7. Dworkin, *The Theory and Practice of Autonomy*, 108.
8. Dworkin, *The Theory and Practice of Autonomy*, 19.
9. Dworkin, *The Theory and Practice of Autonomy*, 20.
10. Gerald Dworkin, review of *Liberation from Self: A Theory of Personal Autonomy* by Bernard Berofsky, *Journal of Philosophy* XCIV, no.5 (May 1997): 214.
11. Dworkin, *The Theory and Practice of Autonomy*, 21.
12. Dworkin, *The Theory and Practice of Autonomy*, 29.
13. Dworkin, *The Theory and Practice of Autonomy*, 23.
14. Dworkin, *The Theory and Practice of Autonomy*, 129.
15. Dworkin, *The Theory and Practice of Autonomy*, 129.
16. Dworkin, *The Theory and Practice of Autonomy*, 22.
17. Dworkin, *The Theory and Practice of Autonomy*, 23.
18. Dworkin, *The Theory and Practice of Autonomy*, 23.
19. Dworkin, *The Theory and Practice of Autonomy*, 30.
20. Dworkin, *The Theory and Practice of Autonomy*, 111.
21. Dworkin, *The Theory and Practice of Autonomy*, 29, 109.
22. Dworkin, *The Theory and Practice of Autonomy*, 29.
23. Dworkin, *The Theory and Practice of Autonomy*, 108.
24. Dworkin, Review of *Liberation from Self*, 215.
25. If we value autonomy highly (a separate issue) the reason for respecting the Witness's wishes can be explained in terms of a descriptive psychological view.
26. Dworkin, Review of *Liberation from Self*, 215.
27. Dworkin, *The Theory and Practice of Autonomy*, 15–23; see also Christman, *The Inner Citadel*, 6–11; Irving Thalberg, "Hierarchical Analyses of Unfree Action," in *The Inner Citadel*, ed. J. Christman, 123–36; Marilyn Friedman, "Autonomy and the Split-Level Self," *Southern Journal of Philosophy* 24, no. 1 (1986); Jay Katz, *The Silent World of Doctor and Patient* (London: Collier, Macmillan Publishers, 1984); Benjamin H. Levi, *Respecting Patient Autonomy* (Urbana, University of Illinois Press, 1999); Richard Lindley, *Autonomy* (London: Macmillan, 1986).
28. John Christman, "Autonomy and Personal History," *Canadian Journal of Philosophy* 21, no. 1 (March 1991): 2, 4–5.
29. John Christman, "Defending Historical Autonomy: A Reply to Professor Mele," *Canadian Journal of Philosophy* 23, no.2 (June 1993): 281.
30. Christman, "Autonomy and Personal History," 10.
31. Christman, "Autonomy and Personal History," 10–11.

32. Christman, "Autonomy and Personal History," 21.
33. Christman, "Autonomy and Personal History," 14.
34. Christman, "Autonomy and Personal History," 14–15.
35. Christman, "Autonomy and Personal History," 14, referring to Richard Brandt, *A Theory of the Good and the Right* (Oxford: Oxford University Press 1979), 72ff.
36. Brandt, *A Theory of the Good and the Right*, 72–73.
37. Christman, "Autonomy and Personal History," 15.
38. Christman, "Autonomy and Personal History," 12.
39. Christman, "Autonomy and Personal History," 15.
40. Christman, "Autonomy and Personal History," 17.
41. Christman, "Autonomy and Personal History," 17, 11–12, and 12n20. Christman notes that his notion of transparency may be resisted by those who are influenced by Freudian theories, who believe in the existence of unconscious desires which are not generally transparent to us without undergoing therapy. He claims this is something he does not want to dispute. He says, his 'only claim here' is that '*insofar as* a person's motives are subject to reflective consideration by the agent under normal conditions, she is autonomous. If therapy is necessary to make this possible, then therapy is necessary to make autonomy possible.'
42. Christman, "Autonomy and Personal History," 17.
43. Christman, "Autonomy and Personal History," 18.
44. Christman, "Autonomy and Personal History," 18.
45. Christman, "Autonomy and Personal History," 19.
46. Christman, "Autonomy and Personal History," 20.
47. Christman, "Autonomy and Personal History," 21.
48. Alfred Mele, "History and Personal Autonomy," *Canadian Journal of Philosophy* 23, no.2 (June 1993): 272; Christman, "Defending Historical Autonomy," 282.
49. Christman, "Defending Historical Autonomy," 288.
50. Christman, "Defending Historical Autonomy," 284, 289.
51. Christman, "Autonomy and Personal History," 22–23.
52. Alfred R. Mele, *Autonomous Agents: From Self-Control to Autonomy* (New York: Oxford University Press, 1995), 145–260; Alfred Mele, "History and Personal Autonomy," 271–80. Alfred Mele has a 'history-sensitive' account of autonomy. Mele is interested in the place of agents' histories. By way of a thought experiment involving a team of 'new-wave brainwashers' he explains that even though there may be a stretch of time when two agents are 'psychological twins' and equally autonomous or nonautonomous with respect to their desires and values, we would view the brainwashed agent as having her autonomy violated and as being significantly heteronomous. According to Mele, given the psychological similarities of the two agents, the difference in current status regarding psychological autonomy is in how the agents '*came* to have certain psychological features.' One agent was compelled to possess her desires and values and that is something

'external' to the agent's psychological constitution. He argues therefore, that autonomy is in some way 'history bound.'

53. Mele, "History and Personal Autonomy," 275–76.

54. Christman, "Defending Historical Autonomy," 284–87.

55. Christman, "Defending Historical Autonomy," 287.

56. Christman, "Defending Historical Autonomy," 284.

57. I owe this point to Peter Singer (personal communication).

58. Christman, "Defending Historical Autonomy," 286.

59. Christman, "Defending Historical Autonomy," 286.

60. Marina Oshana, "Autonomy Naturalized," *Midwest Studies in Philosophy* xix (1994): 94n40.

61. Shelley E. Taylor and Jonathon D. Brown, "Illusion and Well-Being: A Social Psychological Perspective on Mental Health, *Psychological Bulletin* 103, no. 2 (1988): 193.

62. Christman, "Defending Historical Autonomy," 285.

63. Christman, "Defending Historical Autonomy," 287–88.

64. Christman, "Defending Historical Autonomy," 281.

65. Christman, "Defending Historical Autonomy," 283.

66. Christman, "Defending Historical Autonomy," 2–3.

67. Christman, "Defending Historical Autonomy," 3.

68. Dworkin, review of *Liberation from Self*, 216.

69. Bernard Berofsky, *Liberation from Self: A Theory of Personal Autonomy* (Cambridge: Cambridge University Press, 1995), 9.

70. Berofsky, *Liberation from Self*, 8, 1.

71. Berofsky, *Liberation from Self*, 3.

72. Berofsky, *Liberation from Self*, 212.

73. Berofsky, *Liberation from Self*, 13.

74. Berofsky, *Liberation from Self*, 16.

75. Berofsky, *Liberation from Self*, 16.

76. Berofsky, *Liberation from Self*, 210.

77. Berofsky, *Liberation from Self*, 3, 212.

78. Berofsky, *Liberation from Self*, 213.

79. Berofsky, *Liberation from Self*, 212.

80. Berofsky, *Liberation from Self*, 14.

81. Berofsky, *Liberation from Self*, 190.

82. Berofsky, *Liberation from Self*, 191.

83. Berofsky, *Liberation from Self*, 184.

84. Berofsky, *Liberation from Self*, 117, 255n10.

85. Berofsky, *Liberation from Self*, 184.

86. Berofsky, *Liberation from Self*, 248–49.

87. Dworkin, *The Theory and Practice of Autonomy*, 30.

88. Dworkin, review of *Liberation from Self*, 215.

89. Dworkin, review of *Liberation from Self*, 215.

90. Berofsky, *Liberation from Self*, 183, 1.
91. Berofsky, *Liberation from Self*, 211.
92. Berofsky, *Liberation from Self*, 8, 14.
93. Berofsky, *Liberation from Self*, 212.
94. Berofsky, *Liberation from Self*, 25–26.
95. Berofsky, *Liberation from Self*, 11.
96. Berofsky, *Liberation from Self*, 10.
97. Berofsky, *Liberation from Self*, 11.
98. Berofsky, *Liberation from Self*, 214.
99. Berofsky, *Liberation from Self*, 216.
100. Tomis Kapitan, review of *Liberation From Self* by Bernard Berofsky, *International Philosophy Quarterly* 37, no. 3 (September, 1997): 370.
101. Berofsky, *Liberation from Self*, 2.
102. Berofsky, *Liberation from Self*, 25.
103. Berofsky, *Liberation from Self*, 249.
104. Young, *Personal Autonomy*, 109.
105. Young, *Personal Autonomy*, 5.
106. Young, *Personal Autonomy*, 8.
107. Young, *Personal Autonomy*, 109.
108. Young, *Personal Autonomy*, 34.
109. Young, *Personal Autonomy*, 34, 55.
110. Young, *Personal Autonomy*, 8.
111. Young, *Personal Autonomy*, 14.
112. Young, *Personal Autonomy*, 10, 33.
113. Young, *Personal Autonomy*, 33.
114. Young, *Personal Autonomy*, 33.
115. Young, *Personal Autonomy*, 17.
116. Young, *Personal Autonomy*, 12.
117. Young, *Personal Autonomy*, 12.
118. Young, *Personal Autonomy*, 16–17.
119. Young, *Personal Autonomy*, 16.
120. Julian Savulescu and Richard W. Momeyer, "Should Informed Consent Be Based on Rational Beliefs?" *Journal of Medical Ethics* 23, no. 5 (October 1997): 282–88.
121. Young, *Personal Autonomy*, 6.
122. Young, *Personal Autonomy*, 6.
123. Young, *Personal Autonomy*, 17.
124. Young, *Personal Autonomy*, 39, 16–17, 19.
125. Young, *Personal Autonomy*, 38–39.
126. Young, *Personal Autonomy*, 39.
127. Young, *Personal Autonomy*, 41.
128. Young, *Personal Autonomy*, 109.
129. Young, *Personal Autonomy*, 40.

130. Young, *Personal Autonomy*, 51. Young endorses the Dworkin, Frankfurt view with the 'proviso that it not involve running together the reflective self-evaluation manifested in the formation of second-order desires and the process of making one's desires one's own by identifying with them.' This is in the previous chapter pages 40–42.

131. Young, *Personal Autonomy*, 68.

132. Young, *Personal Autonomy*, 65.

133. Young, *Personal Autonomy*, 78–79.

134. Young, *Personal Autonomy*, 40.

135. Young, *Personal Autonomy*, 49.

136. Young, *Personal Autonomy*, 55.

137. Young, *Personal Autonomy*, 62.

138. Young, *Personal Autonomy*, 56.

139. Young, *Personal Autonomy*, 56.

140. Meyers, *Self, Society and Personal Choice*, 52.

141. Meyers, *Self, Society and Personal Choice*, 52–53.

142. Marilyn Friedman, "Autonomy and Social Relationships," in *Feminists Rethink the Self*, ed. Diana Tietjens Meyers (Colorado: Westview Press, 1997), 59.

143. Meyers, *Self, Society and Personal Choice*, 43–44, 53.

144. Meyers, *Self, Society and Personal Choice*, 53. But Meyers is referring to an older account of Dworkin—that is, a 1976 article. In *The Theory and Practice of Autonomy*, p. 17, Dworkin does include this additional aspect. Dworkin's account involves more than critical reflection. He is also concerned with the actual exercise of autonomy because that is where the reflective procedures of an autonomous person manifest, and that is where we see evidence of, autonomy. To be an autonomous person is: 'to have a certain capacity and exercise it. . . . Autonomy, conceived of as a second-order capacity of persons to reflect critically upon their first-order preferences, desires, wishes, and so forth and the capacity to accept or attempt to change these in light of higher-order preferences and values,' 20.

145. Dworkin's account too is more than just a hierarchical account.

146. Meyers, *Self, Society and Personal Choice*, 45, 51–53.

147. Meyers, *Self, Society and Personal Choice*, 49–50.

148. Meyers, *Self, Society and Personal Choice*, 48.

149. Meyers, *Self, Society and Personal Choice*, 48.

150. Meyers, *Self, Society and Personal Choice*, 51.

151. Meyers, *Self, Society and Personal Choice*, 50–51.

152. Meyers, *Self, Society and Personal Choice*, 49.

153. Meyers, *Self, Society and Personal Choice*, 54.

154. Meyers, *Self, Society and Personal Choice*, 54–55.

155. Meyers, *Self, Society and Personal Choice*, 47.

156. Meyers, *Self, Society and Personal Choice*, 52.

157. Meyers, *Self, Society and Personal Choice*, 50–52.

158. Meyers, *Self, Society and Personal Choice*, 52.

159. Meyers, *Self, Society and Personal Choice*, 46–47.

160. Meyers, *Self, Society and Personal Choice*, 50.

161. Jay Katz, *The Silent World of Doctor and Patient* (London: Collier, Macmillan Publishers, 1984); Benjamin H. Levi, *Respecting Patient Autonomy* (Urbana: University of Illinois Press, 1999); Richard Lindley, *Autonomy*, (London: Macmillan, 1986).

162. Lindley, *Autonomy*, 66–67, argues (in reference to Harry Frankfur's hierarchical account) that a higher order preference is 'not sufficient' for autonomy. He claims: 'For a person's will to be autonomous, it must be as he wants it to be; but it must be in accordance with what he judges to be best.'

163. Gerals Dworkin, "Autonomy and Informed Consent," in *Making Health Care Decisions* (President's Commission for the Study of Ethical Problems in Medicine and Biomedical and Behavioural Research, 1982), 74. This later becomes chapter 7 of Dworkin, *The Theory and Practice of Autonomy*, 121.

164. Katz, *The Silent World of Doctor and Patient*, 121.

165. Levi, *Respecting Patient Autonomy*, 45, 47, 124, 194n11, 195n14.

166. Levi, *Respecting Patient Autonomy*, 45–49.

167. Katz, *The Silent World of Doctor and Patient*, 115. Katz refers to 'traditional notions of autonomy' but not specifically to a 'hierarchical' account.

168. Katz, *The Silent World of Doctor and Patient*, 115.

169. Katz, *The Silent World of Doctor and Patient*, 115.

170. Katz, *The Silent World of Doctor and Patient*, 142.

171. Katz, *The Silent World of Doctor and Patient*, 113.

172. Katz, *The Silent World of Doctor and Patient*, 117–20.

173. Katz, *The Silent World of Doctor and Patient*, 111.

174. Katz, *The Silent World of Doctor and Patient*, 123, quoting Mill, *On Liberty*.

175. Katz, *The Silent World of Doctor and Patient*, 123.

176. Katz, *The Silent World of Doctor and Patient*, 124, 155.

177. Katz, *The Silent World of Doctor and Patient*, 122.

178. Katz, *The Silent World of Doctor and Patient*, 128.

179. Katz, *The Silent World of Doctor and Patient*, 205.

180. Katz, *The Silent World of Doctor and Patient*, 174–75.

181. Katz, *The Silent World of Doctor and Patient*, 193.

182. Katz, *The Silent World of Doctor and Patient*, 128.

183. Katz, *The Silent World of Doctor and Patient*, 113.

184. Katz, *The Silent World of Doctor and Patient*, 157, referring to a case in M. Siegler, "Critical Illness: The Limits of Autonomy," *Hastings Center Report* 12 (October, 1977): 7.

185. Katz, *The Silent World of Doctor and Patient*, 156.

186. Katz, *The Silent World of Doctor and Patient*, 156–59.

187. Katz, *The Silent World of Doctor and Patient*, 157–58.

188. Katz, *The Silent World of Doctor and Patient*, 160.

189. Katz, *The Silent World of Doctor and Patient*, 164.

190. Levi, *Respecting Patient Autonomy*, 177.
191. Levi, *Respecting Patient Autonomy*, 7, 177–78.
192. Levi, *Respecting Patient Autonomy*, 13–14.
193. Levi, *Respecting Patient Autonomy*, 7–9.
194. Levi, *Respecting Patient Autonomy*, 9–10.
195. Mill, *On Liberty*, 31, 32.
196. Lindley's account has been categorized as a hierarchical account of autonomy.
197. Lindley, *Autonomy*, 47.
198. Lindley, *Autonomy*, 48.
199. Lindley, *Autonomy*, 50.
200. Lindley, *Autonomy*, 50–51.
201. Lindley, *Autonomy*, 51, quoting Mill, *On Liberty*.

7

SOME TEST CASES FOR THEORIES OF AUTONOMY

In this section I am going to present some very different sorts of clinical context. I will discuss some situations faced by a person who receives a devastating diagnosis, a question about consent given by a Jehovah's Witness, the case of Mr. M in which it is difficult to make sense of the notion of a true or authentic self, and I will also consider the possible enhancement of autonomy brought about by taking Prozac. I will try to determine what is an autonomous act in these circumstances according to the various descriptive psychological accounts of autonomy. I am not setting out to provide an exhaustive analysis covering every possibility but to provide an illustrative sketch of how each approach would handle these cases. I have chosen the cases in order to provide distinct, but realistic, challenges to each theory and when I have done that I will try to decide which is the best, most defensible psychological account of autonomy.

JEHOVAH'S WITNESSES, QUEENSLAND

In Queensland the Jehovah's Witness church is taking advantage of a state law which allows adults to give legally binding directions on their health care in advance of illness.

Jehovah's Witnesses have been asked to sign a document which forbids doctors and hospitals giving them blood transfusions in an emergency. All

12,000 adult members of the church in Queensland have been sent a twenty-four-page form with key answers already filled in. Members had been told to return the signed forms to their religious elders or risk 'defellowship.'

One Jehovah's Witness said signing it was like 'signing my death warrant.'[1]

On the different psychological accounts of autonomy how can we decide if the decision to sign indicated by the testimony of this Witness is an autonomous one? I will examine the decision to sign in light of the different theories and determine the conditions or requirements that would make the decision an autonomous one according to each theory.

Hierarchical Autonomy

Under what circumstances, for this particular Jehovah's Witness, would the signing of the document be an autonomous decision according to a hierarchical account of autonomy?

The fact that the Witness has made a decision to sign indicates a decision to accept rather than reject the consequences of signing. This suggests that there is second-order reflection or an attitude toward an action or preference which in turn suggests that the choice is a reflective or considered choice rather than a coerced one.

Even though Dworkin's concern is with autonomous persons rather than the notion of autonomous acts, in line with his view we could say that the Witness is autonomous because he is engaging in second-order reflection and he has procedural independence.[2] This means that he is not hypnotized or brainwashed and he critically reflects also on the procedural independence of his decision. In other words, even though the threat of 'defellowship' may appear to be coercive and the Witness may not be entirely happy about signing, he has a higher order desire about the kind of life he wants to lead and he is aware of the competing influences at work in his deliberations.

The decision is autonomous on a hierarchical account in the sense that the Witness is using reflective procedures to shape his life. He understands fully the implications of signing. This means that initially he might have felt alarmed and horrified by the document and his first reaction or first-order desire may have been to tear it up. However, if he critically reflects upon this desire, his commitment to the church, the kind of life he wants to lead, and any influences on his thinking and then signs the document, his decision reflects a 'fundamental commitment' about how he wants to live his life.[3] It also reflects his ability to alter his first-order preferences—the desire to destroy the document. Signing the document is able to meet the requirements of autonomy according to a hierarchical account.[4]

There are some difficulties with the hierarchical view. For instance—how can we identify a first-order desire? And where do the higher and lower order desires start and stop? Instead of viewing the Witness's desire to destroy the document as a first order desire, we could say that the Witness's first-order desire was to sign because he feared 'defellowship.' In that case, a desire to tear up the document is a second-order desire that comes about as a result of critical reflection and reflection on the effect of fear. We could say the Witness wants to tear up the document so as *not* to be ruled by fear. Furthermore, deliberation does not need to stop after two levels of desire. After asking himself how this fits with the way he wants to live his life and the kind of person he wants to be the Witness can have a third-order desire to live as a 'follower of the way.' Unless the Witness speaks explicitly about this, there is nothing to tell us why a particular episode of critical reflection and the acceptance or rejection of a lower order desire is the act that confers autonomy.

The Queensland Witness case also raises the question of coercion. The Witness is not coerced in the sense that he has a gun pointed at his head. His options have been reduced but he still has a choice. Initially he had three options: (1) to remain a member of the church and not sign the document, (2) to remain a member of the church and sign the document, or (3) to leave the church. The threat of defellowship reduces the options to two. We know that his preferred option (1) to remain but not sign is no longer available. Is this coercion and does the threat result in a violation of autonomy?

The answer seems to depend on what caused the Witness to sign. It seems not to be a violation of autonomy if we view the matter in terms of an exclusion policy of an organization and the Witness has critically reflected on his options. He can embrace the church, or he can leave. However, we might feel that he is not signing autonomously if we think he signs because he cannot face the idea of exclusion from his community. It is difficult to know if, and at what point, a reduction in options infringes on autonomy and whether the ease or difficulty in changing some desires makes a difference. Someone might want to argue that a higher degree of commitment to something, such as the Witness's commitment to his church, is more difficult to give up because the higher degree of commitment brings with it a sense that there is more to lose. There is some evidence to suggest that decisions involving a heavy investment of time and emotion are more difficult to change and people can be reluctant to find fault with a plan of action in which they have invested much. Changing a course of action can lead to social disapproval, loss of self-esteem, and to the 'stigma of being known as erratic and unstable.' This creates a 'powerful negative incentive' to adhere to a decision.[5]

On a hierarchical account, autonomy is about the right sort of reflection, and that reflection must not be manipulated or coerced. Commitment and a reduction in options are not incompatible with autonomy if a decision is arrived at freely and backed by reasons. Legal sanctions and the act of promising also restrict our options but they do not limit our autonomy. Dworkin argues that the nature of commitment or loyalty or devotion to a cause may mean that a person is no longer self-sufficient but these values are not inconsistent with autonomy if a person is living the kind of life they want to live.[6] In the case we have been discussing, signing the document is confirmation of the Witness's commitment.

Charges of coercion and infringements on autonomy would be less sustainable if the church had a policy of getting members to sign the form when joining the church—before the threat of defellowship represents a price too high for some to contemplate. Some decisions seem to be incremental in nature with a stepwise increase in commitment locking a person into something they have not made a definite decision about.[7] This stepwise increase in commitment can be compared to techniques of coercive persuasion or brainwashing. Once a person is forced to make some concessions, no matter how trivial, it becomes more difficult to resist further ones.[8] We can argue that this is not what happens to the Queensland Witness. When he comments that signing the document was like 'signing my death warrant' but signs anyway, it seems that he still has a second-order capacity to reflect critically and his decision reflects his commitment to the way he wants to live his life. In arguing that the Queensland Witness is autonomous on a hierarchical account of autonomy we are concerned with determining whether the Witness has the right sort of reflection—that he is critically reflecting upon his first-order desires.

Historical Autonomy

If we are more concerned with the process that led to a particular desire we need to look at a historical account of autonomy rather than a hierarchical account.

If we judge the Witness's decision to sign an autonomous one on a historical account, on what grounds is it autonomous? We saw earlier that an indoctrinated cult member is the paradigm case of a lack of autonomy on a historical account. Nevertheless, it is not impossible for someone to autonomously commit to a religious sect on a historical account. To begin with, the assessment of autonomy is made at the level of preference formation; it is not a question of what it means to be an autonomous person. But like the hierarchical account, the historical account is not meant to be an analysis of autonomous acts. In the case of the Queensland Witness the question of autonomy will depend on how much the person knew about the church before he joined. We need to start by examining this person's preference to be a Jehovah's Witness and the circumstances in which he joined the church. The test for autonomy on a historical account is a hypothetical one. It centers on the idea that the Witness would not have rejected the *development* of his preference, which involves his commitment to the church, if he had reflected upon that.

The signing of the document is autonomous if the Witness had an open mind prior to joining the church and he did not reject his allegiance to the church in light of the processes that gave rise to his allegiance. It is conceivable that he observed the church intimidating people and stifling independent thought while believing that this is the right thing to do. It is plausible that he thinks the church is right to discourage the discussion of critical religious issues because that is an effective way to save wayward souls from being lost and from the tragedy of Armageddon and annihilation. In this way he meets the requirements of the historical condition.

The requirements for minimal rationality and self-awareness are met in the sense that the Jehovah's Witness was not under the influence of manipulating factors affecting his ability to assess the manner in which he came to have his preferences. He is also rational in the occurrent sense if, despite the fact that he refers to the document as a 'death warrant,' he has no manifest conflicts of desire or beliefs which affect his behavior. His readiness to sign is evidence that any uncertainties are subsumed under his otherwise rational plan of action—his preference for the Jehovah's Witness way of life.

Even if we think that, in general, Jehovah's Witnesses' beliefs about blood transfusions are irrational, it does not follow that the decision to sign the document is the product of irrationality or self-deception. There may be inconsistencies in the Jehovah's Witness blood doctrine, but the Jehovah's Witness way of life need not fail the rationality test according to a historical account of autonomy—it can be considered an 'otherwise rational' way to live. Occurrently conflicting desires however, those severe enough to fracture and divide a person, would fail the rationality test. The Queenslander's decision to sign can be viewed as an affirmation of the way he wants to live his life. He may be prepared to accept some inconsistent beliefs. We saw earlier that many Christians hold some apparently inconsistent beliefs, e.g., the idea that God is omnibenevolent and omnipotent but there is evil in the world. On a historical account, according to John Christman, determinations of autonomy are essentially the point of view of the agent.[9] If the Jehovah's Witness has the ability to reflect and to resist the Jehovah's Witness way of life but decides not to, his decision to sign the document is an autonomous one.

It might seem like I have been referring to identification with a desire rather than the formation of a desire, but the formation of the desire can be interpreted as the desire or the decision to be a Jehovah's Witness. In other words, the decision to become a Jehovah's Witness is the process that led to the signing of the document. Someone might want to object that the historical account does not avoid the regress after all. There may be some truth in that but it seems to go back several stages only—not infinitely.

The historical account of autonomy is evaluatively neutral with respect to the content of a person's preferences. Judgments of autonomy are centrally concerned with the *origin* of the desire or preference rather than identification with a particular desire. '*Any* preference,' even 'evil, self sacrificing, or slavish' preferences can be autonomously formed. An agent just needs a '*good reason*' to have such a preference.[10] In the Queensland Witness case our concern is with the manner in which the preference for a way of life has developed. Signing the document can be viewed as a component of a way of life. If we assess the signing of the document in terms of a preference for 'no-blood' treatment we are simply concerning ourselves with a person's identification with a desire—we are not applying the historical test.

In keeping with a historical account, someone may object that if we focus on the apparent conflict the Witness is experiencing, his decision to sign the document lacks autonomy. In referring to the document as his 'death warrant' we are aware that even though the Witness did sign he was not happy to do so. This could be interpreted as a conflict of desires and on a historical account a person who is fractured and divided is not autonomous. Nevertheless we *cannot* conclude from the fact that there is some ambivalence that the Queensland Witness is 'fractured' and divided and lacks autonomy. We need to work out whether the conflict is something that can be reconciled within his overall preferences 'under some otherwise rational plan of action' or if it is something more disruptive which affects his ability to reflect and change. Someone who is thoroughly manipulated, brainwashed, or hypnotized is obviously not autonomous but being ambivalent or mildly conflicted does not rule out autonomy on this account.

We should also recognize the fact that if the other 11,999 members of the Queensland Jehovah's Witness church signed without any conflict at all, the lack of conflict does not mean that we can assume they are autonomous. A historical account alerts us to the fact that the process of desire formation may be corrupt. The other 11,999 members could have been intimidated and indoctrinated to the extent that they believe it is right to reject blood transfusions but they may not have reflected on or autonomously chosen the Jehovah's Witness way of life. If they had been intimidated and indoctrinated they would fail the hypothetical historical test for autonomy because presumably they would resist the process of development if that were attended to.

A historical account of autonomy can overcome Bernard Berofsky's criticism in which he argues that Jehovah's Witnesses are non-autonomous because they are 'rigid' persons who are not responsive to the objective relevant features of the world.[11] In signing the document, the Queensland Witness might seem to be applying principles rather than testing his convictions but that does not mean that he has not autonomously chosen his principles and convictions. Berofsky's critique does, however, raise the question of whether autonomy should be regularly assessed. On a historical account, one of the requirements for autonomy is the ability to assess a preference or commitment from a view outside of the commitment but repeatedly subjecting one's commitments to objective scrutiny in order to defend or revise our preferences is not necessary and would be deemed excessive.[12] Nevertheless, the historical account does not tell us when and in what circumstances it is necessary to reflect upon and reevaluate our preferences.

Life-Plan Autonomy

On the life-plan view of autonomy, we can say that the Queensland Witness's decision to sign is autonomous in the sense that it demonstrates personal integrity or authenticity which is constitutive of the person the Witness wants to be. The signing of the document suggests that the Witness has made a decision to accept rather than reject the commands of the Jehovah's Witness way of life; It is autonomous because the Witness is following through on his life-plan and he seems to be taking steps to advance the more important comprehensive sense of autonomy (dispositional autonomy). His resolute determination to abide by the commands of his religion which he has internalized means that the principles he adheres to are his own. They define the person he chooses to be.

Someone might want to say that signing the document threatens the Witness's dispositional (long-term) autonomy and is therefore not autonomous on a life-plan view. In other words, even if it is agreed that signing the document is in some way autonomous, there are grounds, in terms of a life-plan account of autonomy for overriding the decision.

The proponent of a life-plan view can respond by saying the document facilitates autonomy rather than violates autonomy as it is conceived on this view. Dispositional autonomy (which focuses on a person's life as a whole) is viewed as more important than autonomy of the moment (occurrent autonomy) and the crucial thing on the life-plan view is the 'following through' on a plan or conception relating to a person's life style and dominant pursuits. As mentioned already, it is the 'following through' on dispositional interests, which provides the basis for judgments about autonomy. The document, therefore, will help to 'ascertain a person's preparedness to follow through' on his or her life-plan.[13] It tests the 'genuineness of professed motivations.'[14] What is more, on a life-plan view the document is an advance directive which serves 'to protect individuals against giving in to aberrant (occurrent) desires.'[15]

Signing the document can be viewed as autonomous (on the life-plan view) even when death results. Life in this life is only a preliminary to the eternal life for a Jehovah's Witness. Because the Jehovah's Witness's life-plan does not end with death, we can argue that death is not something that thwarts dispositional autonomy. Robert Young's argument that a life-plan view is compatible with voluntary euthanasia supports the view that death does not thwart dispositional autonomy. The document distributed by the Jehovah's Witness church is similar to a living will containing a request for euthanasia—it sets out circumstances in which 'the fulfilment of further aspects' of a Jehovah's Witness's life-plan are blocked. Given that a blood transfusion amounts to destruction at Armageddon and eternal annihilation, we could say that for the Jehovah's Witness like the person requesting euthanasia, death is a benefit and it does not thwart significant further choices.[16]

The document also gives protection for the Witness in a situation in which his dispositional autonomy may be out of reach. It can be relied on to protect his dispositional interests should he become ill and not able to deliberate or order his thoughts because of pain or distress.

In a life-plan view, advance directives have more weight to some extent than contemporaneous choices. The consent on this kind of document attests to the 'genuineness of professed motivations' and the documentation of preferences helps establish a person's preparedness to follow through with his (or her) declared preference.'[17] Enduring preferences are well catered for on a life-plan view of autonomy.

A difficulty arises for the life-plan view if a person autonomously changes their preferences. The difficulty is that there is no criterion for us to decide whether a decision is autonomous or not. We can see the difficulty if we consider a Jehovah's Witness who finds himself in need of a blood transfusion and changes his mind and accepts the blood. It is not hard to imagine how this kind of life and death situation could bring about an abrupt change in values and preferences. We can imagine him deciding that he wants to continue his life in the here and now despite the threat of Armageddon and defellowship. Or perhaps he might decide that he does not believe in Armageddon; being a Jehovah's Witness might lose its appeal and the idea of defellowship might no longer concern him. On a life-plan account of autonomy, Robert Young argues that a life-plan is not an 'inflexible or unchanging set of goals' and that people 'can and do radically alter the courses of their lives without giving up their autonomy.'[18] Nevertheless, he does not explain adequately how we can distinguish between a changing life-plan and a departure from a life-plan on an exercise of the temporary will. The life-plan account does not indicate how we decide whether the Witness's change of mind *is* or *is not* autonomous.

The Authentic-Self Account of Autonomy

life-plans figure in the authentic-self account as well. The idea of autonomy on this view involves a reciprocal and dynamic relationship between life-plans and an evolving self-concept or 'true self.' Deferring to others or automatic conformity to popular conventions (having an 'alien' life-plan) is heteronomy on this view.[19]

I will begin by sketching out how the decision to sign could be considered autonomous on this view. As we saw earlier, the 'core of the concept of personal autonomy' on Meyers' view is 'the concept of an individual living in harmony with his or her authentic self.' The criteria on which the Witness's decision to sign can be deemed autonomous is that it 'facilitates the harmony autonomy requires' so that after considering his options and signing the document the Witness's conduct is 'congruent with [his] authentic self.' He is adhering to a 'well-wrought' life-plan while 'attending to intermittent needs' to adjust the plan.[20] We can argue that he is autonomous because coupled with the fact that he did sign, his comment that signing was like signing his death warrant is evidence of adherence to a life-plan while having the requisite sensitivity to self and the ability to deal with symptoms of discord.

Following an 'alien' life-plan and an 'unwillingness' and 'inability' to reconsider plans is heteronomy on this account. We could declare the Witness's decision to sign heteronomous if he has chosen his life-plan in deference to others or if his life-plan has been imposed on him by others and if he does not reconsider his plans. He may be suffering from 'the psychic dissonance of persistent and irremediable regrets.'[21] A difficulty with the authentic-self account is that we don't really know whether the remark he makes is an expression of 'psychic dissonance' or an expression of sensitivity to self and successful dealing with the symptoms of discord.

The authentic-self account of autonomy accommodates a change in values and preferences better than the life-plan account. We are able to also judge the Queensland Witness autonomous on the authentic-self account if he changes his mind and accepts the blood. We can see how this works if we look at an example Meyers uses to show that a person can retrospectively certify their conduct autonomous by interpreting an out of character action in terms of a revised life-plan or a revised understanding of the self. Nancy, who takes her leadership qualities to be a part of her authentic self, attends an organizational meeting for her church on a day when she is suffering from a debilitating head cold. Uncharacteristically, she finds herself listening to others and being assigned a subservient role in the group. What is more, she does not resign and she continues to attend the meetings without trying to secure her more accustomed position. According to Meyers we can say that 'Nancy has violated her life-plan, but she has not necessarily acted heteronomously.' The fact that Nancy does not feel disgust and dismay and even finds herself 'relishing the intimacy and camaraderie of behind-the scenes committee work' can be interpreted as a first step to giving up a tendency to dominate others. Meyers claims that Nancy's true self seems to be in transition, it makes no sense to declare her action heteronomous and her action is better characterized as 'an autonomous expression of this evolving self.'[22]

In the same way, on an authentic-self account of autonomy we could say that the Witness who accepts blood has a true self that seems to be in transition and his action is an 'autonomous expression of this evolving self.' He discovers his self is changing and he is 'capable of following this lead.' The authentic-self account of autonomy seems to cater well for this kind of change in values and preferences. A person's conduct can express a true self that is evolving or transforming and being created. Meyers argues that it is the ability to reflect on conduct and determine whether or not this is the way a person really wants to act that distinguishes autonomy from heteronomy. A lack of sensitivity to self with an inability to deal with discord in one's self indicates heteronomy.[23]

Again there is a difficulty. In some situations we are not going to know how to distinguish between a self in transition and heteronomy. The Queensland Witness might change his mind and accept the blood because he has an autonomous change of values—or he may be acting heteronomously. The idea of a reciprocal dynamic relationship between life-plans and the self means that almost anything could be rationalised under the heading of an 'evolving self.' In one sense though this does not matter and we can understand why Meyers' claims 'it would make no sense to declare [Nancy's] action heteronomous.' Similarly, it would make no sense to declare the Witness's action heteronomous. Ultimately, on this account, it is it is up to the Witness to decide how he wants to act and to interpret and deal with the relationship between his life-plan and self concept.

Summing Up

How can we decide which is the best psychological account of autonomy in this case? We want it to give a clear indication whether the signing of the document is or is not autonomous. We also want it to tell us what circumstances would justify overriding the Witness's decision to refuse blood.

Each of the four accounts strongly suggests that the Witness is autonomous. Therefore, if we value autonomy we would respect his wishes. As we have seen, more is revealed about the different accounts if we look at what is required for each to justify overriding the Witness's decision and on the whole, the hierarchical account seems to handle the case best. The hierarchical account clearly distinguishes autonomous from heteronomous decisions. It tells us that we could override the decision if the Witness has been coerced or brainwashed by his church or family with the result that he is unable to reflect on his desires. Nevertheless, autonomy on a hierarchical account does not mean that the Witness cannot choose to be a follower who does all that the church tells him. As long as that is how he decides he wants to live his life he will count as autonomous.[24]

On the historical account we could justify giving him blood if the process that led to his allegiance has been corrupted or if he is fractured and divided because of manifest conflicts of desire. He would be heteronomous if he cannot decide because he wants to reject the blood to avoid Armageddon at the same time that he wants to accept the blood in order to live. By focusing on the process of desire formation leading to the Witness's allegiance to his church, the historical account, compared to the hierarchical account, seems to have additional relevant criteria. Nevertheless, this does not seem to make it any easier for us to distinguish an autonomous decision from a heteronomous one. The historical account includes ideas of minimal rationality relating to past processes and to an agent's current state, conflicting desires and the idea of fractured, divided persons. These ideas are open to various interpretations—we can use or manipulate these ideas in support of a claim that the Witness is autonomous or a claim that the Witness is not autonomous. The additional criteria do not really help. By themselves, they do not give a clear indication whether the signing of the document is autonomous or not autonomous.

The life-plan account has no problems while the Witness is 'following through' on his life-plan or acting on enduring preferences but it is less helpful in distinguishing an autonomous from a heteronomous decision. This view supports the idea that if the Witness departs from or does not follow through on his life-plan we could justify overriding his decision—but would we really want to stop him from accepting blood in a situation where he needs a life-saving blood transfusion and that is what he says he wants? The life-plan account allows autonomous departure from a life-plan but it does not give us criteria to recognize what is autonomous departure from a life-plan and what is heteronomous departure from a life-plan.[25]

The authentic-self account is not terribly helpful either. In order to make the Witness have the blood, we would have to argue that he signed the document in deference to the church and he is unable or unwilling to reconsider his plans. Nevertheless, as we have seen, it is also possible to interpret his decision as an expression of his authentic self. There are also situations, irrespective of what he does, in which it makes no sense to declare him heteronomous.

There is nothing to suggest that proponents of any of these accounts would argue conclusively that the Witness in this particular case is clearly heteronomous. Given the nature of the Witness's beliefs, however, one of the things we are left to wonder about is what work a rationality requirement actually does. We may wonder if proponents of these accounts want ways to say the Jehovah's Witness is autonomous so they do not have to override his decision.

PROZAC

Peter Kramer, who is a professor of psychiatry and the author of *Listening to Prozac*, makes the startling claim that Prozac increases personal autonomy. He claims that it has the ability to make patients 'better than well.'[26]

If behavioral problems are treated as neurologically based, medications or mood altering drugs may be an effective and legitimate way to treat mental disorders which interfere with an individual's autonomy. Some people believe that there are mental disorders which have an organic basis in that they involve an excess or deficiency of certain chemicals. If these disorders are 'deficiency' diseases they are analogous to diabetes and insulin deficiency. On this 'disease' or 'medical' model, drug use seems to be 'acceptable' when the purpose is 'to bring a person's physiological or behavioural function up to medically determined levels.'[27] As well as being socially acceptable, it is considered 'ethically justifiable' to prescribe drugs as long as the aberrant behavior meets the criteria for a medical or psychiatric disorder.[28] A familiar example of this kind is the use of stimulants such as Ritalin for behavioral and attentional problems in children and adults. These kinds of drugs are defended on the basis that they reestablish a normal level of behavioral function. The use of Ritalin, specifically, is defended on the grounds that children with an attention deficit disorder learn better after taking it.[29]

The distinction between therapies that are curative and enhancement therapies seems to mark off what is commonly regarded as ethically acceptable and what Carl Elliott calls 'self-transforming therapies.'[30] As well as Prozac and Ritalin, various types of intervention which alter physical appearance, personality, intelligence, and genetic constitution; characteristics which are bound up with a person's identity can be described as self-transforming therapies. Elliott argues that bioethicists generally regard and differentiate between these identity-transforming therapies according to whether they are considered to be curative or enhancement. Curative interventions such as 'growth hormone for growth-hormone deficiency' and 'gene therapy for metabolic disorder' are acceptable while enhancement interventions such as 'gene therapy for one's looks, or Prozac for shyness' are not. Enhancing or changing one's identity 'is thought to be ethically questionable.'[31]

According to Elliott, however, our concern with what is at stake with self-transforming therapies and the ease with which we shift between the language of identity and illness shows that 'our concepts are contingent'—they could be otherwise.[32] Elliott argues that the distinction between cure and enhancement is difficult to sustain.[33] Our common use of language shows that our identities are tied up with our illnesses. A person who has diabetes is called a diabetic and someone with schizophrenia is called a schizophrenic.

Over time and in different cultures or locations, concepts of identity and illness that seemed fixed do change:

> We used to have a very rich vocabulary, albeit a somewhat backward one. . . . One spoke of dwarves, lunatics, imbeciles, mongoloids—a vocabulary that has now been transformed into one of illness. A person with three copies of chromosome 21 is no longer a mongoloid; she has a genetic disease, Down's syndrome. Whereas we used to think of her as a different type of human being, now we think of her as sick. And of course, we also slide easily in the other direction, from illness to identity. A person who is sexually attracted to others of his own sex is not considered mentally ill, as he once was. Homosexuality is simply part of a person's identity, a constituent part of the way some people are.[34]

Because we move so easily between the province of identity and that of illness, in areas of medicine these shifts of language tend to blur the distinction between cure and enhancement. New technology and the development of new therapies can also alter the boundaries of what constitutes illness. Before the advent of new reproductive techniques, infertility was seen as a 'fact of nature.' Now that it can be treated, it is considered a medical problem. Mental illness now includes phobias, obsessions, compulsions, and personality disorders whereas before the development of psychotherapy mental illness indicated a psychotic disorder.[35]

Kramer's book shows us how psychiatry may come to recognize illness in terms of the drugs that treat them: 'you must have depression because antidepressants work for you.' More specifically, you are depressed 'because your brain has a chemical imbalance—and one proof of that is that Prozac rectifies it.'[36]

People who use drugs, especially mind-altering drugs are generally viewed as the paradigm of the nonautonomous person. Dan Brock describes a popular image of someone who uses drugs for pleasure and claims that the image is probably clearest when we think of a heroin user. The heroin user is addicted, unable to resist the desire for the drug and so much under the control of the drug as to be the paradigm of the nonautonomous person.[37] According to Brock, the empirical facts concerning the consequences of drug use are the basis for the disapproval of pleasure that is produced by drugs. Disapproval comes from the idea that such drug use is bad rather than being based on philosophical issues.

Brock lists the following components as 'part of the good for persons' on any of the usual theories of the good for persons:

1. participation in social relations of friendship, love, and intimacy;
2. development and exercise of certain distinctive human capacities, especially intellectual capacities;
3. being responsible in one's relations to other persons;
4. being an active person, actively participating in a full array of activities and experiences; and
5. being autonomous, at least in the sense of having and exercising the capacity to act in a manner that on reflection one values or most wants to act.[38]

Following Brock, it seems reasonable to suggest that objections to chemical intervention or what Kramer calls 'cosmetic psychopharmacology'[39] are disputes over empirical facts. Furthermore, on the basis of what Brock lists as part of the good for persons it is plausible to argue that Prozac increases autonomy.

Kramer's interest is in the way that Prozac 'goes beyond treating illness.' He does not just sing the praises of Prozac; his book also includes reports of adverse events and risks and he details the way Prozac has been treated in the media. Kramer raises interesting ethical and philosophical questions. The book has become an international best-seller.[40]

Kramer discusses the wider issues such as the idea that biochemistry underpins not just mental illness but temperament as well.[41] He claims that despite all of the attention Prozac has received, the media 'missed the main story' which is about the way Prozac enters 'into our struggle to understand the self.' Prozac is a drug that 'acts on personality.' It transforms longstanding character problems and it 'can induce the sort of widespread change ordinarily brought about by psychotherapy.'[42] Robert Wright supports this view. Wright also argues that Prozac 'isn't the issue' in the Prozac debate. He claims that Prozac:

> is just an emblem for a new age of psychopharmacology in which mental health and mental illness will lose their current meanings. Major depression, minor depression, a dour outlook, occasional moodiness, a short attention span, vocationally costly standoffishness—all these (the scenario goes) will be subject to swift and clean chemical intervention. "Cosmetic pharmacology" will let us custom-build minds and personalities.[43]

There are countervailing claims about the powers and effects of Prozac.[44] Admittedly, Kramer's claims about Prozac's transformative powers apply only to a small number of cases. A minority of people are transformed while most merely recover from their depression.[45] With any treatment however, no one drug is right for everyone. The 'premise' of the Prozac debate, according to Wright, is that 'as the future unfolds, more and more people will have a drug that's right for them.'[46] Wright suggests that the reported gains for patients taking Prozac are indistinguishable from and as legitimate as those gained in psychotherapy: 'although any given drug may have bad effects, and thus be undesirable, any good effects are valid—as valid as if earned arduously by lying on a couch and chatting. Pharmacology is not *inherently* suspect.'[47] According to another commentator, the 'predilection for psychotherapy over psychopharmacology' by the critics of Prozac is 'simply "no pain, no gain" snobbery.'[48]

Raised self-esteem is a frequent effect of Prozac.[49] How does this come about? Prozac raises the level of serotonin insofar as it 'inhibits re-uptake' of serotonin by the brain cells.[50] Neurologists believe that raising the level of serotonin raises self-esteem. According to Wright, there is 'tentative evidence' that the level of serotonin rises when self-esteem increases 'through conventional means—when say, someone gets a promotion or otherwise gains respect at the office.' It is thought that talk-therapists who provide feedback that has a positive effect on self-esteem may be raising the serotonin levels. This is what Prozac does. Talk therapists may argue that any rise in serotonin is incidental—change occurs because the patient has come to believe in himself. Wright asks how we can know which comes first—or if either does.[51]

Wright claims that, in developing its health care plan, the Clinton administration blurred the lines between psychotherapy and pharmacology: 'the very fact that pharmacology works, they have said, is evidence that mental maladies are bona fide, diagnosable diseases, not just vague and elusive discomforts.' Wright then asks how it is that successful chemical treatment is considered 'the hallmark of a disease,' but not everything that is treated by 'cosmetic pharmacology' is considered a disease: ' If pharmacology can make us less impaired, and happier, and if there is indeed nothing wrong with chemical intervention in principle, then what's the problem? Why is this not a cure?'[52]

The information about Prozac given here is derived from Kramer's book. For the purpose of this discussion I will assume that Kramer is right and even if these claims are not true of Prozac we could assume we are talking about a hypothetical mood-altering drug.[53]

It is the positive 'side-effects' that some patients experience in the process of having other symptoms treated that Kramer is interested in. He reports that on Prozac some people are 'transformed'; without distortions of perception they become confident, socially capable and they gain in 'emotional resilience.' These patients do not *just* recover from their depressions and their obsessional disorders, they become what Kramer calls 'better than well.' Prozac changes 'illness and temperament.'[54]

The effects of Prozac are consistent with the components referred to by Brock as what is good for persons. Prozac allows people to participate in and enjoy social relations. It can make patients 'socially attractive' and it lends them courage so that they can participate more fully in life. They can enjoy activities that are both social and productive because they are freed from barriers such as low self-worth, competitiveness, jealousy, or shyness that may have prevented ordinary interactions and activities.[55]

Prozac does not distort perception.[56] Patients seem to have a new 'surety of judgment.' What is more, their judgment seems to be sound. There are no signs of mania or euphoria.[57] On Prozac, one of Kramer's patients reports that she feels 'clearheaded' and she no longer tortures herself with inner conflicts such as wondering if she is being too demanding or too lenient.[58] Prozac also seems to promote better concentration. Because of this, mental or intellectual agility seems to improve.[59] Better critical reflection suggests that autonomy is promoted—at least on accounts of autonomy requiring critical reflection.

Prozac does not seem to have the side effects that accompany other mood-altering drugs such as alcohol, marijuana, heroin, or LSD. It is not addictive and it does not encourage self-absorption.[60] People seem to be less obsessional when they are taking the drug.[61] None of this fits Brock's picture of the drug user.

According to Kramer, Prozac helps us to see what is biologically determined and what is acquired in a person's character—hence the title of his book *Listening to Prozac*. He tells of Sam, an architect, who was cured of a prolonged bout of depression and declared himself 'better than well.' As well as feeling more vitally alive and less pessimistic Sam found his memory became more reliable and his concentration improved. He appeared 'more poised, more thoughtful,' and 'less distracted.' Sam's work also went more smoothly after trying Prozac. In the past he sketched and sketched but now he could complete a project in one draft. He could also now speak at professional gatherings without notes.

Sam experienced another change that was a kind of loss. His interest in pornographic videos had been the cause of great conflict in his marriage. On medication he felt freed of an addiction and less driven. Although he enjoyed sex as much as before, he no longer had any interest in pornographic videos. The attitude he had 'nurtured and defended' now seemed 'not a part of him but an illness.' Prozac seemed to redefine what was 'essential and what contingent about his own personality.' Kramer adds that in seeing the way patients respond to Prozac: 'I had come to see inborn, biologically determined temperament where before I had seen slowly acquired, history-laden character.'[62]

Kramer also refers to the case of Ms. B.

> Ms. B is prescribed Prozac for trichotillomania, a syndrome in which a person cannot help pulling out her own hair. Hair pulling in moderation is a sign of anxiety but the need to pull hair relentlessly, to the point of disfigurement, is recognized as an illness, related to obsessive-compulsive disorder.
>
> Ms. B has another concern: she is unmarried at age thirty-six, despite her 'appropriate, if somewhat strenuous, efforts to meet eligible men.'
>
> On Prozac, Ms. B's hair-pulling diminishes, but so does her feeling of urgency about meeting men. Though still interested in men, she is no longer driven. . . . For the first time in memory she feels perfectly relaxed and happy sitting at home reading books or listening to music and feels less of the free-floating anxiety that was previously quelled by going out. . . . Ms. B does not isolate herself; on the contrary, she now enjoys time spent with people, such as her parents, with whom she argued in the past. She is now more content with life and she considers that maybe marriage isn't in her future—but she feels that is not necessarily bad. She will make her life happy in other ways.[63]

This case is different to many of the Prozac success stories which have led to the concern that Prozac seems to make people 'too social.' Kramer argues that Ms. B's drive—her strenuous social efforts—have been ineffectual and her more 'measured approach' may work better. He makes a distinction between 'driveness' in the sense of 'inner drive' which is a desirable characteristic and 'being driven' which suggests alien forces, neurotic compulsion, and compromised autonomy.[64] Off Prozac, Ms. B bar-hopped in search of men, but on Prozac she was spared the 'pain of social desperation.' Kramer declares that an ethical clinician might have to inform a patient: 'We can diminish your hair pulling, but I must warn you, you may feel more contented.'[65]

Kramer asks: 'Who is Ms. B?' There seems to be two people, one discontented and driven, the other contented and complacent. 'Whose autonomy are we out to preserve?' Kramer thinks that we may intuitively want to say that the 'unmedicated woman has priority.' The idea that Ms. B has been 'opiated into a cocoon' makes us think this way. But then he asks:

> How would we see the matter if we considered her driveness to be the result of a deficiency state—If we believed she "needed" more serotonin in the brain

> the way some people need vitamins or insulin or thyroid hormone? In that case we would associate personhood with the medicated self. How would we understand Ms. B if she were . . . to "discover" on Prozac that her man-chasing had been compulsive?[66]

If, as we become more accustomed to Prozac and similar drugs that help people with mental illness we become comfortable with the idea that these drugs enhance autonomy, then it will be instructive to see how we fit this into our various accounts of autonomy.

Hierarchical Autonomy

The claim that Prozac promotes better concentration and makes people 'clearheaded'[67] suggests that, on a hierarchical conception of autonomy, taking Prozac is consistent with being an autonomous person. However, it is a legitimate question to ask if taking Prozac interferes with a person's capacity for second-order reflection. The answer seems to be no if we think of Ms. B. She is content with her first-order desires but that does not mean that she is 'opiated into a cocoon' by Prozac. We will see this in more detail if we look at Kramer's other patient Sam who clearly has not lost the ability to critically reflect and to have a preference about a preference. Sam loses his interest in pornographic videos and decides that the attitude he had 'nurtured and defended for years now seemed not a part of him but an illness.' He does not accept this change passively however. Sam, is grateful for the relief from his depression, and he believes that the drug distinguishes the 'essential' from the 'contingent' in his personality in the sense that he now believes what he had 'touted' as 'independence of spirit' was in fact a 'biological tic.' Nevertheless, Sam is disconcerted by the fact that what the drug seems to be telling him is what his wife criticizes about him, so any suggestion that he is palliated or under the influence of a psychic anaesthetic is not substantiated—his discomposure prevents us from drawing such a conclusion. Sam continues to rent the videos, 'to save face in the marriage' (something that seems very important to him) and this can be construed as evidence of second-order reflection—according to Sam's value structure.[68]

On a more general level someone might want to argue that the underlying reasons for depression are often situational things such as poverty, being out of work, being oppressed or abused and Prozac simply numbs people to these facts.[69] Prozac might make patients feel cured of their personality disorders, and it may make them feel 'better than well' but it could be interfering with a person's critical capacities and procedural independence in the sense that they stop worrying about the state of their world.

If Prozac is as Kramer describes it, the objection that Prozac numbs the poor and makes people passively accept their world does not seem sound. From what we have seen Prozac seems to makes people better equipped mentally to earn a living.

Nevertheless, David Rothman contrasts Prozac with the sedatives of the 1950s and 1960s and claims that while Prozac may not accommodate people to the monotony and drudgery of their lives nor make them 'comfortable in a setting that should have been uncomfortable' Prozac is a form of social control and he views the cosmetic use of Prozac as medication 'in the service of conformity to social values' and maintains that Prozac emerges in Kramer's book as a 'male-gendered' and a 'quintessentially American' drug enforcing values of aggression and self-seeking ambition. He describes Prozac as an 'office drug' which 'enhances the social skills necessary in a post-industrial, service-oriented economy.' [70]

Again, if Prozac is as Kramer describes it, the objection is not a good one. There is a paradox in asserting that Prozac induces conformity with American values by increasing assertiveness, since, as Kramer objects in turn, 'assertiveness can be in the service of social reform of the sort ordinarily understood as nonconformity or rebellion.'[71]

The concerns about Prozac expressed by Rothman and others[72] pose no problem for a hierarchical account of autonomy. The important thing on a hierarchical account is that a person is leading the kind of life he or she thinks is valuable, is doing what he or she wants to do and arrives at decisions freely, backed by reasons. Autonomy on a hierarchical account is quite compatible with the fact that someone may be taking Prozac.

It is possible on a hierarchical account of autonomy to see some truth to the claim that Prozac can make a person more autonomous. Suppose a person knows that he lacks confidence, has low self-esteem, and retreats from situations that could lead to advancement at work because he finds them difficult and intimidatory, i.e., his first-order desire is to withdraw and his second-order desire is to be in the running with his colleagues for promotion. If Prozac gives him courage enough to participate he has lost his first-order desire to withdraw. On Prozac he still has a second-order desire. He has a second-order desire that he thinks it is better to be the way he is now. In a case like this, it seems that Prozac can even overcome the regress problem of the hierarchical account of autonomy.

Historical Autonomy

The historical account of autonomy is about the processes which lead to a particular desire. This suggests that we need to look at the development of a person's desire to take Prozac or to continue taking Prozac. On a historical account, the idea of 'participation' in the development of the desire to take Prozac is important. In order to declare that person (i.e., the Prozac taker) autonomous we need to know that the individual was in a position to reflect upon and resist the development of the desire but did not.[73] Kramer's patients who willingly take or who ask to be prescribed Prozac seem to be autonomous according to the historical account of autonomy.

Rothman objects that 'listening to Prozac obviates listening to the patient.' This suggests that taking Prozac and a historical account of autonomy are not compatible. Rothman claims that Kramer 'invokes an explanatory model for mental illness that looks to the biology of the species' rather than to the life history of the patient. [74] This objection is not a good one. The doctor should listen to the patient regardless of whether the patient's condition can be explained in terms of biology or life history. What is more, it is plausible to argue that a person who wants to bring about self change, with Prozac as the means, is autonomous.[75] Even though Prozac works directly on a person's biochemistry rather than indirectly, like the practice of psychotherapy which some people may regard as more 'natural,' admirable, and laborious, the decision to take Prozac can still meet the requirements of a historical account of autonomy. If a person is in a position to reflect on and resist the development of the desire to take Prozac but did not resist it we can declare that person autonomous.

According to the historical account of autonomy a person would not count as autonomous if Prozac was put into her drink or fed to her surreptitiously. And she is certainly not autonomous if, like a willing addict, she initially chooses to take Prozac then comes upon new reasons to stop but cannot do so.[76]

The *continued ingestion* of Prozac, however, is consistent with being autonomous according to a historical account if, as Kramer claims, Prozac does not distort perception and seems to give a new surety of judgment—assuming the initial desire to take Prozac was autonomous.

The historical account of autonomy has difficulties where there is no prior state of autonomy. When we make assessments about autonomy it seems that we rely on some kind of natural default position. The idea that Prozac makes us autonomous suggests that the normal state for a lot of people is not autonomous. The historical account seems able to explain cases where there is a loss of autonomy such as the indoctrinated cult member who undergoes a process that we would criticize or reject, but as we shall see, the account has greater difficulties when the loss of autonomy is internal in a person's own make up.

It is not clear what the historical account would say about a situation where someone in a normal psychological state is given Prozac without their knowledge or against their wishes, yet comes to have reason to continue taking Prozac. The point at which the process of desire development begins (from which we make our assessment of autonomy)[77] is not clear. If a person did not want the drug we would probably want to say that the development of the desire begins with that person's reasons for not wanting to take it. But we might also think that the development of the desire begins with a person's newfound reasons to take Prozac. We have seen (by way of the willing addict example) that new reasons to stop taking a drug are considered relevant on the historical account. Suppose one of Kramer's patients was given the drug without their knowledge. We can imagine the development of newfound reasons to take Prozac if the patient says I am now much better off and want to continue taking Prozac. It seems hard to deny that this is not an autonomous decision. However, this creates problems for the historical account because, rather than historical conditions, it seems to be patient's final state and their undamaged sense of judgment that prompts us to say this person is autonomous.

Life-Plan Autonomy

Young describes autonomy as something that 'has to be worked at.'[78] We might want to ask if this means that taking Prozac is not compatible with the life-plan account because Prozac makes autonomy too easy. The point of Young's claim however, is to distinguish autonomy from negative liberty. He is trying to show that autonomy is a more complex issue which concerns people and actions rather than 'freedom from' something. His claim therefore, does not rule out the use of Prozac on the grounds that taking it might make autonomy more effortless.

On a life-plan account, Prozac seems to facilitate autonomy by helping a person follow through on his or her plan of life. We have seen with the example of Kramer's patients that it gives some people the boost needed to thrive in areas of career, lifestyle, and 'dominant pursuits':

> There has always been the occasional patient who seems remarkably restored by one medicine or another, but with Prozac I had seen patient after patient

become, like Sam, 'better than well.' Prozac seemed to give social confidence to the habitually timid, to make the sensitive brash, to lend the introvert the social skills of a salesman. Prozac was transformative for patients in the way an inspirational minister or high-pressure group therapy can be.[79]

The Authentic-Self Account of Autonomy

According to Meyers, autonomy is doing what we really want and that is something that originates in the true or the authentic self which, as noted earlier, can be an evolving self. We are autonomous when we live in harmony with our authentic self. It is plausible therefore, to argue that Prozac promotes autonomy in the sense that it helps a person institute a program of self-change in order to become the persen they really want to be.

Kramer refers to the case of a forty-four-yea- old woman who is not clinically depressed but requests Prozac to help her on her 'down days' when she feels apathetic and unable to complete her usual tasks. After taking Prozac she has more energy, optimism and self-confidence. She claims: 'This is the way I have always wanted to feel.' [80] We might wonder if this is really an authentic response or an euphoric side effect like that which might accompany the mood elevators of abuse. On the other hand, if we accept what Kramer says we could concede that this is her authentic or 'true' self.

According to Kramer, this patient does not meet the criteria for any of the depressive disorders but she appears to have 'a "personality disorder" characterized by dependency and passive aggression.' Psychotherapy was recommended as the more effective treatment but the patient insisted on Prozac. [81] If Prozac is as Kramer says, there is nothing to suggest that taking Prozac robs us of authenticity or prevents us living in harmony with our authentic self.

The critics of Prozac and cosmetic pharmacology suggest that Prozac might preclude authenticity in the sense that it might 'decrease true autonomy' by 'reinforcing dehumanizing cultural expectations such as the requirement always to be happy and productive' even when that is not appropriate. They argue that Prozac distances 'man from an aspect of his humanity—his legitimate despair.'[82]

Kramer responds that rather than robbing people of emotional growth, the 'edifying potential for tragedy' and in turn authenticity, Prozac lends people courage and facilitates participation in a full array of experiences and relationships: 'it catalyzes the precondition for tragedy' he claims. Further to this, he argues that the idea that bad feelings are useful leads to 'ghastly conclusions.' It implies we should ban analgesia and anesthesia and that the downtrodden should be glad of their depression.[83]

Carl Elliott is one of Prozac's critics. He argues that deliberately changing one's personality with Prozac is *inauthentic* because even if it were to give me a 'better' personality, it is not 'my' personality.'[84] This argument does not rule out the idea that (on an authentic-self account of autonomy) someone can autonomously take Prozac. Elliott's argument involves the idea of the self as something that is 'given' or 'static.' In response, David DeGrazia argues that '[A] person can be true to oneself even while transforming and even creating the person one is. One's self is not something merely waiting to be discovered, after all.' DeGrazia acknowledges that Elliott is not embracing the image of a self that is 'given' but claims that his argument about Prozac promotes that idea.[85]

Some people think that psychotherapy rather than chemical intervention is more consistent with the idea of an authentic or 'true' self. David Rothman calls into question the idea that a drug can improve character and suggests that courage gained through understanding is different in quality than courage gained with 'cosmetic psychopharmacology.' He admits there is no way to be certain whether a drug-induced rise in serotonin level could not produce the same results as psychotherapy, but concludes: 'we know we are in the presence of someone who has achieved an authenticity of self in a way that no dose of a pill is likely to achieve,' after reading the memoir of a woman who 'got better' with sixteen months of psychotherapy.[86]

Rothman's observation brings to mind Wright's argument which was referred to earlier—that the gains from taking Prozac are as legitimate as those gained in psychotherapy: 'as valid as if earned arduously by lying on a couch and chatting.'[87] The raising of self-esteem by a talk therapist is not in itself the thing that gets someone a promotion or raises the amount of respect he gets. Prozac and psychotherapy do the same thing; they both convince the patient that he deserves respect. That belief and an apparent rise in serotonin levels may make him more likely to get a promotion and more respect. To the extent that psychotherapy raises a person's self-esteem and their capacity to do what they really want, Prozac does the same. If Prozac is an artificial intervention so is psychotherapy—but they are artificial interventions initially only.[88] Prozac is therefore consistent with the idea of authenticity because it enables a person to do what they really want to do.

It does not present a problem for Meyers' account if someone wants to argue that the claim 'this is the way I always wanted to feel' is not the same as the authentic self. On Meyers' view, the true self is an 'evolving self' and the true self can be in transition.[89] What matters, is that individuals deal with symptoms of discord. Both the woman who insists on Prozac and the contented Ms. B seem to have the autonomy competency that makes the difference between autonomy and heteronomy on Meyers' account. It is plausible to argue that both have an ongoing sensitivity to the self and while neither has symptoms of discord, there is no evidence to suggest that either lacks the ability to deal with discord if it was present. Both appear to be individuals living in harmony with an authentic self.

Summing Up

Taking Prozac seems to be consistent with being autonomous on the hierarchical, life-plan and authentic self accounts of autonomy. Prozac does not interfere with the ability to critically reflect—there is even some suggestion that it aids critical reflection; it helps people follow through on their life-plans; and it is an aid to becoming authentic—taking Prozac helps a person to become the person they want to be. Taking Prozac is also consistent with being autonomous on a historical account as long as the person (were they to understand the process) would not take action to counteract the development of the desire to take Prozac.[90]In order to work out which account is most helpful in distinguishing an autonomous decision from a heteronomous one we also need to consider what would justify intervening in or overriding a person's decision when they are taking Prozac. In particular, we are looking at Prozac's enhancement of autonomy—the situation when a person feels 'better than well.'

As noted previously, things like hypnotic suggestion, deception, coercive persuasion, and subliminal influences affect a person's reflective and critical faculties and rule out autonomy on a hierarchical account. Prozac will not ward off threats to autonomy of this kind. What is more, these influences or threats originate from things outside of the person and have no connection to the fact someone is taking Prozac. On this account being 'better than well' is not something that affects autonomy in any adverse way. In other words, Prozac will not guarantee autonomy, but it is compatible with it.

On a life-plan account of autonomy we are justified in intervening in a person's choice on the grounds of preserving autonomy, e.g., we may intervene to stop a person from 'giving in to aberrant (occurrent) desires.'[91] But, how do we tell if a person taking Prozac is giving into aberrant desires? Perhaps it is more relevant to ask what it would take, on this account, for us to think that someone taking Prozac lacks autonomy. The answer to this is when someone starts to act in ways that depart from a previously held life-plan and which interfere with 'dominant pursuits,' career, and life-style.

These are the pursuits that count in the assessment of autonomy on a life-plan account and they are the pursuits that Prozac promotes. Someone might argue that we are looking in the wrong place and that the thing that led a person to want or need Prozac requires scrutiny. Nevertheless, as we saw earlier, the life-plan account has nothing to say about the development of the desire. We saw this in Robert Young's support for the view that Jehovah's Witnesses imprisoned by the Nazis held on to their integrity and their autonomy:

> It does not matter so much how one came to have one's particular desires, but whether one matches up effective and reflective preferred motivations. . . .[92]
> However dimly we regard the inculcatory processes which led them to internalise the set of values they followed, and however unreasonable their continued adherence to those values may appear to us, in their conduct they clearly made them their own.[93]

This suggests that on a life-plan account of autonomy a person taking Prozac is autonomous. If a person's actions in some way rule out that judgment, it is due to something other than Prozac.

The authentic-self account of autonomy is similar to the life-plan account in the sense that a person taking Prozac seems to be an exemplar of autonomy. And again, it seems that anything that would justify overriding a decision is not connected to the fact that the person is taking Prozac. Added to this there are the situations, as we saw earlier, in which it makes no sense to declare a person heteronomous on an authentic-self account because we do not know how to distinguish between a self in transition and heteronomy. The enhancement of autonomy brought about by Prozac is, on this account, autonomous. There is nothing that compels us or suggests we could say that 'better than well' is not autonomous.

The historical account of autonomy is a bit different in the case of Prozac. Prozac creates a problem for this account. Ultimately, the things that prompt us to say someone is autonomous seem to depend on an individual's final state and the fact that their judgement has not been damaged rather than the process which led to the desire to take Prozac. We think differently about someone taking Prozac and someone taking heroin not because of the process leading to the desire to take the respective drug but because the person taking heroin seems to be under the control of the drug; in a state where he or she is unable to resist the desire for heroin. The person taking Prozac on the other hand is not suffering from this kind of distorted judgment. On Prozac, a person seems better able to act without conflicts of desire.

The difference between a person taking Prozac and a person taking heroin helps illustrate the need for a nonhistorical minimal rationality requirement but the need for the nonhistorical condition raises the question of whether we really need the historical condition—and whether we need the historical account of autonomy. The nonhistorical condition obscures the distinguishing features of this account of autonomy and consequently undermines the usefulness of the historical account in the case of Prozac. Therefore on the grounds that its usefulness is not as a historical account of autonomy, we can rule out this account as a contender for the best psychological account of autonomy when we consider the case of a person taking Prozac.

It is not clear which of the other three accounts of autonomy is the best in this case. There is nothing to suggest that a person cannot be autonomous in deciding to take Prozac on the remaining three accounts. A better question may be to ask how well the accounts explain why a person can be autonomous in taking Prozac and how that might differ from taking, for example, heroin when one is addicted.

The hierarchical account is helpful. It seems unlikely that a person addicted to heroin, when under the influence of the drug or when craving the drug, could critically reflect upon and endorse their first-order desires and the procedural independence of the desire for heroin. Further to this, the hierarchical account shows us that the heroin addicted person lacks autonomy because typically, he or she would not have the ability to alter preferences. If this person had the capacity to alter preferences and to make them effective in action they would count as autonomous—and be seen as having cast off the addiction. Taking Prozac on the other hand is consistent with autonomy. A different sort of reflection (e.g., reflection that is manipulated or coerced) indicates a lack of autonomy. In other words, the hierarchical account seems well able to judge what is an autonomous act. It can differentiate between drugs which affect autonomy and those which do not.

The life-plan account is also helpful. We have seen how a person taking Prozac can demonstrate autonomy on this account; the heroin user though, would surely fail. The addicted heroin user exemplifies the antithesis of 'a life that is unified, orderly, and free from self-defeating conflicts.'[94]

The authentic-self account of autonomy gives us some interesting insights into what can count as autonomy but it is not that useful in distinguishing autonomy from heteronomy. This account lets a Prozac user count as autonomous. We have seen that Prozac is consistent with the idea of authenticity. The difficulty with this account however, is that we cannot distinguish between a self in transition and heteronomy. On this account it makes no sense to say that a person taking Prozac lacks autonomy because the charge of heteronomy can be countered with the claim that the self is an evolving self. This raises the question of whether we should argue that the addicted heroin user is autonomous—a self in transition. We could argue for that but the idea of the addicted heroin user seems incompatible with the authentic self account of autonomy in other ways. Intuitively we are unlikely to think that the addict is an individual living in harmony with his or her authentic self and the addict does not fit the picture of a person with the ability to deal with symptoms of discord. Proponents of the authentic-self account of autonomy are able to argue for autonomy for Prozac users in terms of a self in transition and to argue in terms of a lack of authenticity that addicted heroin users are heteronomous. However, there is a certain arbitrariness that seems to have crept into these judgments. Notions of what counts as a good life may have also crept in—and these ideas are not part of a descriptive psychological account of autonomy.

When we consider the possible enhancement of autonomy brought about by taking Prozac, only the hierarchical account and the life-plan account remain as contenders for the best, most defensible psychological theory of autonomy. The hierarchical account seems to be the best in the sense that it is more responsive. It has reasonably clear, identifiable criteria for judging what is autonomous and what is not.

MR. M

Consider the case of Mr. M, a case discussed by Tony Hope in 'Personality Identity and Psychiatric Illness.'[95] Mr. M is a man who is mildly manic and acts differently in important ways from when he is not manic. He is not cognitively impaired in any significant way and when manic he is not incompetent. His manic state is considered abnormal only because of the existence of an alternative state. In fact, it is really not clear why Mr. M's mildly manic state is regarded as an illness at all. It is equally plausible to suggest that the unmedicated Mr. M is the normal healthy one while the medicated Mr. M is a sufferer of mild depression.

Mr. M (Mania) Case History

> Mr. M was forty-three years old. He is married and has two teenage daughters. He is a schoolteacher in French. He is a tall, thin man with dark hair. His speech comes in rapid slightly jerky sentences. His wife says that he has always

tended to be moody with periods when he seems somewhat depressed and then periods when he is happy and energetic. Until three years ago these swings in mood had not been so marked as to cause concern and have not put strain on the marriage. They appear to have been a happy couple.

Three years ago he experienced what was diagnosed as a manic episode. At home his wife had become concerned because he had been charging ahead with arranging a major new extension to their house which they couldn't afford. He had also bought an expensive car without discussing this with her and he got angry and upset when she did not show the enthusiasm for his purchase which he expected her to feel. At work there had been considerable concern that he was not teaching his students properly. Following a car accident in which no one was hurt but there was some question of his driving unusually fast, he agreed to be seen by a psychiatrist. Manic illness was diagnosed.

He started treatment with lithium carbonate and soon returned to his normal self. Lithium is the standard medication used to reduce the likelihood of another episode of mania. He took lithium for one year following the diagnosis and then stopped taking it. He restarted it on medical advice six months later, came off it again a year later and restarted it again about six months after that. There is a clear relationship between his state and whether or not he is taking lithium. He has never, however, even when off the lithium had another florid manic episode.

When off lithium he feels full of energy. He finds his wife and family boring, and says that the marriage has never been good. He began an affair with a Spanish teacher who is a few years younger than his wife. He says he intends to divorce his wife and marry this person. He says he is more creative when off lithium and he composes songs although none has been published. His colleagues have the impression that his teaching is not as good, because he makes little allowance for the knowledge level of his students. Nevertheless there isn't the concern that there was three years ago. Some colleagues find him more stimulating when he is not taking lithium, but although he seems full of ideas his written output at work is lower. All those who have known him a long time say that he is clearly more irritable off lithium than he used to be and all are concerned for his marriage, because close friends say that he and his wife have always been devoted to each other.

In a letter to his hospital doctor he wrote that since coming off the lithium he felt he had been living a double life, both aspects of which seemed real: one was his life with his wife and children, the other his life with his girlfriend and song-writing. He then went on to write that he feared that the latter was a 'post-lithium high.' Eventually, when off lithium he wants to go back to it.

When he is taking lithium he is somewhat different. He says that his relationship with his girlfriend is superficial and he stops seeing her. He says that he wants to stay with his family and that this has always been important to him. He is less immediately stimulating than when off lithium, but more reliable,

> and in terms of written output, more productive. He denies, when on lithium, that he has ever contemplated leaving his wife, and he dismisses his affair as being of no importance. For a short time, he accepts both his family's and his doctor's advice to stay on lithium, and then he decides to stop, saying that it reduces his creativity.
>
> His girlfriend says that she is confused. Off lithium he seems to care for her, and they have been planning for their marriage. On lithium he virtually ignores her, and behaves as though she is a colleague who has fallen in love with him and is making a nuisance of herself.[96]

This case poses questions as to whether we should respect the treatment decisions of someone who is like Mr. M. Do we respect his wishes when he is manic or when he is depressed—when he is medicated or unmedicated?

Hierarchical Autonomy

On this account there does not seem to be any doubt about the autonomy of Mr. M in either his manic or his depressed state or when he is medicated or unmedicated. He has second order reflection and he uses rational deliberation. Even the influence of medication does not pose a problem because when he takes the lithium he chooses to take it and he still has the right kind of reflection. His reflection is not manipulated or coerced.

We might think that there is a problem when Mr. M is off lithium and starts thinking that he wants to go back to it, or when he is on it and starts thinking about stopping the lithium because he feels that his creativity is being reduced. When this happens, he seems to be at a stage in which he is not leading the kind of life he thinks is worth leading. It is not clear how long he can remain in this state without being deemed *not* autonomous.[97] When he is in this state of unease and discontent we may think that his disorder (bipolar disorder) is affecting his reflective and his critical faculties—not in the sense that his thinking is muddled and he lacks procedural independence, but in the sense that his critical reflection varies. Nevertheless, for most of the time (according to a hierarchical account), Mr. M seems to be the very model of autonomy. He obviously has *second-order reflection* and he demonstrates a capacity to accept or change his preferences and to make them effective in action.[98] Even when Mr. M is off lithium and life with his girlfriend and song writing is his first-order desire, he is able to critically reflect upon this life. When he finds himself with a higher order desire that doubts his first-order desire, he is able to choose to go back on the lithium which takes him back to his wife and children. Back on medication and with his wife and children (now his first-order desire) Mr. M has not lost the ability to critically reflect on the life he is leading. For a time his first- and second-order desires coincide but because he values creativity and he feels the lithium is reducing his creativity he develops a second-order preference which entails going off the lithium. Because Mr. M. attributes value to creativity his decision to stop the lithium reflects a fundamental commitment to how he wants to live his life and the kind of person he wants to be. Equally when he critically reflects on life with his girlfriend and song writing, and fears that it is a 'post-lithium high,' his decision to go back on the lithium also reflects a fundamental commitment to how he wants to live his life and the kind of person he wants to be.

On a hierarchical account of autonomy Mr. M is clearly autonomous but we are likely to feel that this is a matter of luck because of the mildness of his condition and the fact that the manic and the nonmanic phase seem to have some permanence or constancy associated with them.

Historical Autonomy

If we look to the development of Mr. M's desires, would we have to say that he is not autonomous on a historical account? Would we be compelled to say that although he does not seem irrational, '*in light of* the processes that gave rise' to his desires (that is, in light of a psychiatric disorder), his preferences in the manic state and the nonmanic slightly depressed state are the product of a disorder and 'but for the disorder' he *would* reject his desires?[99] Some people might want to argue that the nature of the illness—bipolar disorder—means that we must say that Mr. M is not autonomous in either state. It would not help even if we tried to argue that one of Mr. M's states represents autonomy and only one of his states is the product of illness. Complications arise because when he is on medication he wants to stop medication and when he is off medication he wants to go back to it. This means, (e.g., when we assume the manic state is the product of the illness), that when he is on lithium he autonomously acts in a way that takes him to a state we call heteronomous and when he is in this state (off lithium, in the manic phase and heteronomous), he acts in a way that embraces autonomy.

Despite these problems there is a way in which the historical account of autonomy can be used to defend Mr. M in both his manic phase and in the nonmanic phase as an autonomous individual. This is by way of a minimal rationality requirement. On a historical account someone who has 'manifestly conflicting desires'; a person who is 'fractured and divided' is deemed not autonomous. This kind of incompatibility of desires is deemed to have a noticeable effect on behavior.[100] However, Mr. M's conflict of desires do not effect his behavior in a way that would make us want to say there is a loss of autonomy. He has not become a slave to an original desire nor is he victimized by the continued presence of an original desire.[101] Mr. M is able to overcome the conflicts he experiences and to act on his preferences. When he is not happy with the way his life is going he goes back to his medication or he stops his medication—which ever is needed to resolve the conflict in his desires.

The problem is that the minimal rationality requirement is a nonhistorical condition. We can say that he is autonomous but the historical condition, the crucial part of the historical account seems to have become superfluous. In other words, Mr. M can be autonomous on a historical account of autonomy—but only when it disqualifies itself as a historical account.

Life-Plan Autonomy

In each phase, his life with his wife and children and his life with his girlfriend and song writing, Mr. M seems to be acting according to a conception of his life that is expressive of his will. Nevertheless, there does not seem to be any convincing way for us to argue that Mr. M is autonomous on a life-plan account of autonomy. He 'follows through' on things like career and lifestyle for only a short time and then abandons his apparent life-plan. What is more, to the extent that he is able to choose in ways expressive of his preferences or his life-plan is a matter of luck that depends on things external to Mr. M. There is little about Mr. M's life that suggests 'following through' and that we could call autonomous (according to a life-plan account of autonomy). If Mr. M or another person had been hurt in the car accident during his manic episode, if he had lost his job because of his poor teaching, or if his wife and girlfriend were not so patient in letting him pick up his life from where he left off six or twelve months earlier he would appear less autonomous. This does not mean that a person can only be autonomous if their life goes well but in this case it seems to be that Mr. M's autonomy does not depend on his own efforts. Recalling Young's claim that autonomy 'has to be worked at' and that an autonomous person's actions are self-directed or self-determined, we have to conclude that Mr. M's actions are not consistent with a life-plan account of autonomy.

I may seem to be dispensing with the life-plan account too hastily—someone might want to argue that the life-plan account can cope with altered life-plans. According to Young: 'People can and do radically alter the courses of their lives.'[102] Nevertheless, on a life-plan account, the basis of judgments about autonomy focus on 'life as a whole.'[103] While Mr. M swaps between two different phases he cannot be autonomous on this view; we cannot say that his life is 'unified, orderly, and free from self-defeating conflict over fundamentals.'[104] Even if the life-plan account of autonomy does not condemn Mr. M as nonautonomous because he leaves his wife and children and takes up with his girlfriend and song writing, it does not give us criteria to judge whether he is autonomously altering the course of his life or whether he lacks autonomy by not 'following through.'

Authentic-Self Account of Autonomy

In the case of Mr. M it is difficult to make sense of the notion of a true or authentic self but Mr. M is attending to signs of internal discord. Although we may not be able to say which is the authentic Mr. M, he is constantly working toward being an authentic person. In some ways, he is certainly doing what is required of an autonomous person on an authentic-self account of autonomy:

> Autonomous people must be disposed to consult their selves, and they must be equipped to do so. More specifically, they must be able to pose and answer the question "What do I really want, need, care about, value, etcetera?"; they must be able to act on the answer; and they must be able to correct themselves when they get the answer wrong.[105]

A lack of autonomy is indicated by a lack of sensitivity to self and an inability to deal with discord. Despite the fact that Mr. M does not lack these things, he never seems to reach what Diana Meyers' considers the 'core concept of personal autonomy.' We do not seem able to say that Mr. M is an individual 'living in harmony' with his 'authentic self'[106] because (1) he does not seem to reach a state of harmony and (2) it is not clear what is the authentic self.

There is no suggestion that Mr. M's life-plan has been adopted in deference to others. However, someone might want to argue that he has an alien life-plan imposed by his disorder and this indicates heteronomy. Nevertheless, this does not help us determine which of Mr. M's personalities is due to the disorder. As noted earlier, Mr. M is not cognitively impaired and cannot be considered incompetent in either state. The authentic-self account of autonomy gives us no guidance in these matters.

Summing Up

How can we decide which is the best psychological account of autonomy in this case? What do we want it to tell us in the case of Mr. M? Presumably we want it to tell us which of Mr. M's choices we should respect. If we think any of his wishes should be respected, do we respect his wishes when he is manic or when he is depressed—when he is medicated or unmedicated? Or do we respect his wishes at both times?

On the hierarchical account, we might wonder what it would take (apart from incompetence or cognitive impairments) for us to declare Mr. M not autonomous. There seems to be no obvious problem but there must surely be some relevance to time and change. How much time is Mr. M allowed to be in a state of discontent before we declare him not autonomous and how often and how much time between changes should we allow? How often can a person make a fundamental commitment and be deemed autonomous rather than vacillating or unstable?—something that does not seem to fit with the idea of autonomy on any of the psychological accounts. Mr. M may be OK but this might not be the case if his wife and girlfriend were not so patient; if his changes meant he did not get what he wanted in either state. Also, someone who changes more often or who has more than two distinct states would pose problems for this account.

It is plausible on a hierarchical account of autonomy to argue that we should respect Mr. M's choices and his changes even though they may lead to disaster. On this account, Mr. M is not incompetent. We can presume that he will be able to factor in to his deliberations the consequences of his choices which turn out badly. Beyond that, there is a point where constant changes would surely amount to cognitive impairment. When that point is reached, we would have to say that unlike Mr. M, the person suffering from this disorder is incompetent.

The hierarchical account of autonomy is the most useful account in the case of Mr. M. The historical account is a non-contender because it deals with Mr. M's situation by disqualifying itself as a historical account of autonomy. The life-plan and the authentic-self accounts give insufficient guidance. There are no criteria for Mr. M to defend himself as autonomous on the life-plan account and the authentic-self account is close to nonsensical in this situation.

A DEVASTATING DIAGNOSIS

A devastating diagnosis is one of the most frightening experiences a person can go through. It often involves having to make decisions in the face of dramatically changed circumstances and sometimes, in that kind of situation, a person may act contrary to his or her physician's recommendation. A person may also act in a way that could be interpreted as a departure from a previously held life-plan or stable values. In this section I look at two kinds of devastating diagnosis: the diagnosis of a chronic condition and the diagnosis of a life-threatening illness.

The first case involves Mrs. Pinelli a thirty-five-year-old divorcee with three children who seeks treatment for severe headaches and chest pains which are caused by dangerously high blood pressure. She has a blood pressure reading of 240/120.[107] The consequences of untreated hypertension, or high blood pressure as it is commonly called, can be 'dramatic' and 'sometimes fatal.' [108] Heart or kidney failure, heart attack, and stroke are the possible consequences.[109]

Hypertension is unusual in the sense that in the early stages there are often no symptoms, it requires lifetime management, and it is usually the treatment rather than the disease that causes problems for patients.[110] Mrs. Pinelli's condition cannot be controlled by lifestyle changes and it cannot be corrected by surgery. [111] Drug therapy is therefore, the recommended treatment for her.

Mrs Pinelli is devastated by the diagnosis. The sudden onset of a chronic condition can be devastating in the sense that it means submitting to a lifelong regime of medication or treatment. And accompanying this, there can be an altered sense of self. Apart from the debilitating effects of a disease, seeing oneself as 'sick' or not well is often devastating in itself.

Medication—the treatment that is recommended for Mrs. Pinelli—has a number of side effects. Extreme drowsiness is the most common side effect. Other frequent undesirable effects caused by the standard drugs for treating high blood pressure include; nausea, diarrhoea, faintness, pins and needles, cramps, itchy rashes, dryness of the eyes, painful joints and muscles, rapid heart beat, tremors and abnormal muscular movement, headaches, mouth ulcers, muscle cramps, and depression.[112] The choice for Mrs. Pinelli is between drug treatment and the accompanying side effects or doing nothing and living with the consequences. Her way is to steer a path somewhere between these two options but this is a course of action that is not to her doctor's liking. She takes the treatment only when symptoms appear, despite the fact that hypertension is a condition that, without proper control, can progress silently and do damage at the same time. There is a limit to what she is prepared to endure even if it is for the good of her future health: 'There are just some things I can't tolerate. Like walking around being drowsy all the time. I've got to work to support my family.'[113]

When the side effects of her medication become troublesome, she stops taking it and does nothing until symptoms reappear. Her symptoms appear only when her blood pressure is dangerously high. Mrs. Pinelli's way of dealing with her condition is not the method that her physician recommends. Her attitude is: 'I'll chance what happens later.'[114]

A life-threatening illness is another kind of devastating diagnosis. Through literary examples we can observe the way in which a person experiences this kind of sudden life-shattering event. Sometimes, paradoxically, literary accounts of a traumatic event can seem more vivid and life-like than personal testimonials.[115] Literature draws us into the world of a particular character and 'allows us to participate, in imagination and with empathy' in the character's experience.[116] Aleksandr Solzhenitsyn draws us into the world of a cancer victim with his vivid sense of what it is like to experience the devastation of a sudden illness:

> the hard lump of his tumour—unexpected, meaningless and quite without use—had dragged him in like a fish on a hook and flung him on to this iron bed—a narrow, mean bed, with creaking springs and an apology for a mattress. Having once undressed . . . said goodbye to the family and come up to the ward, you felt that the door to all your past life had been slammed behind you.[117]

As well as the sudden disruption to his life, Rusanov experiences an altered sense of self: 'In a matter of hours he had as good as lost all his personal status, reputation and plans for the future—and had turned into eleven stones of hot, white flesh that did not know what tomorrow would bring.'[118]

Francoise Sagan gives us a similar insight. At thirty-nine, Paul Casavel is diagnosed with cancer and the prognosis is that he has at best six months to live. We get insight into the havoc this inflicts on his life:

> In the space of one brief hour he had distanced himself from a project that had long been the focal point of his professional life, a project that, only yesterday, had excited him and fired his imagination . . . he had become a man without a future, a man without any plans or projects, a man henceforth stripped of all desire . . . it was safe to say that there was nothing romantic about not having a future. The charm of living, of life itself, was built on the notion of time with a capital T.[119]

From Tolstoy's *The Death of Ivan Ilyich* we get an insight into the way in which the jolt from a devastating diagnosis can lead a person to reassess their life. Tolstoy's Ivan Ilyich is shaken by the sudden thought:

> "What if in reality my whole life has been wrong. . . . It occurred to him that what had appeared utterly impossible before—that he had not lived his life as he should have done—might after all be true. . . . And his professional duties, and his ordering of his life, and his family, and all his social and official interests might all have been false. . . . He lay flat on this back and began going over his whole life entirely anew. In the morning when he saw first the footman, then his wife, then his daughter, then the doctor, every movement they made, every word they uttered, confirmed for him the awful truth that had been revealed to him during the night. In them he saw himself—all that he had lived for—and saw plainly that it was all wrong, a horrible, monstrous lie.[120]

On the different psychological accounts of autonomy, how can we decide whether a decision made by someone like Ivan Ilyich is an autonomous one given that in the face of a devastating diagnosis he has reassessed his whole life? And how can we decide whether Mrs. Pinelli's way of dealing with her illness is autonomous given that she unexpectedly gets a very serious diagnosis and then takes a course of action not to her doctor's liking?

Hierarchical Autonomy

We can imagine that Ivan Ilyich's doctor offers him a treatment which Ivan Illyich refuses. We can say he is autonomous if we think his decision reflects a fundamental commitment to how he wants to live his life (what remains of it) and the kind of person he wants to be (for the duration of his life). He may even be depressed (given his circumstances), but if he arrives at a decision which is backed by reasons he is autonomous on a hierarchical account.

Ivan Ilyich's reassessment that his life until now has been wrong does not create immediate problems if we are assessing his autonomy on a hierarchical account of autonomy. His abrupt change is not significant in itself because his autonomy will be judged according to the kind of reflection he engages in and on his having or not having procedural independence. If Ilyich considers the available options and refuses a recommended treatment, the important thing (the conditions for autonomy according to a hierarchical account) is that he has reflected critically, he understands the implications of refusing treatment and he is not manipulated or coerced, or choosing from depression. He can be depressed, but not to the extent that his depression prevents his ability to think critically. If these conditions are met his refusal of treatment is autonomous. His reassessment of his life may affect what he chooses but in itself, his reassessment and what he chooses do not impact on the assessment of his autonomy.

Mrs Pinelli too, is easily declared autonomous on a hierarchical account. She has obviously engaged in second-order reflection: 'There are just some things I can't tolerate. . . . I'll chance what happens later.' And her procedural independence is not in question. The decisions of Mrs. Pinelli and Ivan Ilyich may reflect a change of values but they can still be regarded as autonomous on a hierarchical account of autonomy.

Historical Autonomy

What counts as an autonomous decision for Ivan Ilyich on a historical account of autonomy? Despite his devastating diagnosis and sudden reassessment of his life—that it had all been wrong—we can declare a refusal of treatment by Ivan Ilyich as autonomous. On this account we assess a decision on the basis of the process that led to the choice. In the case of Ivan Ilyich however, we may wonder where the process that led to his choice begins and where our assessment ought to begin.

We can take Ivan Ilyich's devastating diagnosis and his reassessment as the starting point of the process that led to the choice. The test for autonomy is that Ivan Ilyich *himself* would not have rejected the *development* of his preference to refuse treatment *if he had reflected upon that*. The determination of autonomy does not depend on any concerns we may have about when the process began or what caused the process. The recent catastrophic events in Ivan Ilyich's life mark the beginning of the development of his desire. Given these circumstances and his insight that all he had lived for had been wrong, it seems that Ivan Ilyich understands and accepts the development of his desire to refuse treatment even though the desire is of short duration. It can be deemed autonomous even if, prior to these events and for a longer period of his life, we and even Ivan Ilyich himself think he would have embraced treatment and rejected the formation of his current preference to refuse treatment. If he is not inhibited in his ability to reflect on his own mental states and the forces that affect them; if there is nothing to suggest that his devastating diagnosis or his illness has destroyed his ability to reflect and nothing to suggest that he lacks minimal rationality, Ivan Ilyich's refusal of treatment is autonomous. The 'illegitimate factors' just mentioned must be absent for autonomy to be established.

On the historical account the point of view of the agent plays a central role in the determination of autonomy. Ivan Ilyich's current situation, his devastating diagnosis and subsequent reassessment of his life make up his point of view. In contrast with the hierarchical account of autonomy, his devastating diagnosis and reassessment of his life play a part in the determination of autonomy. We can say that Ivan Ilyich's refusal of treatment is autonomous on both the hierarchical and the historical accounts of autonomy but we have arrived at these determinations differently. Here, on the historical account, we seem to have factored in the effect of the devastating diagnosis (we had to in order to account for the short duration of the desire), whereas the devastating diagnosis has no part at all to play (it was not needed), in the determination of autonomy on a hierarchical account.

Mrs. Pinelli too, can count as autonomous on the historical account. Given the reality and the constraints of her situation she is nevertheless in a position to reflect on and resist the development of her preference to 'chance what happens later.' But she does not resist the desire—she is taking a considered calculated risk. Mrs. Pinelli is a bit like Mr. M in the sense that any conflict of desires she experiences do not effect her behavior in a way that would make us want to say there is a loss of autonomy. She is not victimized by desires that no longer serve her situation. She goes without medication until symptoms reappear but when the side effects become troublesome, she stops taking it and does nothing again until symptoms reappear. She does what is necessary at the time to resolve the conflict between her desire to work and take care of her family and her desire to avoid illness. On the historical account, for Mrs. Pinelli like Ivan Ilyich, there may be doubt as to where the process that led to her choice begins. But, again we should take the starting point of the process as the point where she learns of her condition. There is nothing in this account to suggest that we need to go back earlier than that.

Life-Plan Autonomy

On a life-plan account of autonomy, Ivan Ilyich's decision to refuse treatment and Mrs. Pinelli's course of action seem to be acts of occurrent autonomy (autonomy of the moment) rather than dispositional autonomy which is viewed as more important. Perhaps we can say that Mrs. Pinelli's decision to 'chance what happens later' is a kind of plan; a conception of her life that is expressive of her will, but it would not be easy to say the same of Ivan Ilyich's decision. Made in the face of a devastating diagnosis and a reassessment of his whole life, Ivan Ilyich's decision is not in keeping with past actions or prior plans. The absence of his 'following through on a plan' suggests his decision is heteronomous rather than autonomous. Proponents of the life-plan view, however, want to defend the idea that someone like Ivan

Ilyich in these circumstances can be autonomous. Robert Young argues that people 'can and do radically alter the course of their lives without giving up their autonomy.'[121] The trouble is, it is not clear how this can be assessed for someone like Ivan Ilyich or even Mrs. Pinelli. The life-plan account has no criteria for us to judge what is a changing or changed life-plan and what is a temporary or capricious departure from a life-plan in these circumstances. Young can only offer: 'There is a legitimate sense in which a person can occurrently act autonomously. But judgments about personal autonomy are centrally dispositional; they relate to a person's following through on a plan or conception of his (or her) life.'[122]

Autonomy on an Authentic-Self Account

What counts as autonomous for Mrs. Pinelli and Ivan Ilyich on an authentic-self account of autonomy? We could say that Mrs. Pinelli is autonomous because she is being true to herself by attending to signs of internal discord in her life-plan. Ivan Ilyich can be declared autonomous on this account too. Even though it seems his life-plan has been violated we can take the view that his true self is in transition—not that he has acted heteronomously. Heteronomy on this view is following an 'alien' life-plan and being unwilling and unable to reconsider plans. Ivan Ilyich's reassessment of his whole life suggested that the old life-plan has become the 'alien' life-plan. Given the dramatically changed circumstances accompanying a devastating diagnosis it is reasonable to attribute 'following through' on the old plan to desperation or fear rather than autonomy. The old plan is no longer suited to the new radically altered circumstances.

Summing Up

Having considered what counts as autonomous for Mrs. Pinelli and Ivan Ilyich on the different accounts, in order to work out which of the different accounts is the most useful, I will now consider what it would take to declare Ivan Ilyich and Mrs. Pinelli not autonomous on these accounts. When considering the decisions of someone faced with a devastating diagnosis we want an account of autonomy to give a clear indication of whether a decision is or is not autonomous. It needs to provide us with criteria so that when Ivan Ilyich refuses treatment we can judge whether he is deluded and disturbed, acting out of fear or depression or whether he is making an autonomous decision. And we need to know if there is, or why there is not, some point at which Mrs. Pinelli's course of action which is not to her doctor's liking indicates a lack of autonomy. In the clinical context, given the ways that a devastating diagnosis can affect different people, we want an account of autonomy that will tell us if there are circumstances that justify overriding a person's decision.

On the hierarchical account we could declare someone not autonomous if they lacked procedural independence—if they were depressed for instance. But how do we tell? To some extent we can't. If a person can critically reflect on their first order desires and critically reflect on their own procedural independence, on a hierarchical account we should declare that person autonomous. What would it take to declare Ivan Ilyich not autonomous on a hierarchical account? On the basis of his reassessment alone we wouldn't say he is not autonomous, but if he was in a state of despondence and unable to give reasons for a refusal of treatment we could say that he lacks autonomy. Or, if he were cognitively impaired we would declare him not autonomous.

The hierarchical account recognizes severe cases of depression but it seems that we give the benefit of any doubt to the agent. We are more likely to respect a decision that lacks autonomy than intervene in a decision that is autonomous. Where giving the benefit of the doubt entails respecting the desires of patients, some people think this is good, but some may not—for example, if the benefit of the doubt entails allowing a depressed person to refuse treatment. Proponents of a hierarchical account could respond that the lack of an easy solution in determining the severity of a person's depression need not be regarded as a defect. It is *severe* depression only that provides justification for overriding a decision because depression that is not severe does not necessarily interfere with decision making. While severe depression is likely to be obvious to others, it is important to note that we are only entitled to assess autonomy in terms of the sort of reflection the depressed person engages in or fails to engage in—we do not assess on the basis of the choice. In other words we are not entitled to say Ivan Ilyich must be severely depressed because he refused treatment.

On the hierarchical account we cannot justify interfering with Mrs. Pinelli's decision even if we think she is not acting in her own interests; even if we think the situation she is in has made her choose poorly—that she would choose differently in better circumstances. Mrs. Pinelli is autonomous because she has the right kind of reflection and her reflection is not manipulated or coerced.

What would justify intervening in Mrs. Pinelli or Ivan Ilyich's decision on a historical account of autonomy? We have already seen that we could declare these two people autonomous on a historical account and now, with the same evidence before us, we see that we could justify intervening in the same decisions by claiming (according to the historical account) that Ivan Ilyich and Mrs. Pinelli are not autonomous. If we wanted to we could argue that they are fractured and divided because they have manifest conflicts of desire. They do not pass the test for autonomy. We could say that Ivan Ilyich is fractured and divided with his past, more stable self and we could compare Mrs. Pinelli to Alex (the character introduced by Alfred Mele).[123] We could say that although she has not been the subject of reflection-constraining factors, she suffers from similar internal conflict to Alex who wanted both to have time for his family and to do a lot of work. We saw how, with the addition of a nonhistorical condition to allow 'mildly conflicted individuals' to remain autonomous but rule out those with 'manifestly conflicting desires' Christman declared Alex not autonomous. He claimed that Alex had desires 'both to work relentlessly and also not to do so in order to spend more time in other pursuits'[124] On the historical account we could interpret Mrs. Pinelli's desires in the same way: Mrs. Pinelli has desires to take care of her health and also not to do so (to neglect her health) in order to work and take care of her children. On the historical account, disappointingly, the determination of autonomy seems to be a matter of interpretation—based on nothing more than a preconceived view of whether Mrs. Pinelli is autonomous or not autonomous. Furthermore, as we have seen with some of the other cases, the historical requirement (the defining feature of this account), seems superfluous. In the end, that which prompts us to decide whether a decision is autonomous or not seems more to do with the requirements for minimal rationality and self-awareness. Ultimately, the historical account is unhelpful because determinations of autonomy are to some extent arbitrary.

The life-plan account, as we have seen, does not provide proper criteria for us to judge in a devastating diagnosis situation when someone acts in a way that could be interpreted as a departure from a previously held life-plan or stable values. There is a similar problem with the authentic-self account of autonomy. On that account, although Mrs. Pinelli and Ivan Ilyich can be declared autonomous, it makes no sense to declare them heteronomous—even if we had reason to think they lacked autonomy. We have no criteria to distinguish between an autonomous self in transition and heteronomy. We may think that Mrs. Pinelli is choosing from desperation but it could be countered that Mrs. Pinelli is simply dealing with symptoms of discord. We might think that Ivan Ilyich is choosing from depression but the authentic-self account does not tell us how to distinguish autonomous expressions of the 'evolving self' from heteronomy or how to identify illegitimate influences on an evolving self.

The hierarchical account of autonomy seems to be the most useful in a situation where someone is faced with a devastating diagnosis. Overall, the hierarchical account seems to have emerged as the best, most defensible psychological account of autonomy.

NOTES

1. Chris Griffith, "Blood Oath Death Risk," *Sunday Mail*, Queensland, 7 March 1999, 3.

2. Dworkin, *The Theory and Practice of Autonomy*, 18.

3. Dworkin, Review of *Liberation from Self*, 215.

4. I am looking at the circumstances that make this decision autonomous on a hierarchical account.

5. Irving L. Janis and Leon Mann, *Decision Making: A Psychological Analysis of Conflict, Choice, and Commitment* (New York: Free Press, 1977), 284–86. See ch. 11. Studies cited include, e.g., of what makes a parachutist go through with a jump. As the time nears, the parachutist may want to avoid the jump but the 'psychological momentum provided by the difficulty of reversing the decision, particularly as a result of the social commitment, which, if broken, would lead to a loss of face' acts as an incentive for the parachutist to jump. In a study of the effect of public commitment on adherence to a decision, some home owners were told that the results of research into natural gas consumption would be published in the newspaper listing the names of those who agreed to attempt energy conservation. It was found that these people had significantly lower energy consumption than a control group and those who were told they would not be personally identified.

6. Dworkin, *The Theory and Practice of Autonomy*, 23–24.

7. Janis and Mann, *Decision Making*, 35. For example, the decision to marry and career choices including the careers of lawbreakers can be arrived at in a 'stepwise, drifting fashion,' without any single stage at which the person makes a definite choice

8. Janis and Mann, *Decision Making*, 296–97.

9. Christman, "Autonomy and Personal History," 24. The idea of agents assessing their own autonomy may seem impractical and unhelpful in the clinical context but we need to remember that Christman's test for autonomy is a hypothetical historical test. If the process of desire formation is corrupt, presumably the agent would resist the development of the desire. This hypothetical test also involves the agent subjecting his or her commitments to 'objective' scrutiny

10. Christman, "Autonomy and Personal History," 22–23.

11. Berofsky, *Liberation from Self*, 184.

12. Christman, "Defending Historical Autonomy," 286.

13. Young, *Personal Autonomy*, 78–79.
14. Young, *Personal Autonomy*, 40.
15. Young, *Personal Autonomy*, 40.
16. Young, *Personal Autonomy*, 78–79.
17. Young, *Personal Autonomy*, 40.
18. Young, *Personal Autonomy*, 8.
19. Meyers, *Self, Society and Personal Choice*, 45–53.
20. Meyers, *Self, Society and Personal Choice*, 49–50.
21. Meyers, *Self, Society and Personal Choice*, 50.
22. Meyers, *Self, Society and Personal Choice*, 54.
23. Meyers, *Self, Society and Personal Choice*, 54–55.
24. Dworkin, *The Theory and Practice of Autonomy*, 21.
25. I have not dealt with the way a hierarchical or historical account of autonomy handles a change of values or preferences in the Jehovah's Witness case because that is the main focus of one of the test cases to come.
26. Peter D. Kramer, *Listening to Prozac* (London: Fourth Estate, 1993), x, 265.
27. Willard Gaylin, "Feeling Good and Doing Better" in *Feeling Good and Doing Better: Ethics and Nontherapeutic Drug Use*, ed. Thomas H. Murray, Willard Gaylin, and Ruth Macklin (New Jersey: Humana Press, 1984), 1–10.
28. Lawrence H. Diller, "The Run on Ritalin: Attention Deficit Disorder and Stimulant Treatment in the 1990s," 26, *Hastings Center Report* (March–April, 1996): 15.
29. Gaylin, "Feeling Good and Doing Better," 4–7.
30. Carl Elliott, "Hedgehogs and Hermaphrodites: Toward a More Anthropological Bioethics," in *Philosophy of Medicine and Bioethics: A Twenty-Year Retrospective and Critical Appraisal*, ed. Ronald A. Carson and Chester R. Burns (Netherlands: Kluwer Academic Publishers, Dordrecht, 1997), 197–211.
31. Elliott, "Hedgehogs and Hermaphrodites," 200.
32. Elliott, "Hedgehogs and Hermaphrodites," 202.
33. Elliott, "Hedgehogs and Hermaphrodites," 201.
34. Elliott, "Hedgehogs and Hermaphrodites," 201.
35. Elliott, "Hedgehogs and Hermaphrodites," 202.
36. Roy Porter, "Is Dr. Feelgood Here to Stay," review of , *Listening to Prozac* by Peter D. Kramer, *Times Literary Supplement* .4747 (March 25, 1994): 28.
37. Dan Brock, "The Use of Drugs for Pleasure: Some Philosophical Issues," in *Feeling Good and Doing Better: Ethics and Nontherapeutic Drug Use*, ed. Thomas H. Murray, Willard Gaylin, and Ruth Macklin (New Jersey: Humana Press, 1984), 103–104.
38. Dan Brock, "The Use of Drugs for Pleasure," 83–84, 102–103.
39. Kramer, *Listening to Prozac*, xvi; Peter Kramer, "The Valorization of Sadness: Alienation and the Melancholic Temperament" *Hastings Center Report* 30, no.2 (2000): 13. 'Cosmetic psychopharmacology' is Kramer's term for the effect of a medication that makes patients 'better than well.' Elsewhere Kramer describes it

as the 'potential' of 'a medication that can move a person from a normal psychological state to another normal psychological state that is more desired or better socially rewarded.'

40. Elliott, "Hedgehogs and Hermaphrodites," 209; David Healy, "Good Science or Good Business?" *Hastings Center Report* 30, no.2 (2000): 19.

41. Jerrold F. Rosenbaum, "Clinical Trial by Media: The Prozac Story" in *Psychiatric Practice Under Fire: The Influence of Government, the Media, and Special Interests on Somatic Therapies*, ed. Harold I. Schwartz (Washington, D.C.: American Psychiatric Press Inc. 1994), 25; Roy Porter, "Is Dr. Feelgood Here to Stay," 28.

42. Kramer, *Listening to Prozac*, xvii–xviii, 267–68.

43. Robert Wright, "The Coverage of Happiness: When Prozac Meets Universal Coverage," in *The New Republic*, (March 14, 1994), reprinted in *Ethical Issues in Modern Medicine*, 5th. ed. eds. John D. Arras and Bonnie Steinbock (California: Mayfield Publishing Co., 1999), 693.

44. Peter R. Breggin and Ginger Ross Breggin, *Talking Back to Prozac* (New York: St. Martin's Press, 1994); Jerrold F. Rosenbaum, "Clinical Trial by Media," 3–28.

45. Kramer, *Listening to Prozac*, 11.

46. Wright, "The Coverage of Happiness," 696.

47. Wright, "The Coverage of Happiness," 694.

48. Porter, "Is Dr Feelgood Here to Stay," 28.

49. Wright, "The Coverage of Happiness," 694; David J. Rothman, "Shiny Happy People: The Problem with 'Cosmetic Psychopharmacology,'" *New Republic* (February 14, 1994): 35.

50. This has been the conventional thinking but it seems that the mechanism by which Prozac actually works is not clear. The conventional view that anxiety, panic, and anxiety-related depression are caused by a lack or underactivity of serotonin and that selective serotonin reuptake inhibitor (SSRI) drugs increase serotonin has been challenged in a study by researchers at the Baker Medical Research Institute, Melbourne. The finding was made inadvertently by a team of cardiologists investigating the link between panic disorder and heart attack. The researchers found that patients with panic disorder had eight times the amount of serotonin of healthy patients. It appears that SSRIs are effective because they decrease serotonin. It is not important in the context of this work, or for the claims Wright is making, whether Prozac increases serotonin or decreases serotonin. Critics of Prozac often refer to the fact that some patients experience increased anxiety in their first weeks of treatment. One of the researchers claims that the finding that SSRIs decrease serotonin could lead drug companies to create drugs that stop serotonin directly rather than decreasing it over time. The findings may explain the problem of "serotonin agitation"—the fact that Prozac and similar drugs sometimes make the problem worse before they make it better—Mary-Anne Toy, "Closing in on Prozac's Secrets," *The Age*, 26 February 2000, A16; Steve Dow, "Dramatic Reversal in Research on Anxiety," *The Sunday Age*, 14 May 2000, A6.

51. Wright, "The Coverage of Happiness," 694.
52. Wright, "The Coverage of Happiness," 694–95.
53. Richard S. Schwartz, "Mood Brighteners, Affect Tolerance and the Blues," *Psychiatry* 54 (November 1991): 397. Schwartz responds to a challenge by a colleague who argues that we need to consider the implications of a hypothetical medication—a mood brightener without side effects, etc. His colleague also argued that Fluoxetine (Prozac) is a significant step in that direction.
54. Kramer, *Listening to Prozac*, 11, 258, 267.
55. Kramer, *Listening to Prozac*, .258, 265.
56. Kramer, *Listening to Prozac*, 265.
57. Kramer, *Listening to Prozac*, 12.
58. Kramer, *Listening to Prozac*, 8–9.
59. Kramer, *Listening to Prozac*, x.
60. Kramer, *Listening to Prozac*, 265.
61. Kramer, *Listening to Prozac*, 259.
62. Kramer, *Listening to Prozac*, ix–xv.
63. Kramer, *Listening to Prozac*, 265–67. This account is from Kramer's report of a case used by Aranow, Schwartz and Sullivan combined with an account of Ms. B's recovery from the psychiatrist who treated her—also reported by Kramer.
64. Kramer, *Listening to Prozac*, 265–66.
65. Kramer, *Listening to Prozac*, 267.
66. Kramer, *Listening to Prozac*, 268.
67. Kramer, *Listening to Prozac*, x, 8–9.
68. Dworkin, *The Theory and Practice of Autonomy*, 29.
69. Porter, "Is Dr. Feelgood Here to Stay," 28.
70. Rothman,, "Shiny Happy People," 36.
71. Kramer, "The Valorization of Sadness," 15.
72. Carl Elliott, "Pursued by Happiness and Beaten Senseless: Prozac and the American Dream," *Hastings Center Report* 30, no. 2 (March–April 2000): 7–12; Schwartz, "Mood Brighteners," 397–403.
73. Christman, "Autonomy and Personal History," 10–11.
74. Rothman, "Shiny Happy People," 36.
75. David DeGrazia, "Prozac, Enhancement, and Self-Creation," *Hastings Center Report* 30, no.2 (March–April 2000): 38.
76. Christman, "Defending Historical Autonomy," 283–84.
77. Although we may be making an assessment about autonomy, determinations of autonomy on a historical account remain the point of view of the agent.
78. Young, *Personal Autonomy*, 9.
79. Kramer, *Listening to Prozac*, xv.
80. Kramer, *Listening to Prozac*, 252.
81. Kramer, *Listening to Prozac*, 252.
82. Kramer, *Listening to Prozac*, 256–57. Kramer is referring to the arguments of Randolph M. Neese, "What Good Is Feeling Bad? The Evolutionary Benefits of

Psychic Pain," *The Sciences* (November–Decmber 1990): 30–37; Schwartz, "Mood Brighteners," 397–403; Robert B. Aranow, Richard S Schwarts, and Mark D. Sullivan. "Mood Brighteners," *American Journal of Psychiatry* n.d. (referred to in Kramer, *Listening to Prozac* as "(in press) draft of March 19, 1992").

83. Kramer, *Listening to Prozac*, 258, 254–55.

84. Carl Elliott, "The Tyranny of Happiness: Ethics and Cosmetic Psychopharacology," in *Enhancing Human Traits: Ethical and Social Implications*, ed. E. Parens, (Washington: Georgetown University Press, 1998), 182, 186.

85. DeGrazia, "Prozac, Enhancement, and Self-Creation," 34–36.

86. Rothman, "Shiny Happy People," 36–37.

87. Wright, "The Coverage of Happiness," 694.

88. Wright, "The Coverage of Happiness," 694.

89. Meyers, *Self, Society, and Personal Choice*. 54.

90. Christman, "Autonomy and Personal History," 13.

91. Young, *Personal Autonomy*, 40.

92. Young, *Personal Autonomy*, 41.

93. Young, *Personal Autonomy*, 16.

94. Young, *Personal Autonomy*, 8.

95. Tony Hope, "Personal Identity and Psychiatric Illness," in *Philosophy, Psychology, and Psychiatry*, ed. A. Phillips Griffiths (New York: Cambridge University Press, 1994), 131–43.

96. Hope, "Personal Identity and Psychiatric Illness," 138–40.

97. I do not mean that he is not autonomous because his life is not exactly as he wants it to be—it is because (with the options he has available to him) he is not living according to the one he prefers.

98. Dworkin, *The Theory and Practice of Autonomy*, 20, 108.

99. Eric Matthews, "Autonomy and the Psychiatric Patient," *Journal of Applied Philosophy* 17, no. 1 (2000): 67.

100. Christman, "Defending Historical Autonomy," 287.

101. Mele, "History and Personal Autonomy," 275–76.

102. Young, *Personal Autonomy*, 8.

103. Young, *Personal Autonomy*, 5.

104. Young, *Personal Autonomy*, 8.

105. Meyers, *Self, Society, and Personal Choice*, 52–53.

106. Meyers, *Self, Society, and Personal Choice*, 49–50.

107. Bursztajn, Feinbloom, Hann, and Brodsky, *Medical Choices, Medical Chances: How Patients, Families, and Physicians Can Cope with Uncertainty* (New York: A Merloyd Lawrence Book, 1981), 122.

108. Caroline Shreeve, *Lower Your Blood Pressure in 4 Easy Stages* (Wellingborough, Northamptonshire: Thorsons Publishing Group, 1989), 37; E. B. Blanchard, J. E. Martin, Patricia M. Dubbert, *Non-Drug Treatments for Essential Hypertension* (New York: Pergamon Press, 1988), 4; Bursztajn, Feinbloom, Hann, and Brodsky, *Medical Choices, Medical Chances*, 121.

109. Bursztajn, Feinbloom, Hann, and Brodsky, *Medical Choices, Medical Chances*, 70.

110. Shreeve, *Lower Your Blood Pressure*, 37.

111. Bursztajn, Feinbloom, Hann, and Brodsky, *Medical Choices, Medical Chances*, 123–30. Hypertension can often be controlled by lifestyle changes and can sometimes be corrected by surgery but Mrs Pinelli's condition is not responsive to these interventions.

112. Shreeve, *Lower Your Blood Pressure*, 13–16.

113. Bursztajn, Feinbloom, Hann, and Brodsky, *Medical Choices, Medical Chances*, 158.

114. Bursztajn, Feinbloom, Hann, and Brodsky, *Medical Choices, Medical Chances*, 144.

115. Merle Spriggs, "Autonomy in the face of a devastating diagnosis," *Journal of Medical Ethics* 24, no. 2 (April, 1998): 123–26. Reports of how people experience life-threatening illnesses are usually written retrospectively after the crisis has lessened and the focus is on rebuilding one's life. This can create a 'distance' or a sense of remoteness.

116. Femi Oyebode and Christina Pourgourides, "Literature and Medicine," (Letter to the editor) *The Lancet* 348, no. 9,031 (September 28, 1996): 894.

117. Aleksandr Solzhenitsyn, *Cancer Ward*, trans. Nicholas Bethall and David Burg (London, Penguin Books, 1971), 17.

118. Solzhenitsyn, *Cancer Ward*, 19.

119. Francoise Sagan, *A Fleeting Sorrow*, trans. Richard Seaver, (New York: Arcade Publishing, 1995), 35.

120. Leo Tolstoy, *The Death of Ivan Ilyich and Other Stories* (London: Penguin Books, 1960), 157.

121. Young, *Personal Autonomy*, 8.

122. Young, *Personal Autonomy*, 109.

123. Mele, "History and Personal Autonomy," 275–76.

124. Christman, "Defending Historical Autonomy," 284.

8

CONCLUSION: PRELIMINARY IDEAS FOR A BETTER, MORE USEFUL THEORY FOR THE CLINICAL CONTEXT

THE BEST, MOST DEFENSIBLE PSYCHOLOGICAL ACCOUNT OF AUTONOMY

A descriptive psychological account of autonomy is the most applicable in the clinical context and the hierarchical account of autonomy has emerged as the best, most defensible, psychological account. Before I propose an improved version for the clinical context I will briefly recap the first part of this work to show how the hierarchical account fits into the overall picture.

I have argued that current usage of the term autonomy is muddled. I identified various notions of autonomy which are being run together and I assessed the applicability of these notions in the clinical context. We saw Kant's idea of autonomy that comes with a whole metaphysics from which it cannot be detached, the descriptive psychological view which helps us to identify an autonomous person or an autonomous choice without telling us how to act, the procedural approach which avoids social strife and resolves conflict without force, and the evaluative notion which, when we say someone or something is autonomous, makes a moral judgment rather than describes. Having decided that a descriptive psychological account was the most applicable in the clinical context I then categorized and assessed various psychological theories.

The hierarchical account (one category of psychological theories) seems to be the one account that provides appropriate criteria on which to judge a person's decisions as autonomous or lacking in autonomy. It also seems to be the one account in which judgments about autonomy are not sometimes empty or arbitrary. The sketch of an account I am proposing for the clinical context is a hierarchical account but it is not simply a wholehearted endorsement of Gerald Dworkin's hierarchical account. There are some aspects of that account that I want to clarify or make more explicit and some aspects that I reject. I introduce additional criteria also.

From my earlier analysis I will present preliminary ideas and suggest criteria for what I think could be a better, more useful theory of autonomy in the clinical context and one that is also philosophically defensible. It will be a *revised* hierarchical account of autonomy. The criteria will give us a specific idea of autonomy—a descriptive psychological conception of autonomy for the clinical context, but it will not tell us how to act. Why we should value or respect autonomy is a separate question which I will address after sketching the criteria.

CRITERIA FOR AUTONOMOUS CHOICES AND A BETTER THEORY OF AUTONOMY

The following headings are not meant to suggest a recipe for autonomy, but they may help the reader.

The Right Kind of Thinking

On the hierarchical version of a descriptive psychological account of autonomy, a person who chooses autonomously has the right kind of thinking. This means that autonomy is assessed according to the way a person reasons. We look at the content of the choice but only in so far as 'content' refers to psychological considerations such as the right kind of thinking. We do not assess the choice itself by looking at the specific content—for example, the refusal of a recommended medical procedure. Content may come into the assessment if we think a decision is irrational but assessments about autonomy and assessments about rationality do not depend on a substantive idea of the good life. As we saw earlier, responses such as 'Paul McCartney, nothing to zero' are not the right kind of thinking. That response fails because of psychological considerations; it lacks understanding and rationality. In order for a decision to be called autonomous, a patient needs to be able to understand and appreciate the circumstances of the decision. The right kind of thinking raises questions about the role of rationality and questions about what kind of rationality autonomy requires. A philosophically defensible theory which is useful in the clinical context must address these questions and I will deal with these questions separately after I have sketched out the criteria for autonomous choices.

The Right Kind of Thinking Involves Critical Reflection, Which Involves Having Reasons and Higher Order Desires

A person who chooses autonomously reflects critically and makes decisions backed by reasons. This involves higher order reflection; having desires about desires. When questioned, a person who is making an autonomous decision is able to critically reflect about whether that decision fits in with the kind of life he or she wants to lead. This person is able to defend their choices in terms of their own values. This is not necessarily the same thing as a life plan as referred to in the life-plan account of autonomy—it could involve briefly held values.

Autonomous Decisions Reflect a Fundamental Commitment about How We Want to Live

This means that in assessing a particular decision we *do* look at the content but only to the extent that we want to see that a decision has this feature. We *look for the 'fundamental commitment'* but we do not concern ourselves with *how* someone wants to live. Making decisions that reflect a fundamental commitment about the way a person wants to live is a psychological feature which amounts to a kind of rationality. This will figure in the discussion to come.

Autonomous Choices Do Not Have to Be Good Choices

Autonomous choices do not have to be prudent (e.g., we might think Mrs Pinelli's choice is not prudent) and autonomous choices do not have to be palatable (e.g., a restricted range of options can result in a choice that is not ideal or not to our liking, e.g., the Queensland Jehovah's Witness and Mrs Pinelli). Nevertheless, choices (including those just mentioned) do have to meet other criteria such as some kind of rationality to satisfy a judgment of autonomy.

Obstacles to Autonomous Choice

Things that prevent critical reflection obstruct the making of autonomous decisions. A person cannot choose autonomously if they are cognitively impaired, brainwashed, coerced, deluded and disturbed, if they lack understanding or if they are choosing from fear or depression that is severe enough to prevent critical reflection.

A Person Who Makes an Autonomous Decision Is Aware of Influences on Their Deliberation

Dworkin uses the idea of procedural independence to rule out influences that can interfere with a person's reflective and critical faculties. I noted earlier that Dworkin's notion of procedural independence is not consistently clear. I am concerned with the same ideas but will treat them differently. Like Dworkin, I want to rule out influences which seriously interfere with critical thinking, but, instead of grappling with and trying to understand Dworkin's notion of procedural independence I will focus on a more practical approach. I will give a role to conversation by utilizing Jay Katz' idea of the 'imposition of dialogue' which gets people to engage in second order reflection. This will also help people to act with an awareness of any influences affecting their thinking.

In order to explain my approach I will discuss a point where my view differs from Dworkin's. Dworkin thinks there is something wrong with autonomy that comes about by changing one's higher order preferences whereas I think that changing a higher order preference can amount to an expression of autonomy. Dworking says: 'Say one is envious but does not want to be an envious person. One way of becoming autonomous is by ceasing to be motivated by envy. But another way . . . is to change one's objections to envy, to change one's second-order preferences.'[1] According to Dworkin, procedural independence limits this to some extent but he suggests changing one's second-order preferences is not an appropriate way to seek autonomy:

> it wouldn't do to have one hypnotized into identifying with one's envious motivations. But even if the procedures used were "legitimate," there seems to be something wrong with the idea that one becomes more autonomous by changing one's higher-order preferences.[2]

We can compare this with Isaiah Berlin's discussion about one way of becoming autonomous which is also viewed as questionable or problematic:

> It is as if I had performed a strategic retreat into an inner citadel . . . It is as if I were to say; 'I have a wound in my leg. There are two methods of freeing myself from pain. One is to heal the wound. But if the cure is too difficult or uncertain, there is another method. I can get rid of the wound by cutting off my leg.'[3]

In contrast, in the clinical context from the observations of a person who becomes disabled and the observations of a person who develops cancer, we see how a change of higher order preferences can demonstrate autonomy—how patients' ideas about what is acceptable can change:

> When I was young and physically strong, to live life from a wheelchair was unthinkable. When I became disabled it was unacceptable, but gradually, over the years, not only did it become acceptable, but I found it satisfying as well.[4]

> Cancer . . . has a disarming way of bargaining downward, beginning with your whole estate and then letting you keep the game warden's cottage or the badminton court; and by the time it has tried to frighten you to death and threatened to take away your very existence, you'd be amazed at how little you're willing to settle for.[5]

Changing one's higher order preferences does not have to be as extreme as Berlin's example of cutting off a leg to get rid of the wound. The point I am making is that if a person has suffered a loss they can accept or reject the limitation and either response can be an expression of autonomy. Accepting a limitation by changing a higher order desire can be an autonomous act—though I am not suggesting that autonomy demands acceptance of a situation.

Alternatively, when loss occurs, autonomous choices can also involve keeping a second-order preference. An example of autonomy in this kind of situation is the case of Chris Hill who demonstrates autonomous action by taking his own life. Hill, a journalist who has led an extremely active and satisfying life, is left paralyzed from the chest down after a tragic hang gliding accident. He describes his life as a 'grey void of bleak despair' which involves 'unbearable abominations that made [him] feel less than human.' His life has become 'painful, frustrating and completely unsatisfying' and he writes 'I accepted death—embraced it eagerly . . . without fear or regret.'[6] A different person might adjust by changing their view of what is acceptable—as we saw in the example of the person who manages to live a satisfying life from a wheelchair.

Hill maintained his view that the kind of life available to him was not what he wanted. Even though he takes his own life his choice is autonomous and he is 'more than a passive spectator'—just as much as the person who accepts and finds satisfaction in life from a wheelchair.

Either way, it is not always clear in terms of the higher and lower order desires of a hierarchical account how we can decide what it is that indicates autonomy.[7] The point is that reflection must undergo scrutiny and conversation or dialogue can play an important role in this.

The Role of Conversation

We have seen how the role of conversation assists patients in going second-order about their wishes and helps patients act with an awareness of the influences on their thinking. The imposition of conversation is a practical way to address Dworkin's concerns about procedural independence and the need for subjecting one's preferences and desires to critical reflection.[8]

The imposition of dialogue or conversation also overcomes Beauchamp and Childress's criticism of hierarchical accounts of autonomy.[9] Beauchamp and Childress think that hierarchical accounts lack a way for allowing ordinary persons to qualify as deserving respect when they have not reflected on their preferences at a higher level. The imposition of conversation however, does provide a way for ordinary persons to qualify as deserving respect because it gets them to critically reflect—to go second-order with their choices—at least on important matters. And this is surely desirable in the clinical context. Those who have already reflected at a higher level might consolidate their second-order preferences or they may go third-order, but there is no need to keep going higher. There need be no problem with an infinite regress. At some point desires become brute facts. Giving conversation a role in critical reflection can eliminate the problem of an infinite regress because by questioning the person we recognise that the critical reflection or a particular higher order desire is autonomous.

A particularly reflective person can have higher order preferences, beyond second-, third-, or fourth-order preferences. If we are simply talking about living autonomously it is not inconceivable for a person to have a number of preferences about their preferences—but the clinical context is different. In the clinical context, decisions are required and there is a limit to the number of preferences about preferences or at least there is a limit to the length of time that can be spent on critical reflection before a preference must be selected. Conversation helps in the sense that it helps ascertain that the preference settled on is autonomous—that it meets certain criteria and it is the preferred preference in the circumstances.

Task Related

On my revised hierarchical account, autonomy is viewed as task specific rather than being about what it means to be an autonomous person. Autonomy on this account involves psychological capacities in relation to particular decisions or acts but the focus is not on the character of the person with those characteristics. In his discussion of the nature of autonomy, Dworkin asks whether autonomy is to be assessed over relatively long stretches of a person's life or brief stretches and whether it is about autonomous *persons* or particular *choices*.[10] Nevertheless, these considerations seem somewhat confused and conflated in his original account of autonomy. In a later article Dworkin makes these ideas more explicit by drawing our attention to the importance of identifying how the idea of autonomy in a particular context is being used or defined. He claims that autonomy is 'a term of art' and that 'given various theoretical purposes' theorists must 'construct a concept' but the construction of the concept 'must be relative to a set of problems and questions.' He suggests that when we are looking at the way a particular theorist uses, defines or characterizes the term we should ask: 'Of what is the term predicated? Is it of a person? If so is it a term that can apply to a moment of time, a span of time, a life? Is it of his actions? Is it of his beliefs, values, desires?'[11]

In the clinical context it makes sense for us to assess the autonomy of choices, decisions or acts rather than persons. We might say a *person* is autonomous as a kind of shorthand when we think the person in question has made an autonomous decision and we may refer to the autonomy *of the person* when we are wondering about whether the person has the capacity to make an autonomous decision. However, it is not necessary to assess the *whole person* or their *whole life* to see if a particular *decision* is autonomous. It is not obviously the case that an autonomous choice only flows from a person we can describe as autonomous in the ways just mentioned. We need to look at specific choices. And if a particular choice passes as autonomous we should not assume that a *person* is autonomous in the sense that they always make autonomous choices or that they are autonomous over an extended period or in terms of their whole life. And someone considered not autonomous in these senses can make an autonomous decision in some things on some occasions. Someone with dementia who no longer always recognizes family and friends and cannot remember the immediate past can still have a strong preference with supporting reasons about certain important things, e.g., to be buried or cremated.

Similarly, even if we were to say that someone is autonomous, they can make a decision that is not autonomous. We could refer to Mrs Pinelli as an autonomous *person* on a hierarchical account but individual decisions still need to be assessed. If in the future we ask Mrs Pinelli why she chooses a particular course of action and instead of saying 'There are just some things I can't tolerate . . . I'll chance what happens later,' she said something nonsensical like 'Paul McCartney, nothing to zero' or her decision was constrained by the threats of another,[12] we would say the decision lacked autonomy—but, apart from this decision, we may not want to say that Mrs Pinelli is not autonomous.

The idea that autonomy is task related does not restrict us to considerations of what Young calls occurrent autonomy (autonomy of the moment)—nor what appears to be a similar idea when Dworkin claims that autonomy seems to be a 'global' rather than a 'local' concept. Making judgments about a particular decision does not mean that we only consider brief periods of time—we can look at choices in the context of an extended period of that person's life but it may be the case that only a brief period is relevant or necessary for a judgment about autonomy, e.g., we only had to consider the time from Ivan Ilyich's diagnosis rather than his whole life.[13]

Dworkin says he 'is not trying to analyze the notion of autonomous acts, but of what it means to be an autonomous person, to have a certain capacity and exercise it'[14] and he claims that 'intuitively' autonomy seems to be a 'global' rather than a 'local' concept in the sense that it is about a 'whole way of living one's life.' It is not clear however, where his emphasis lies—in the way one lives or in consistency over time.

Dworkin's claim about what it means to be an autonomous person and his suggestion that autonomy is global, are in response to an objection concerning acts of critical reflection and an attempt to get around the infinite regress problem. It is in response to the question: 'why is a first-order motivation evaluated by a nonautonomous process itself autonomous?' Dworkin says:

> I do claim that the process of reflection ought to be subject to the requirements of procedural independence, but if a person's reflections have not been manipulated, coerced, and so forth and if the person does have the requisite identification then they are, on my view, autonomous. There is no conceptual necessity for raising the question of whether the values, preferences at the second order would themselves be valued or preferred at a higher level, although in particular cases the agent might engage in such higher-order reflection.'[15]

Having the 'requisite identification' seems to require having a higher order desire about the kind of life that a person wants to lead. As noted, this seems to be Dworkin's attempt to avoid the infinite regress. I do not disagree with the idea that having a higher order desire about the kind of life that a person wants to lead should be a requirement for autonomy, but I do not think that the focus needs to be on *persons*. I think that the issue is rationality, e.g., about the right kind of thinking—and this will become more apparent in the discussion to come.

Dworkin makes a distinction between autonomy and identification by saying that autonomy 'is a feature that evaluates a whole way of living one's life and can only be assessed over extended portions of a person's life, whereas *identification* is something that may be pinpointed over short periods of time.'[16] On Dworkin's account it seems that being an autonomous *person* is a byproduct of the following:

> Autonomy is conceived of as a second-order capacity of persons to reflect critically upon their first-order preferences, desires, wishes, and so forth and the capacity to accept or attempt to change these in light of higher-order preferences and values. By exercising such a capacity, persons define their nature, give meaning and coherence to their lives, and take responsibility for the kind of person they are.[17]

The ending of this could be changed. It could read:

> By exercising such a capacity, persons define their nature, give meaning and coherence to their lives and take responsibility for their choices. Ultimately, the kind of person they become is a result of these choices—and that could mean that they are an autonomous, mostly autonomous, sometimes autonomous or never autonomous person.

Dworkin refers to 'the condition of being a chooser' and may be saying something like this but it is not clear enough for us to be sure.[18]

I do not think we need the distinction Dworkin makes between autonomy and identification. In making the distinction, Dworkin says identification is not the crucial thing and he introduces the idea that autonomy is global rather than local. I also do not think we need autonomy to be a global concept. As we saw earlier, it is plausible on a hierarchical account of autonomy to argue that we should respect Mr. M's choices and his changes even though they may lead to disaster. On a hierarchical account Mr. M is autonomous in the sense that he has the right kind of thinking. We can presume that he will be able to factor in to his deliberations the consequences of his choices which turn out badly. Constant changes would rule him out as incompetent on the grounds of cognitive impairment.

Dworkin's requirements for autonomy give content to the notion of an autonomous *person* but we do not have to view autonomy in terms of *persons* or their *whole lives*. A hierarchical account does not need to be construed in this way. As I have noted, it seems that Dworkin has introduced this idea into his account to deal with the problem of the infinite regress—but it is not necessary. The main emphasis of a hierarchical account is critical reflection or the right kind of thinking. Putting the emphasis on *persons* and *whole lives* makes it resemble a life-plan account. On a hierarchical account we can view autonomy as primarily task related—but in terms of the agent's psychology.

States That Are Consistent with Autonomy

A number of states that are consistent with autonomy on a hierarchical account are considered *in*consistent with autonomy by some commentators.[19] On a hierarchical account, devotion to a cause, loyalty, commitment including family commitment, making promises, and obeying laws do not restrict autonomy. A *decision* can be autonomous (and in a nontrivial way—that is, more than choosing meals) even though we are unfree. Our decisions can be autonomous though we are influenced by unconscious forces and irrational thought,[20] when we are faced with a devastating diagnosis and even when we are dying. We can be a follower but still make autonomous decisions and our decisions can be autonomous when we are taking Prozac, when a patient, and when we are ill. They can be autonomous even when they reflect a sudden dramatic change in our values. That kind of decision will be autonomous if there is a reason for the change such as a devastating diagnosis or some other life-changing event. These are often the times when we are prompted to 'reflect upon, reassess, and restructure' our values and change our minds.[21]

WHAT IS THE ROLE OF RATIONALITY?

As we have seen, rationality of some kind is a requirement for autonomy. However, a rationality requirement poses problems. Without a certain amount of rationality autonomy seems meaningless but if we emphasize rationality it becomes easier for health professionals to justify intervening in or overriding decisions. If we emphasize rationality a lot, decisions that we generally think of as autonomous are likely to be undervalued or overridden. On the other hand, our wanting to respect people's autonomous choices can come at a cost if they are foolish or badly thought out choices.

The hierarchical account of autonomy is more than a minimalist account in which autonomy is whatever a person chooses as long as they do not use faulty reasoning. A hierarchical account does not just exclude faulty reasoning. It requires the *right kind of reasoning*—and that is something extra. A certain amount of rationality is necessary for autonomy and for consent to have meaning.

WHAT KIND OF RATIONALITY?

There are different kinds of rationality. Rationality can be instrumental in the sense that it involves the optimal pursuit of a person's preferences or goals whatever they may be. Then there is another kind or rationality in which certain ends have importance. Instrumental rationality does not prevent acts from being 'in the end absurd, lawless' or 'unintelligible.'[22] Dependence on absurd or unintelligible ends suggests that instrumental rationality and pursuing desired ends is not the whole thing. Consider the case cited by John Rawls about a man 'whose only pleasure is to count blades of grass in various geometrically shaped areas such as park squares and well-trimmed lawns. He is otherwise intelligent and actually possesses unusual skills, since he manages to survive by solving difficult mathematical problems for a fee.'[23]

On Dworkin's view, there is nothing about Rawls' example that is inconsistent with autonomy. One of the reasons why 'autonomy is a relatively weak and contentless notion' according to Dworkin is 'because people can give meaning to their lives in all kinds of ways: from stamp collecting to taking care of one's invalid parents.' He claims 'there is no particular way of giving shape and meaning to a life.'[24] In the medical setting however, even if a decision demonstrates instrumental rationality, we may not want to accept a decision based on absurd or unintelligible motives. Typical of many suicides is the combination of 'basically sound reasoning' (from the agent's viewpoint) and 'nonrational motives.'[25] The act may demonstrate instrumental rationality but the act may be, in the end, absurd or unintelligible. It seems counterintuitive to count these actions as autonomous. In a revised hierarchical account there seems to be a need for another requirement (in terms of certain ends) that should be met—something to do with rational ity. And this is where conversation has a role.

Earlier on, I rejected a substantive notion of the good life as part of a theory of autonomy but a substantive notion of rationality is something different. A substantive notion of rationality can be one that rules out obviously absurd or unintelligible ends and desires based on false or irrational beliefs.

In the Jehovah's Witness case, given the nature of the Witness's beliefs, we were left to wonder what work a rationality requirement really does and whether proponents of most psychological accounts wanted ways to say Jehovah's Witnesses are autonomous so they did not have to override their decisions. So, how do we give a role to rationality?

R. B. Brandt's idea of cognitive psychotherapy can be linked to the role Katz gives to conversation. As we saw in an earlier chapter, Brandt's idea of cognitive psychotherapy is one way in which decisions involving desires can be considered rational. According to Brandt, although desires can be irrational they are also open to rational criticism. And when desires are subject to and survive the rational criticism of cognitive psychotherapy (in which dialogue or conversation obviously has a role) they can be considered rational. Brandt's argument about cognitive psychotherapy illustrates the way in which conversation and rationality are linked. The role of conversation can test and enhance the rationality and the autonomy of decisions.

On Brandt's view, a choice that includes desires could be called autonomous if it is a choice that is responsive to facts and logic (or desires subject to Katz idea of enforced reflection with self and others). Because it is responsive to facts and logic it could also be called rational choice. Brandt argues that there are intrinsic desires and aversions and claims that if we were given all available relevant information and we are repeatedly confronted with it 'in an ideally vivid way, and at an appropriate time,' our desires will be affected.[26] He claims that an irrational desire is one that extinguishes after cognitive psychotherapy. For instance, there are appropriate times such as when a person is about to light a cigarette or is having thoughts that make the idea of smoking appealing, and at those times reflection on the bad consequences of the habit could remove the desire to smoke. Irrational desires extinguish under cognitive psychotherapy and any desire which will not extinguish is not an irrational desire. A desire that does not extinguish is a rational desire.

A rationality requirement on the revised hierarchical account of autonomy involves critical reflection or the right kind of thinking. That may involve conversation or the 'imposition of dialogue' and something like Brandt's cognitive psychotherapy.

WHY SHOULD WE RESPECT AUTONOMOUS CHOICES?

The main focus of this work has been identifying what we are referring to when we talk about autonomy in the clinical context and finding a useful account of autonomy for that context. Now, with an improved hierarchical descriptive psychological account of autonomy we can look at the question: What is there about autonomy and autonomous choices that is valuable?

Gerald Dworkin says his concept of autonomy 'which has no particular content, that allows for the possibility of a patient granting complete authority to a doctor, seems too formal to be of great value.'[27] There is no content that we can justify as worthy of admiration, e.g., the 'self-sufficient, independent, person relying on his own resources' that we can justify as worthy of admiration. Instead, his concept of autonomy that has no particular content 'emphasizes self-definition in abstraction from the self that is so defined.'[28] Nevertheless he argues that this conception of autonomy has value.[29] I agree that the concept of autonomy as described in his account has value and a hierarchical concept of autonomy has no content in the sense of a substantive notion of the good life. On the other hand, content can be attributed to my revised hierarchical account of autonomy. It has content in the sense that it is a descriptive psychological account and that includes a substantive notion of rationality.

The way the value of autonomy will be interpreted will depend on an underlying ethical theory. Autonomy can be instrumentally valuable (it leads to something else that is good) or intrinsically valuable (it is good in itself or for its own sake) or it can be both instrumentally and intrinsically valuable. In the clinical context it seems to be primarily instrumental value that we are concerned with. Instrumental value is easy to recognize while intrinsic value, if autonomy has intrinsic value, is not as obvious or as readily detectable. However, the question of intrinsic value may come up in discussions about promoting autonomy or if we choose to save the lives of autonomous beings rather than ones that are not autonomous.

On an instrumental/Millian account of value, autonomy is good because it leads to things such as preference satisfaction or pleasure which are intrinsically valuable.[30] On a Millian view,[31]as we saw earlier, some of the value of autonomy seems to reside in the critical reflection that encourages us to question ourselves and our understanding and to learn the grounds of our own opinions:

> It is better to be a human being dissatisfied than a pig satisfied, better to be Socrates dissatisfied than a fool satisfied. And if the fool, or the pig, are of a

> different opinion, it is because they only know their own side of the question. The other party to the comparison knows both sides.[32]

Dworkin argues that our lives are more likely to be satisfying if we are able to shape our own choices and values. We should not overlook the fact that, apart from the results, 'the process of thinking about, reflecting upon, choosing among preferences is a source of satisfaction to individuals.'[33] On Dworkin's view 'autonomy is a capacity that is (partly) constitutive of what it is to be an agent . . . the exercise of the capacity is what makes a life *mine.*'[34] This is not inconsistent with the idea that autonomy should be *assessed* as a property of particular acts or decisions. On my revised hierarchical account of autonomy the focus does not have to be on persons or lives or autonomy as a character ideal.

I am in agreement with Dworkin's view that although autonomy is important and it is important to respect autonomy it is also important to respect a person's 'welfare, or their liberty, or their rationality.'[35] Dworkin claims that autonomy does not always have value and 'more autonomy' is not 'always better than less.' He points out that as well as the instrumental gains of exercising autonomy there are instrumental losses: 'With responsibility comes blame and punishment.'[36]

Dworkin argues that autonomy also has intrinsic value—that 'there is value connected with being self-determining that is not a matter either of bringing about good results or the pleasures of the process itself. He says:

> This is the intrinsic desirability of exercising the capacity for self-determination. We desire to be recognized by others as the kind of creature capable of determining our own destiny. Our own sense of self-respect is tied to the respect of others—and this is not just a matter of psychology'[37]

Whether autonomy on my revised hierarchical descriptive psychological account has intrinsic value can be left open. The answer to that would depend on the kind of underlying ethical theory one holds.

Some will say that to talk about the value of autonomy, whether instrumental or intrinsic, is to assume a consequentialist view. Assessing actions as good or right by reference to means to an end or by reference to an end in itself is to view morality simply as a matter of ends. The importance of autonomy, they will argue, is clearer in a rights-based ethic where the issue is not the value of autonomy but the role autonomy has in defining what one has a right to do to another person and this seems especially pertinent in the clinical context. On this view autonomy is a procedural constraint reflecting the idea that we are different individuals with separate lives and we may not be sacrificed or used as a resource for the benefit of others without our consent.[38] This is a view that has been employed by Robert Nozick in libertarian political philosophy and by H. Tristram Engelhardt in biomedical ethics.[39]

The view that the ethical significance of autonomy lies in seeing it as a side constraint that we ought not to violate, rather than as a value that we ought to maximize seems to fit most naturally with a Kantian idea and principle. Nevertheless, someone could have a descriptive psychological view of autonomy and hold to the ethical principle that it is wrong to violate someone's autonomy, and the wrongness consists in violating a side constraint, not in failing to maximize a value. On this view, autonomy should be honoured rather than promoted.[40]

Autonomy can be regarded as an absolute or inviolable side constraint in which it trumps all other moral considerations or it can be viewed as a constraint that is only prima facie. Autonomy as an absolute side constraint has added to the muddle in contemporary discussions. Adhering to the idea that it is wrong to violate a side constraint makes people want to label some decisions as nonautonomous so they can justify overriding some decisions, or labeling a decision autonomous so it will be respected even though it is clearly not autonomous on a descriptive psychological account. As a side constraint however, autonomy is probably more likely to be viewed as a prima facie side constraint. On this view there is a point at which autonomy should be infringed.[41] For instance, it is prima facie wrong to incarcerate an innocent person but the wrongness can be overridden if it is the only way to prevent the spread of a life-threatening disease. It would not be wrong to incarcerate 'Typhoid Mary' on this view.

These views are compatible with a descriptive psychological account of autonomy, and do not require the adoption of a procedural account. Indeed, these views do not even really make sense on a procedural account of autonomy because of its lack of descriptive content.

My revised descriptive psychological account of autonomy is compatible with both conseqentialist and rights-based ethics. Autonomy can be regarded as good because it helps bring about particular ends, or because it is intrinsically good, or it can be seen as a side constraint that we ought not to violate except in exceptional circumstances. Deciding what is the correct ethical theory is a task that requires substantial discussion of the choice between consequentialist and rights-based ethical theories and this is a task for another occasion.

SOME DECISIONS WON'T MEASURE UP

Given the tensions in wanting to respect autonomy, the need for a rationality requirement and the question of how high or how low to set the rationality requirement, some decisions we generally think of as autonomous may not measure up.The Jehovah's Witness may not measure up but we may still think that it is better for us to respect their decisions regarding blood transfusions.

RECOGNIZING AN EVALUATIVE ASPECT

Autonomy can be a purely descriptive notion but, as we saw earlier, the characteristics of psychological autonomy tend to be something that we regard as an ideal. There tends to be an implicit assumption that autonomy ought to be respected and that it is a desirable quality in persons and choices. This seems to make the idea of autonomy both descriptive and evaluative but not evaluative by definition.[42]

The term 'autonomy' has evaluative meaning but its descriptive meaning is more firmly tied to it than its evaluative sense. In order to see this more clearly we can compare it to the term 'courage' which also has this characteristic. 'Courage' is something that we are generally in favor of. We admire and encourage 'courage' though it may not always be conducive to human well-being and we may not always want to praise it.[43]

The point I am making is that in response to the question 'What is autonomy?' the best account is a descriptive psychological account but we need to acknowledge that a descriptive psychological notion of autonomy has a secondarily evaluative sense. The descriptive meaning of autonomy has a laudatory force and there is a pejorative force when we say something is not autonomous. The evaluative meaning comes with the characteristics of psychological autonomy, i.e., the characteristics of someone who chooses autonomously (although I argue that the *assessment* of autonomy should be task related in the clinical context). These characteristics tend to be things we regard as desirable (e.g., rationality and self-awareness and having a fundamental commitment to the kind of life a person wants to live) and therefore there is an implicit assumption that a decision made by someone with these characteristics should be protected and respected.

When we acknowledge the existence of the evaluative meaning we can also acknowledge the fact that we are not committed to the evaluative meaning; we do not have to be 'prisoners of our own conceptual apparatus'[44] We can, if we want to, explicitly reject the evaluations encapsulated in the term. We can give moral instruction to counteract any moral instruction that is implicit in the term. We can be explicit and say: 'This decision is not autonomous but it is better to respect it than not.' We could argue that decisions of a Jehovah's Witness or decisions based on Christian beliefs[45] are not autonomous but it is better to respect them than not. It is not the case that simply using the word autonomy commits us to a particular evaluation. The evaluation can be eliminated. We can also say that 'This decision is autonomous but it is better not to respect it.' We could argue that deciding to experiment with addictive drugs, entering a risky clinical trial or entering a cult that uses brainwashing techniques may well be autonomous but it is better to intervene.

This approach allows paternalism in certain situations but the fact that we acknowledge the evaluative meaning of autonomy and the fact that we can be explicit and reject that meaning makes this an open, transparent approach. We are not pressured to say that a decision is autonomous or nonautonomous because we think it is better not to intervene in a decision or because we think there is reason to intervene. Recognition of an evaluative element in a descriptive psychological account of autonomy allows other values to figure but it does so without disparaging or discounting the idea of autonomy.

SUMMING UP

We have covered a lot of ground. I began by trying to work out what we are really referring to when we talk of autonomy and I identified different strands of the idea and found that current usage is muddled. I have isolated and critically examined different notions of autonomy and argued that a revised hierarchical descriptive psychological account is the best and the most defensible account for the clinical context. I have done what I set out to do—I have an account of autonomy that is applicable and useful for the clinical setting. It gives us criteria that explain why we should respect autonomous choices and we are able to justify some interventions without disposing of or discrediting the notion of autonomy. This account is philosophically defensible. We can be clear about the concept we are defending and we can use it in a consistent way.

NOTES

1. Dworkin, *The Theory and Practice of Autonomy*, 16.

2. Dworkin, *The Theory and Practice of Autonomy*, 16.

3. Isaiah Berlin, "Two Concepts of Liberty" 135.

4. Carl E. Schneider, *The Practice of Autonomy: Patients, Doctors, and Medical Decisions* (New York: Oxford University Press, 1998), 90–91, quoting Arnold R. Beisser, *Flying Without Wings* (New York: Doubleday, 1989), 135.

5. Schneider, *The Practice of Autonomy*, 91, quoting Wilfrid Sheed, *In Love With Daylight: A Memoir of Recovery* (New York: Simon & Schuster, 1995), 13–15.

6. Helga Kuhse, ed., *Willing to Listen, Wanting to Die* (Ringwood: Penguin Books 1994), 12, 15–16.

7. Even though, of the various psychological accounts assessed the hierarchical account was found to be the most appropriate for the clinical context.

8. As noted earlier, Benjamin Levi also advocates something similar to Katz' role for conversation.

9. Beauchamp and Childress, *Principles of Biomedical Ethics*, 1994, 4th ed., 121–22 and; Beauchamp and Childress, *Principles of Biomedical Ethics*, 2001, 5th ed. 58–59.

10. Dworkin, *The Theory and Practice of Autonomy*, 13.

11. Gerald Dworkin, "Autonomy," in *A Companion to Contemporary Political Philosophy*, eds. Robert E. Goodin and Philip Pettit (Oxford: Blackwell, 1993), 359–60.

12. Dworkin, *The Theory and Practice of Autonomy*, 18.

13. It is important to note that Ivan Ilyich reassesses his life in light of the relatively recent past, i..e., his devastating diagnosis, and may reject the long-term or stable values that he previously held.

14. Dworkin, *The Theory and Practice of Autonomy*, 19–20.

15. Dworkin, *The Theory and Practice of Autonomy*, 19–20.

16. Dworkin, *The Theory and Practice of Autonomy*, 15–16.

17. Dworkin, *The Theory and Practice of Autonomy*, 20.

18. Dworkin, *The Theory and Practice of Autonomy*, 18.

19. For example, communitarian objections and feminist objections and critiques by European and other non-American ethicists. See Soren Holm, "Autonomy," in *Encyclopedia of Applied Ethics*, vol. 1 (Academic Press, 1998), 272–73; Lawrence C. Becker and Charlotte B. Becker, eds., *Encyclopedia of Ethics*, vol. 1, (New York: Garland Publishing, Inc., 1992), 74; Marilyn Friedman, "Autonomy and Social Relationships: Rethinking the Feminist Critique," in *Feminists Rethink the Self*, ed. Diana Tietjens Meyers (Boulder, Colo.: Westview Press, 1997), 40–61; Catriona Mackenzie and Natalie Stoljar eds., *Relational Autonomy* (Oxford: Oxford University Press: 2000). Mackenzie and Stoljar's book is a response to critics who view the idea of autonomy as too individualistic and rationalistic (a caricature of autonomy) and their book shows why autonomy is an important concept for feminists

to 'reclaim and reconceptualize.' Understood correctly, however, the hierarchical descriptive psychological theory relied on in this work does not need to be reclaimed.

20. See Katz, *The Silent World of Doctor and Patient.*

21. Levi, *Respecting Patient Autonomy*, 44.

22. O'Neill, *Constructions of Reason*, 76.

23. John Rawls, *A Theory of Justice* (Oxford: Clarendon Press, 1972), 432–33.

24. Dworkin, *The Theory and Practice of Autonomy*, 31.

25. David Heyd and Sidney Bloch, 'The Ethics of Suicide' in *Psychiatric Ethics*, eds., Sidney Bloch and Paul Chodoff (Oxford: Oxford University Press, 1991, 2nd ed.), 259–60.

26. Brandt, *A Theory of the Good and the Right*, 112–13.

27. Dworkin, *The Theory and Practice of Autonomy*, 109.

28. Dworkin, *The Theory and Practice of Autonomy*, 30.

29. Dworkin, *The Theory and Practice of Autonomy*, 109–12.

30. Holm, "Autonomy," 270.

31. Although Mill does not use the word "autonomy."

32. J. S. Mill, *Utilitarianism, On Liberty, and Considerations on Representative Government* (London: Dent, 1910), quoted in Holm, "Autonomy," 269.

33. Dworkin, *The Theory and Practice of Autonomy*, 112.

34. Dworkin, *The Theory and Practice of Autonomy*, 32.

35. Dworkin, *The Theory and Practice of Autonomy*, 32.

36. Dworkin, *The Theory and Practice of Autonomy*, 112.

37. Dworkin, *The Theory and Practice of Autonomy*, 112.

38. Robert Nozick, *Anarchy, State and Utopia* (New York: Basic Books, 1974), 30–33.

39. Holm, "Autonomy," 270–71.

40. Philip Pettit, "Consequentialism" in *A Companion to Ethics*, ed. Peter Singer (Oxford: Blackwell, 1993), 231.

41. Jonathan Dancy, "An Ethic of Prima Facie Duties," in *A Companion to Ethics*, ed. Peter Singer (Oxford: Blackwell, 1993), 227.

42. We saw in the earlier section on the evaluative notion, that when autonomy is an evaluative concept something happens at the level of formulating the concept.

43. R. M. Hare, *Freedom and Reason* (Oxford: Oxford University Press, 1963), 149.

44. Hare, *Freedom and Reason*, 189.

45. As mentioned earlier, many Christians believe that God is omnibenevolent and omnipotent, yet they know that there is evil in the world and they do not have the arguments to reconcile these things.

BIBLIOGRAPHY

Alderson, Priscilla. "Consent to Children's Surgery and Intensive Medical Treatment." *Journal of Law and Society* 17, no. 1 (Spring, 1990): 52–65.

Annas, George J. "The Dominance of American Law (And Market Values) over American Bioethics." Pp. 83–96 in *Meta Medical Ethics: The Philosophical Foundations of Bioethics*, edited by Michael A. Grodin. Dordrecht: Kluwer Academic Publishers, 1995.

Appelbaum, Paul S., Loren H. Roth, Charles W. Lidz, Paul Benson, and William Winslade, "False Hopes and Best Data: Consent to Research and the Therapeutic Misconception." *Hastings Center Report* 17, no. 2 (April 1987): 20–24.

Aranow, Robert B., Richard S. Schwarts, and Mark D. Sullivan, "Mood Brighteners." *American Journal of Psychiatry* [referred to in Kramer 1993 as "(in press) draft of March 19, 1992"].

Beauchamp, Tom L., "The Principles Approach." *Hastings Center Report*, Special Supplement, "The Birth of Bioethics", 23, (6 Suppl), (November–December 1993): S9.

———. "The Origins, Goals, and Core Commitments of *The Belmont Report* and *Principles of Biomedical Ethics*". Pp. 17–46 in *The Story of Bioethics*, edited by Jennifer K. Walter and Eran P. Klein. Washington, D.C.: Georgetown University Press, 2003

Beauchamp, Tom L., and James F. Childress. *Principles of Biomedical Ethics*. 1st ed. New York: Oxford University Press, 1979.

———. *Principles of Biomedical Ethics*. 2nd ed. New York: Oxford University Press, 1983.

———. *Principles of Biomedical Ethics.* 3rd ed. New York: Oxford University Press, 1989.

———. *Principles of Biomedical Ethics.* 4th ed. New York: Oxford University Press, 1994

———. *Principles of Biomedical Ethics.* 5th ed. New York: Oxford University Press, 2001

Beauchamp, Tom L., and Laurence B. McCullough. "The Management of Medical Information: Legal and Moral Requirements of Informed Consent." Pp. 130–41 in *Bioethics: A Collection of Readings,* edited by Edwards and Graber, San Diego: Harcourt brace Jovanovich, 1988.

Beck, Lewis White. *A Commentary on Kant's Critique of Practical Reason.* Chicago: The University of Chicago Press, 1960.

Beck, Lewis W. "Kant and the Right to Revolution." Pp. 399–411 in *Immanuel Kant: Critical Assessments,* Vol.III, edited by Ruth F. Chadwick, London: Routledge, 1992.

Becker, Lawrence C., and Charlotte B. Becker, ed. *Encyclopedia of Ethics,* Volume 1. New York: Garland Publishing, Inc., 1992.

Beecher, Henry K. "Ethics and Clinical Research." *The New England Journal of Medicine* 274, no. 24 (June 1966): 1,354–60.

Beisser, Arnold R. *Flying Without Wings.* New York: Doubleday, 1989. Quoted in *The Practice of Autonomy: Patients, Doctors, and Medical Decisions,* by Carl E. Schneider, New York: Oxford University Press, 1998.

Berlin, Isaiah. "Two Concepts of Liberty" in *Four Essays on Liberty.* London: Oxford University Press, 1969.

Berofsky, Bernard. *Liberation From Self: A Theory of Personal Autonomy,* New York: Cambridge University Press, 1995.

Blanchard, E. B., J. E. Martin, and Patricia M. Dubbert. *Non-Drug Treatments for Essential Hypertension.* New York: Pergamon Press, 1988.

Bloch, Sidney, and Paul Chodoff, ed. *Psychiatric Ethics,* 2nd ed. Oxford: Oxford University Press, 1991.

Brandt, R. B. *A Theory of the Good and the Right,* Oxford: Clarendon Press, 1979.

Breggin, Peter R., and Ginger Ross Breggin. *Talking Back to Prozac: What Doctors Won't Tell You about Today's Most Controversial Drug.* New York: St. Martin's Press, 1994.

Brock, Dan. "The Use of Drugs for Pleasure: Some Philosophical Issues." Pp. 83–106 in *Feeling Good and Doing Better: Ethics and Nontherapeutic Drug Use,* edited by Thomas H. Murray, Willard Gaylin, and Ruth Macklin New Jersey: Humana Press, 1984.

Brody, Baruch A. *The Ethics of Biomedical Research: An International Perspective.* New York: Oxford University Press, 1998.

Brody, Baruch A., and H. Tristram Jr. Engelhardt. *Bioethics Readings & Cases.* Englewood cliffs, New Jersey: Prentice-Hall, Inc., 1987.

Bulger, Ruth Ellen, Elizabeth Meyer Bobby, and Harvey V. Fineberg, ed. *Society's Choices: Social and Ethical Decision Making in Biomedicine.* Washington D.C.: National Academy Press, 1995.

Bursztajn, H. J., R. I. Feinbloom, R. M. Hann, and A. Brodsky. *Medical Choices, Medical Chances: How Patients, Families and Physicians can Cope with Uncertainty.* New York: A Merloyd Lawrence Book, 1981.

Callahan, Daniel. "Autonomy: A Moral Good, Not a Moral Obsession." *Hastings Center Report,* 14 no. 5 (October 1984): 40–42.

Cavalieri, P., and P. Singer, ed. *The Great Ape Project: Equality beyond Humanity,* London: Fourth Estate, 1993.

Charlesworth, Max. *Bioethics in a Liberal Society.* Cambridge: Cambridge University Press, 1993.

Childress, James. "The Place of Autonomy in Bioethics." *Hastings Center Report* 20, no. 1 (January/February 1990): 12–17.

———. *Practical Reasoning in Bioethics.* Bloomington: Indiana University Press, 1997.

Christman, John, ed. *The Inner Citadel: Essays on Individual Autonomy,* Oxford: Oxford University Press, 1989.

———. "Autonomy and Personal History." *Canadian Journal of Philosophy* 21, no. 1 (March 1991): 1–24.

———. "Defending Historical Autonomy: A Reply to Professor Mele." *Canadian Journal of Philosophy* 23, no.2 (June 1993): 281–89.

———. "Liberalism, Autonomy, and Self-Transformation." *Social Theory and Practice* 27, no. 2 (April 2001): 185–206.

Clouser, Danner K. "Common Morality as an Alternative to Principlism." *Kennedy Institute of Ethics Journal* 5, no. 3 (1995): 219–36.

Crittenden, Jack. *Beyond Individualism: Reconstituting the Liberal Self.* Oxford: Oxford University Press, 1992.

Dancy, Jonathan. "An Ethic of Prima Facie Duties." Pp. 219–20 in *A Companion to Ethics,* edited by Peter Singer. Oxford: Blackwell, 1993.

DeGrazia, David. "Prozac, Enhancement, and Self-Creation." *Hastings Center Report* 30, no. 2 (March–April 2000): 34–40.

Devettere, Raymond J. "The Principled Approach: Principles, Rules, and Actions." In *Meta Medical Ethics: The Philosophical Foundations of Bioethics,* edited by Michael A. Grodin. *Meta Medical Ethics: The Philosophical Foundations of Bioethics.* Dordrecht: Kluwer Academic Publishers, 1995b.

———. *Practical Decision Making in Health Care Ethics: Cases and Concepts,* Washington: Georgetown University Press, 1995a.

Diller, Lawrence H. "The Run on Ritalin: Attention Deficit Disorder and Stimulant Treatment in the 1990s." *Hastings Center Report* 26, (March–April 1996): 12–18.

Double, Richard. "Two Types of Autonomy Accounts." *Canadian Journal of Philosophy* 22, no. 1 (March 1992): 65–80.

Downie, R. S., and Elizabeth Telfer. *Respect For Persons.* George London: Allen and Unwin Ltd., 1969.

Dworkin, Gerald. *The Theory and Practice of Autonomy*, Cambridge: Cambridge University Press, 1988.

———. "Autonomy." Pp. 359–65 in *A Companion to Contemporary Political Philosophy*, edited by Robert E. Goodin and Philip Pettit. Oxford: Blackwell, 1993.

———. Review of *Liberation from Self: A Theory of Personal Autonomy* by Bernard Berofsky, *The Journal of Philosophy*, XCIV, no.5, (May 1997): 212–16.

Elliott, Carl. "Hedgehogs and Hermaphrodites: Toward a More Anthropological Bioethics." Pp. 197–211 in *Philosophy of Medicine and Bioethics: A Twenty-Year Retrospective and Critical Appraisal,* edited by Ronald A. Carson and Chester R. Burns. Dordrecht, The Netherlands: Kluwer Academic Publishers, 1997.

———. "The Tyranny of Happiness: Ethics and Cosmetic Psychopharmacology." Pp. 177–88 in *Enhancing Human Traits: Ethical and Social Implications,* edited by E. Parens. Washington: Georgetown University Press, 1998.

———. "Pursued by Happiness and Beaten Senseless: Prozac and the American Dream." *Hastings Center Report* 30, no. 2 (March–April 2000): 7–12.

Engelhardt, H. Tristram. "Basic Ethical Principles in the Conduct of Biomedical and Behavioral Research Involving Human Subjects." National Commission for the Protection of Human Subjects of Biomedical and Behavioral Research, *Appendix: Vol. 1. Belmont Report*, n.d.

———. *The Foundations of Bioethics.* New York: Oxford University Press, 1986.

———. *The Foundations of Bioethics.* 2nd ed. New York: Oxford University Press, 1996a.

———. "Bioethics Reconsidered: Theory and Method in a Post-Christian, Post-Modern Age." *Kennedy Institute of Ethics Journal* 6, no. 4 (December 1996b): 336–41.

———. *Bioethics and Secular Humanism: The Search for a Common Morality.* Philadelphia: Trinity Press International, 1991.

Emanuel, Ezekiel J. "The Beginning of the End of Principlism." *Hastings Center Report* 25, no. 4 (July–August 1995): 37–38.

Frankfurt, Harry G. "Freedom of the Will and the Concept of a Person." *Journal of Philosophy* 68 (1971). Reprinted pp. 63–76 in *The Inner Citadel: Essays on Individual Autonomy*, Oxford: Oxford University Press, 1989.

Frankl, Viktor E. *Man's Search for Meaning.* Translated by Ilse Lasch. London: Hodder and Stoughton, 1964.

Fried, C. *Medical Experimentation: Personal Integrity and Social Policy.* New York: Elsevier, 1974. P. 98 in *The Theory and Practice of Autonomy*, by Gerald Dworkin. Cambridge: Cambridge University Press, 1988.

Friedman, Marilyn. "Autonomy and the Split-Level Self." *Southern Journal of Philosophy* 24, no. 1 (1986): 19–35.

———. "Autonomy and Social Relationships: Rethinking the Feminist Critique." Pp. 40–61 in *Feminists Rethink the Self,* edited by Diana Tietjens Meyers. Boulder, Colo.: Westview Press, 1997.

Fouts, Roger S., and Deborah H. Fouts. "Chimpanzees' Use of Sign Language." Pp. 28–41 in *The Great Ape Project: Equality beyond Humanity,* edited by P. Cavalieri and P. Singer. London: Fourth Estate, 1993.

Gauthier, Candace Cummins. "Philosophical Foundations of Respect for Autonomy." *Kennedy Institute of Ethics Journal* 3, no.1, (1993): 21–37.

Gaylin, Willard. "Feeling Good and Doing Better." Pp. 1–10 in *Feeling Good and Doing Better: Ethics and Nontherapeutic Drug Use,* edited by Thomas H. Murray, Willard Gaylin, and Ruth Macklin. New Jersey: Humana Press, 1984.

Gaylin, Willard, and Bruce Jennings. *The Perversion of Autonomy: The Proper Uses of Coercion and Constraints in a Liberal Society,* Free Press, New York, 1996.

Gert, Bernard, Charles Culver, and K. Danner Clouser. *Bioethics: A Return to Fundamentals,* New York: Oxford University Press, 1997.

Gray, John. *Mill on Liberty: A Defence,* London: Routledge & Kegan Paul, 1983.

Goodall, Jane. "Chimpanzees: Bridging the Gap. Pp. 10–18 in *The Great Ape Project: Equality beyond Humanity,* edited by P. Cavalieri and P. Singer. London: Fourth Estate, 1993.

Gorovitz, Samuel. *Doctors' Dilemmas.* New York: Oxford University Press, 1982.

Griffith, Chris. "Blood Oath Death Risk." *Sunday Mail,* 7 March 1999.

Grodin ,Michael A., ed. *Meta Medical Ethics: The Philosophical Foundations of Bioethics.* Dordrecht: Kluwer Academic Publishers, 1995.

Group for the Advancement of Psychiatry. *A Casebook in Psychiatric Ethics.* New York: Brunner/Maxel Publishers, 1990.

Hare, R. M. *Freedom and Reason.* Oxford: Oxford University Press, 1963.

———. *The Language of Morals.* Oxford: Clarendon Press, (published 1952) 1992.

———. *Sorting Out Ethics.* Oxford: Clarendon Press, 1997.

Haworth, Lawrence. *Autonomy: An Essay in Philosophical Psychology and Ethics.* New Haven: Yale University Press, 1986.

Healy, David. "Good Science or Good Business?" *Hastings Center Report* 30, no. 2 (2000): 19–22.

Herman, Barbara. "Rules, Motives, and Helping Actions." *Philosophical Studies* 45, (1984): 369–77.

Heyd, David, and Sidney Bloch. "The Ethics of Suicide." Pp. 243–64 in *Psychiatric Ethics,* 2nd ed. edited by Sidney Bloch and Paul Chodoff. Oxford: Oxford University Press, 1991.

Hill, Thomas E. "The Kantian Conception of Autonomy." Pp. 91–105 in *The Inner Citadel: Essays on Individual Autonomy,* edited by J. Christman. New York: Oxford University Press, 1989.

Holm, Soren. "Autonomy." Pp. 267–74 in *Encyclopedia of Applied Ethics,* Volume 1, Academic Press, 1998.

Hope, Tony. "Personal Identity and Psychiatric Illness." Pp. 131–43 in *Philosophy, Psychology and Psychiatry,* edited by A. Phillips Griffiths. New York: Cambridge University Press, 1994.

Hurka, Thomas. "Why Value Autonomy?" *Social Theory and Practice* 13, no. 3, (1987): 361–82.

Janis, Irving L., and Leon Mann. *Decision Making: A Psychological Analysis of Conflict, Choice, and Commitment.* New York: The Free Press, 1977.

Jones, Merry Bloch. *Birthmothers: Women Who Have Relinquished Babies for Adoption Tell Their Stories.* Chicago: Chicago Review Press, 1993.

Jonsen, Albert R., and Andrew Jameton. "Medical Ethics, History of: The Americas." Pp. 1,616–32 in *Encyclopedia of Bioethics*, Vol. 3, edited by Warren Thomas Reich. New York: Simon & Schuster Macmillan, 1995.

Jonsen, Albert R., and Stephen Toulmin. *The Abuse of Casuistry: A History of Moral Reasoning.* Berkley: University of California Press, 1988.

Jonsen, Albert. "American Moralism and the Origin of Bioethics in the United States." *Journal of Medicine and Philosophy* 16, (1991): 115–29.

———. *The Birth of Bioethics*, New York: Oxford University Press, 1998.

Kant, Immanuel. *Critique of Practical Reason and Other Writings in Moral Philosophy.* Trans. and edited with an introduction by Lewis White Beck. Chicago: The University of Chicago Press, 1949.

———. *Groundwork of the Metaphysic of Morals.* In H. J. Paton trans. *The Moral Law.* 3rd ed. London: Hutchinson Of London, 1956.

———. In *Immanuel Kant, Lectures on Ethics*, edited by Peter Heath and J.B. Schneewind. Cambridge: Cambridge University Press, 1997.

———. *Lectures on Metaphysics.* Trans. and edited by Karl Ameriks and Steve Naragon. Cambridge: Cambridge University Press, 1997.

———. *The Doctrine of Virtue, Part II of The Metaphysic of Morals.* Trans. Mary J. Gregor. New York: Harper Torchbooks Harper and Row, 1964.

———. *Idea for a Universal History with a Cosmopolitan Purpose.* In *Kant Political Writings*, 2nd ed. Hans Reiss ed. and H. B. Nisbet trans. Cambridge: Cambridge University Press, 1991.

———. "On the Common Saying: 'This May be True in Theory, But it Does Not Apply in Practice.'" Pp. 61–92 in *Kant Political Writings*, 2nd ed. Hans Reiss ed. and H. B. Nisbet trans. Cambridge: Cambridge University Press, 1991.

Kapitan, Tomis. Review of *Liberation From Self: A Theory of Personal Autonomy* by Bernard Berofsky in *International Philosophy Quarterly*. 37, no. 3 (September, 1997): 370–72.

Katz, Jay. *The Silent World of Doctor and Patient.* London: Collier, Macmillan Publishers, 1984.

———. "Informed Consent: Must It Remain a Fairy Tale?" *Journal of Contemporary Health Law and Policy* 10 (1994): 69–91.

King, Nancy M. P., Gail E. Henderson, and Jane Stein Jane ed. *Beyond Regulations: Ethics in Human Subject Research.* Chapel Hill: The University of North Carolina Press, 1999.

King, Petrea. *Spirited Women: Journeys with Breast Cancer.*, Sydney: Random House, 1995.

———. *Quest For Life*. Sydney: Random House, 1992.

Klepper, Howard, Medical College of Winconsin Bioethics Discussion, 21 February, 1997.

Korsgaard, Christine, quoted in Gerald Dworkin. Review of *Liberation from Self: A Theory of Personal Autonomy* by Bernard Berofsky in *The Journal of Philosophy*, XCIV, no. 5 (May 1997): 212–16.

Kortlandt, Adriaan. "Spirits Dressed in Furs?" Pp. 137–45 in *The Great Ape Project: Equality beyond Humanity*, edited by P. Cavalieri and P. Singer. New York: St. Martin's Griffin, 1993.

Kramer, Peter D. *Listening to Prozac*, London: Fourth Estate, 1993.

———. "The Valorization of Sadness: Alienation and the Melancholic Temperament." *Hastings Center Report*, 30, no. 2, (March 2000): 13–18.

Kuflik, Arthur. "The Inalienability of Autonomy." *Philosophy & Public Affairs* 13, no. 4 (1984): 271–98.

Kuhse, Helga, ed. *Willing to Listen–Wanting to Die*, Ringwood: Penguin Books, 1994.

Levi, Benjamin H. *Respecting Patient Autonomy*. Urbana: University of Illinois Press, 1999.

Levine, Andrew. *The Politics of Autonomy: A Kantian Reading of Rousseau's Social Contract*. Amherst: University of Massachusetts Press, 1976.

———. *The General Will: Rousseau, Marx, Communism*. Cambridge: Cambridge University Press, 1993.

Lindley, Richard. *Autonomy*. London: Macmillan, 1986.

Mackenzie, Catriona, and Natalie Stoljar. *Relational Autonomy: Feminist Perspectives on Autonomy, Agency, and the Social Self*. New York: Oxford University Press, 2000.

Macklin, Ruth. *Man, Mind, and Morality: The Ethics of Behaviour Control*. Englewood Cliffs: Prentice Hall, Inc., 1982.

Matthews, Eric. "Autonomy and the Psychiatric Patient." *Journal of Applied Philosophy* 17, no. 1 (2000):59–70.

Meilaender, Gilbert C. *Body, Soul, and Bioethics*. Notre Dame: University of Nortre Dame Press, 1995.

Mele, Alfred. "History and Personal Autonomy." *Canadian Journal of Philosophy* 23, no.2 (June 1993): 271–80.

———. *Autonomous Agents: From Self-Control to Autonomy*. New York: Oxford University Press, 1995.

Meyers, Diana T. *Self, Society and Personal Choice*. New York: Columbia University Press, 1989.

Mill, J. S. *On Liberty*. Pp.1–104 in *On Liberty and Considerations on Representative Government*, edited by R.B. McCallum. Oxford: Basil Blackwell, 1948.

———. *System of Logic: Ratiocinative and Inductive*, Vol. II, 7th ed. London: Longmans, Green, Reader, and Dyer, 1971.

———. *Utilitarianism*. In *Mill: Utilitarianism*, edited by Samuel Gorovitz. Indianapolis: The Bobbs-Merrill Company, Inc., 1971.

———. *An Examination of Sir William Hamilton's Philosophy and of the Principal Philosophical Questions Discussed in His Writings*, Toronto: University of Toronto Press, 1979.

———. *Utilitarianism, On Liberty, and Considerations on Representative Government.* London: Dent, 1910, quoted by Soren Holm pp. 267–74 in "Autonomy" in *Encyclopedia of Applied Ethics*, Volume 1, Academic Press, 1998.

Moreno, Jonathan D. *Deciding Together: Bioethics and Moral Consensus.* New York: Oxford University Press, 1995.

Murray, Thomas H., Willard Gaylin, and Ruth Macklin ed. *Feeling Good and Doing Better: Ethics and Nontherapeutic Drug Use,* New Jersey: Humana Press, 1984.

The National Commission for the Protection of Human Subjects of Biomedical and Behavioral Research. *The Belmont Report: Ethical Principles and Guidelines for the Protection of Human Subjects Research.* DHEW Publication No (OS) 78-0012, 1978.

National Health and Medical Research Council (NHMRC). *National Statement on Ethical Conduct in Research Involving Humans.* Canberra: Commonwealth of Australia, 1999.

National Research Act Sec. 202 (a)(1)(A) July 1974. P.5 in *Practical Decision Making in Health Care Ethics: Cases and Concepts,* Washington: Georgetown University Press by Raymond J. Devettere 1995.

Neese, Randolph M. "What Good is Feeling Bad? The Evolutionary Benefits of Psychic Pain." *The Sciences* (November–Dece,ber 1990): 30–37.

Nishida, Toshisada. " Chimpanzees Are Always New to Me." Pp.24–26 in *The Great Ape Project: Equality beyond Humanity,* edited by P. Cavalieri and P. Singer. London: Fourth Estate, 1993.

Nozick, Robert. *Anarchy, State and Utopia.* New York: Basic Books, 1974.

Nuremberg Code, ohsr.od.nih.gov/guidelines/nuremberg.html (accessed 22 August 2004).

O'Neill, Onora. *Constructions of Reason: Explorations of Kant's Practical Philosophy.* Cambridge: Cambridge University Press, 1989.

———. "Kantian Ethics." Pp. 175–85 in *A Companion to Ethics,* edited by Peter Singer. Oxford: Blackwell, 1993.

Oshana, Marina. "Autonomy Naturalized." *Midwest Studies in Philosophy* XIX, (1994): 76–94.

Oyebode, Femi, and Christina Pourgourides. "Literature and Medicine" (Letter to the editor). *The Lancet* 348 no. 9031 (Sept. 28, 1996): 894.

Parens, E. *Enhancing Human Traits: Ethical and Social Implications.* Washington: Georgetown University Press, 1998.

Pellegrino, Edmund D., and David C. Thomasma. *The Christian Virtues in Medical Practice.* Washington D.C.: Georgetown University Press, 1996.

Pettit, Philip. "Consequentialism." Pp. 230–40 in *A Companion to Ethics,* edited by Peter Singer. Oxford: Blackwell, 1993.

Porter, Roy. "Is Dr. Feelgood Here to Stay." Review of *Listening to Prozac* by Peter D. Kramer. In *The Times Literary Supplement,* .4747, (March 25 1994): 28.

Rawls, John. *A Theory of Justice.* Oxford: Clarendon Press, 1972.

Reiss, Hans, ed. *Kant Political Writings,* translated by H. B. Nisbet, 2nd ed. Cambridge: University Press, 1991.

Richards, David A. J. "Rights and Autonomy." Pp. 203–20 in *The Inner Citadel: Essays on Individual Autonomy,* edited by John Christman. New York: Oxford University Press, 1989.

Rosenbaum, Jerrold F. "Clinical Trial by Media: The Prozac Story." Pp. 3–28 in *Psychiatric Practice Under Fire: The Influence of Government, the Media, and Special Interests on Somatic Therapies,* edited by Harold I. Schwartz. Washington D.C.: American Psychiatric Press Inc., 1994.

Roth, Loren H., Alan Meisel, and Charles W. Lidz. "Tests of Competency to Consent to Treatment." Pp. 201–11 in *Psychiatry and Ethics: Insanity, Rational Autonomy, and Mental Health Care,* edited by Rem B. Edwards. New York: Prometheus Books, 1982.

Rothman, David J. *Strangers at the Bedside: A History of How Law and Bioethics Transformed Medical Decision Making.* New York: Basic Books, 1991.

———. "Three Views of History." Special Supplement, "The Birth of Bioethics" edited by Albert R. Jonsen. *Hastings Center Report* (November–December 1993): S11–S12.

———. "Shiny Happy People: The Problem with 'Cosmetic Psychopharmacology.'" *The New Republic,* (14 February, 1994): 34–38.

Rousseau, J. J., *The Social Contract,* in *The Essential Rousseau,* translated by Lowell Bair. New York: A Mentor Book, 1974.

Sagan, Francoise. *A Fleeting Sorrow,* translated by Richard Seaver. New York: Arcade Publishing, 1995.

Savarirayan, Ravi. "The Long and the Short of It: Ethics of Surgical Limb Lengthening in Dwarfs." (February 2004). Unpublished. Personal communication.

Savulescu, Julian, and Richard W. Momeyer. "Should Informed Consent Be Based on Rational Beliefs?" *Journal of Medical Ethics* 23, no. 5 (October 1997): 282–88.

Schechtman, Marya. *The Constitution of Selves.* Ithaca: Cornell University Press, 1996.

Schneewind, J. B. "Autonomy, Obligation, and Virtue: An Overview of Kant's Moral Philosophy." Pp. 309–41 in *The Cambridge Companion to Kant,* edited by Paul Guyer. Cambridge: Cambridge University Press, 1992.

———. *The Invention of Autonomy: A History of Modern Moral Philosophy.* Cambridge: Cambridge University Press, 1998.

Schneider, Carl E. *The Practice of Autonomy: Patients, Doctors, and Medical Decisions.* New York: Oxford University Press, 1998.

Schwartz, Harold I., ed. *Psychiatric Practice Under Fire: The Influence of Government, the Media, and Special Interests on Somatic Therapies.* Washingtong D.C.: American Psychiatric Press Inc., 1994.

Schwartz, Richard S. "Mood Brighteners, Affect Tolerance and the Blues." *Psychiatry* 54 (November 1991): 397–403.

Secker, Barbara. "The Appearance of Kant's Deontology in Contemporary Kantianism: Concepts of Patient Autonomy in Bioethics." *Journal of Medicine and Philosophy,* 24, no. 1 (1999): 43–66.

Sheed, Wilfrid. *In Love With Daylight: A Memoir of Recovery.* New York: Simon & Schuster, 1995. P.91 quoted by Carl E. Schneider in *The Practice of Autonomy: Patients, Doctors, and Medical Decisions,* New York: Oxford University Press, 1998.

Sher, George. *Beyond Neutrality: Perfectionism and Politics.* New York: Cambridge University Press, 1996.

Shreeve, Caroline. *Lower Your Blood Pressure in 4 Easy Stages.* Northhamptonshire: Thorsons Publishing Group, 1989.

Siegler, M. "Critical Illness: The Limits of Autonomy." *Hastings Center Report* 7 (October, 1977): 12–15.

Siminoff, L. A., and J. H. Fetting. "Factors Affecting Treatment Decisions for a Life-Threatening Illness: The Case of Medical Treatment of Breast Cancer." *Soc. Sci. Med.* 32, no.7 (1991): 813–18.

Sloan, Tod S. *Deciding: Self-Deception in Life Choices.* New York: Methuen, 1987.

Solzhenitsyn, Aleksandr. *Cancer Ward.* Trans. Nicholas Bethel and David Burg. London: Penguin Books, 1st Published 1968, Penguin edition 1971.

Spriggs, Merle. *Autonomy and Shattered Assumptions.* Unpublished manuscript. Submitted for the degree: Master of Bioethics, Centre for Human Bioethics, Monash University, 1995.

———. "Autonomy in the Face of a Devastating Diagnosis." *Journal of Medical Ethics* 24, no. 2 (April 1998): 123–26.

Taylor, Shelley E., and Jonathon D. Brown. "Illusion and Well-Being: A Social Psychological Perspective on Mental Health." *Psychological Bulletin* 103, no. 2 (1988): 193–210.

Ten, C.L. *Mill on Liberty.* Oxford: Clarendon Press, 1980.

Thalberg Irving. "Hierarchical Analyses of Unfree Action." *Canadian Journal of Philosophy* 8 (June 1978). Pp. 123–36 reprinted in *The Inner Citadel: Essays on Individual Autonomy,* edited by John Christman. Oxford: Oxford University Press, 1989.

The Age, 26 February 2000.

The Sunday Age, 14 May 2000.

Tolstoy, Leo. *The Death of Ivan Ilyich and Other Stories.* London: Penguin Books, 1960.

Tooley, Michael. *Abortion and Infanticide.* Oxford: Clarendon Press, 1983.

Toulmin, Stephen. "The National Commission on Human Experimentation: Procedures and Outcomes." In *Scientific Controversies: Case Studies in the Resolution and Closure of Disputes in Science and Technology,* edited by H. Tristram Engelhardt, Jr. And Arthur L. Caplan. Cambridge: Cambridge University Press, 1987.

Urmson, J. O., and Jonathan Ree. *The Concise Encyclopedia of Western Philosophy and Philosophers*. London: Unwin Hyman, 1991.

Walter, Jennifer K., and Eran P. Klein, ed. *The Story of Bioethics*. Washington, D.C.: Georgetown University Press, 2003.

Wolf, Susan M. "Ethics Committees and Due Process: Nesting Rights in a Community of Caring." *Maryland Law Review* 50, no.3 (1991) 798–858.

Wright, Robert. "The Coverage of Happiness: When Prozac Meets Universal Coverage." *The New Republic* (March 14, 1994): 24–26, 28–29. Pp. 693–98 reprinted in *Ethical Issues in Modern Medicine* 5th. ed. Edited by John D. Arras and Bonnie Steinbock. California: Mayfield Publishing Co., 1999.

Young, Robert. *Personal Autonomy: Beyond Negative and Positive Liberty*. London: Croom Helm, 1986.

———. Review of *Self, Society, and Personal Choice* by Diana T. Meyers. *Australasian Journal of Philosophy* 68 (1990): 353–54.

INDEX

ABOUT THE AUTHOR

Merle Spriggs is a bioethicist at the Murdoch Childrens Research Institute in Melbourne, Australia. She received her Ph.D. in 2002 from the Centre for Human Bioethics, Monash University. Her research interests include the ethics of genetics, the ethics of reproductive technologies, addiction, research ethics, autonomy and the development of children's autonomy. She has published widely in bioethics, medical ethics, health consumer and medical journals. She is a past editor of *Monash Bioethics Review* and past associate editor of the current controversy section of the Journal of *Medical Ethics*.